高等教育出版社　中國·北京
Higher Education Press, Beijing, China

英漢實用中醫藥大全

趙樸初題

5

PROCTOLOGY
肛門直腸病學

THE ENGLISH–CHINESE ENCYCLOPEDIA OF PRACTICAL TRADITIONAL CHINESE MEDICINE

Chief Editor   Xu Xiangcai
Assistants   You Ke   Kang Kai
                 Bao Xuequan Lu Yubin

英汉实用中医药大全

主　编　　徐象才
主编助理　尤　可　　康　凯
　　　　　鲍学全　　路玉滨

Higher Education Press
高等教育出版社

15 肛门直肠病学

	中文	英文
主编	黄乃健	方廷钰
编者	黄乃健	许亦群

PROCTOLOGY

	English	Chinese
Chief Editor	Fang Tingyu	Huang Naijian
Editor	Xu Yiqun	Huang Naijian

(京) 112号

The English-Chinese
Encyclopedia of Practical TCM
Chief Editor　　Xu Xiangcai
15
PROCTOLOGY
English Chief Editor　　Fang Tingyu
Chinese Chief Editor　　Huang Naijian

英汉实用中医药大全
主编　徐象才
15
肛门直肠病学
中文　　英文
主编　黄乃健　方廷钰

*

高等教育出版社出版发行
高等教育出版社激光照排技术部照排
国防工业出版社印刷厂印刷

*

开本 850×1168 1/32　印张 13　插页 3　字数 330 000
1994 年12月第 1 版　1994 年12月第 1 次印刷
印数 0 001—3 170
ISBN7-04-004081-6/R·20
定价

The Leading Commission of Compilation and Translation
编译领导委员会

Honorary Director   Hu Ximing
名誉主任委员   胡熙明

Honorary Deputy Directors   Zhang Qiwen   Wang Lei
名誉副主任委员   张奇文   王镭

Director   Zou Jilong
主任委员   邹积隆

Deputy Director   Wei Jiwu
副主任委员   隗继武

Members   Wan Deguang   Wang Yongyan   Wang Maoze
委员   万德光   王永炎   王懋泽
(以姓氏笔划为序)

     Wei Guikang   Cong Chunyu   Liu Zhongben
     韦贵康   丛春雨   刘中本

     Sun Guojie   Yan Shiyun   Qiu Dewen
     孙国杰   严世芸   邱德文

     Shang Chichang   Xiang Ping   Zhao Yisen
     尚炽昌   项平   赵以森

     Gao Jinliang   Cheng Yichun   Ge Linyi
     高金亮   程益春   葛琳仪

     Cai Jianqian   Zhai Weimin
     蔡剑前   翟维敏

Advisers   Dong Jianhua   Huang Xiaokai   Geng Jianting
顾问   董建华   黄孝楷   耿鉴庭

     Zhou Fengwu   Zhou Ciqing   Chen Keji
     周凤梧   周次清   陈可冀

The Commission of Compilation and Translation
编译委员会

Director   Xu Xiangcai
主任委员   徐象才

Deputy Directors 副主任委员	Zhang Zhigang 张志刚	Zhang Wengao 张文高	Jiang Zhaojun 姜兆俊
	Qi Xiuheng 亓秀恒	Xuan Jiasheng 宣家声	Sun Xiangxie 孙祥燮
Members 委员 (以姓氏笔划为序)	Yu Wenping 于文平	Wang Zhengzhong 王正忠	Wang Chenying 王陈应
	Wang Guocai 王国才	Fang Tingyu 方廷钰	Fang Xuwu 方续武
	Tian Jingzhen 田景振	Bi Yongsheng 毕永升	Liu Yutan 刘玉檀
	Liu Chengcai 刘承才	Liu Jiaqi 刘家起	Liu Xiaojuan 刘晓娟
	Zhu Zhongbao 朱忠宝	Zhu Zhenduo 朱振铎	Xun Jianying 寻建英
	Li Lei 李磊	Li Zhulan 李竹兰	Xin Shoupu 辛守璞
	Shao Nianfang 邵念方	Chen Shaomin 陈绍民	Zou Jilong 邹积隆
	Lu Shengnian 陆胜年	Zhou Xing 周行	Zhou Ciqing 周次清
	Zhang Sufang 张素芳	Yang Chongfeng 杨崇峰	Zhao Chunxiu 赵纯修
	Yu Changzheng 俞昌正	Hu Zunda 胡遵达	Xu Heying 须鹤瑛
	Yuan Jiurong 袁久荣	Huang Naijian 黄乃健	Huang Kuiming 黄奎铭
	Huang Jialing 黄嘉陵	Cao Yixun 曹贻训	Lei Xilian 雷希濂
	Cai Huasong 蔡华松	Cai Jianqian 蔡剑前	

Preface

I am delighted to learn that THE ENGLISH-CHINESE ENCYCLOPEDIA OF PRACTICAL TRADITIONAL CHINESE MEDICINE will soon come into the world.

TCM has experienced many vicissitudes of times but has remained evergreen. It has made great contributions not only to the power and prosperity of our Chinese nation but to the enrichment and improvement of world medicine. Unfortunately, differences in nations, states and languages have slowed down its spreading and flowing outside China. At present, however, an upsurge in learning, researching and applying Traditional Chinese Medicine (TCM) is unfolding. In order to maximize the effect of this upsurge and to lead TCM, one of the brilliant cultural heritages of the Chinese nation, to the world for it to expand and bring benefit to the people of all nations, Mr. Xu Xiangcai called intellectuals of noble aspirations and high intelligence together from Shandong and many other provinces in China and took charge of the work of both compilation and translation of THE ENGLISH-CHINESE ENCYCLOPEDIA OF PRACTICAL TRADITIONAL CHINESE MEDICINE. With great pleasure, the medical staff both at home and abroad will hail the appearance of this encyclopedia.

I believe that the day when the world's medicine is fully

developed will be the day when TCM has spread throughout the world.

I am pleased to give it my preface.

Prof. Dr. Hu Ximing
    Deputy Ministerof the Ministry of Public Health of the People's Republic of China,
    Director General of the State Administrative Bureau of Traditional Chinese Medicine and Pharmacology,
    President of the World Federation of Acupuncture —Moxibustion Societies,
    Member of China Association of Science & Technology,
    Deputy President of All—China Association of Traditional Chinese Medicine,
    President of China Acupuncture & Moxibustion Society.

December, 1989

Preface

The Chinese nation has been through a long, arduous course of struggling against diseases and has developed its own traditional medicine—Traditional Chinese Medicine and Pharmacology (TCMP). TCMP has a unique, comprehensive, scientific system including both theories and clinical practice. Some thousand years since its beginnings, not only has it been well preserved but also continuously developed. It has special advantages, such as remarkable curative effects and few side effects. Hence it is an effective means by which people prevent and treat diseases and keep themselves strong and healthy.

All achievements attained by any nation in the development of medicine are the public wealth of all mankind. They should not be confined within a single country. What is more, the need to set them free to flow throughout the world as quickly and precisely as possible is greater than that of any other kind of science. During my more than thirty years of being engaged in Traditional Chinese Medicine(TCM), I have been looking forward to the day when TCMP will have spread all over the world and made its contributions to the elimination of diseases of all mankind. However it is to be deeply regretted that the pace of TCMP in extending outside China has been unsatisfactory due to the major difficulties in expressing its concepts in foreign languages.

Mr. Xu Xiangcai, a teacher of Shandong College of TCM, has sponsored and taken charge of the work of compilation and translation of The English—Chinese Encyclopedia of Practical Traditional Chinese Medicine—an extensive series. This work is a great project, a large—scale scientific research, a courageous effort and a novel creation. I deeply esteem Mr. Xu Xiangcai and his compilers and translators, who have been working day and night for such a long time, for their hard labor and for their firm and indomitable will displayed in overcoming one difficulty after another, and for their great success achieved in this way. As a leader in the circles of TCM, I am duty—bound to do my best to support them.

I believe this encyclopedia will be certain to find its position both in the history of Chinese medicine and in the history of world science and technology.

>Mr. Zhang Qiwen
>Member of the Standing Committee of
>All—China Association of TCM,
>Deputy Head of the Health Department
>of Shandong Province.
>March, 1990

Publisher's Preface

Traditional Chinese Medicine(TCM) is one of China's great cultural heritages. Since the founding of the People's Republic of China in 1949, guided by the farsighted TCM policy of the Chinese Communist Party and the Chinese government, the treasure house of the theories of TCM has been continuously explored and the plentiful literature researched and compiled. As a result, great success has been achieved. Today there has appeared a world-wide upsurge in the studying and researching of TCM. To promote even more vigorous development of this trend in order that TCM may better serve all mankind, efforts are required to further it throughout the world. To bring this about, the language barriers must be overcome as soon as possible in order that TCM can be accurately expressed in foreign languages.

Thus the compilation and translation of a series of English-Chinese books of basic knowledge of TCM has become of great urgency to serve the needs of medical and educational circles both inside and outside China.

In recent years, at the request of the health departments, satisfactory achievements have been made in researching the expression of TCM in English. Based on the investigation into the history and current state of the research work mentioned above, the English-Chinese Encyclopedia of Practical TCM has been published to meet the needs of extending the knowledge of TCM around the world.

The encyclopedia consists of twenty-one volumes, each dealing with a particular branch of TCM. In the process of compilation, the distinguishing features of TCM have been given close attention and great efforts have been made to ensure that the content is scientific, practical, comprehensive and concise. The chief writers of the Chinese manuscripts include professors or associate professors with at least twenty years of practical clinical and / or teaching experience in TCM. The Chinese manuscript of each volume has been checked and approved by a specialist of the relevant branch of TCM. The team of the translators and revisers of the English versions consists of TCM specialists with a good command of English professional medical translators, and teachers of English from TCM colleges or universities. At a symposium to standardize the English versions, scholars from twenty-two colleges or universities, research institutes of TCM or other health institutes probed the question of how to express TCM in English more comprehensively, systematically and accurately, and discussed and deliberated in detail the English versions of some volumes in order to upgrade the English versions of the whole series. The English version of each volume has been re-examined and then given a final checking.

Obviously this encyclopedia will provide extensive reading material of TCM English for senior students in colleges of TCM in China and will also greatly benefit foreigners studying TCM.

The assiduous efforts of compiling and translating this encyclopedia have been supported by the responsible leaders of the State Education Commission of the People's Republic of China, the State Administrative Bureau of TCM and Pharmacy, and the Education Commission and Health Department of Shandong

Province. Under the direction of the Higher Education Department of the State Education Commission, the leading board of compilation and translation of this encyclopedia was set up. The leaders of many colleges of TCM and pharmaceutical factories of TCM have also given assistance.

We hope that this encyclopedia will bring about a good effect on enhancing the teaching of TCM English at the colleges of TCM in China, on cultivating skills in medical circles in exchanging ideas of TCM with patients in English, and on giving an impetus to the study of TCM outside China.

Higher Education Press
March, 1990

Foreword

The English—Chinese Encyclopedia of Practical Traditional Chinese Medicine is an extensive series of twenty—one volumes. Based on the fundamental theories of traditional Chinese medicine(TCM) and with emphasis on the clinical practice of TCM, it is a semi—advanced English—Chinese academic works which is quite comprehensive, systematic, concise, practical and easy to read. It caters mainly to the following readers: senior students of colleges of TCM, young and middle—aged teachers of colleges of TCM, young and middle—aged physicians of hospitals of TCM, personnel of scientific research institutions of TCM, teachers giving correspondence courses in TCM to foreigners, TCM personnel going abroad in the capacity of lecturers or physicians, those trained in Western medicine but wishing to study TCM, and foreigners coming to China to learn TCM or to take refresher courses in TCM.

Because Traditional Chinese Medicine and Pharmacology is unique to our Chinese nation, putting TCM into English has been the crux of the compilation and translation of this encyclopedia. Owing to the fact that no one can be proficient both in the theories of Traditional Chinese Medicine and Pharmacology and the clinical practice of every branch of TCM, as well as in English, to ensure that the English versions express accurately the inherent meanings of TCM, collective translation measures have been taken. That is, teachers of English familiar with TCM, professional medical translators, teachers or physicians of TCM and even teachers of palaeography with a strong command of English were all invited together to co-translate the Chinese manuscripts and, then, to co-deliberate and discuss the English versions. Finally English-speaking foreigners studying TCM or teaching English in China were asked to polish the English versions. In this way, the skills of the above translators and foreigners were merged to ensure the quality of the English versions. However, even using this method, the uncertainty that the English versions will be wholly accepted still remains. As for the Chinese manuscripts, they do reflect the essence, and give a general picture, of traditional Chinese medicine and pharmacology. It is not asserted, though, that they are perfect, I whole-heartedly look forward to any criticisms or opinions from readers in order to make improvements to future editions.

More than 200 people have taken part in the activities of compiling, translating and revising this encyclopedia. They come from twenty-eight institutions in all parts of China. Among these institutions, there are fifteen colleges of TCM:Shandong, Beijing, Shanghai, Tianjin, Nanjing, Zhejiang, Anhui, Henan, Hubei, Guangxi, Guiyang, Gansu, Chengdu, Shanxi and Changchun, and scientific research centers of TCM such as China Academy of TCM and Shandong Scientific Research Institute of TCM.

The Education Commission of Shandong province has included the compilation and translation of this encyclopedia in its scientific research projects and allocated funds accordingly. The Health Department of Shandong Province has also given financial aid together with a number of pharmaceutical factories of TCM. The subsidization from Jinan Pharmaceutical Factory of

TCM provided the impetus for the work of compilation and translation to get under way.

The success of compiling and translating this encyclopedia is not only the fruit of the collective labor of all the compilers, translators and revisers but also the result of the support of the responsible leaders of the relevant leading institutions. As the encyclopedia is going to be published, I express my heartfelt thanks to all the compilers. translators and revisers for their sincere cooperation, and to the specialists, professors, leaders at all levels and pharmaceutical factories of TCM for their warm support.

It is my most profound wish that the publication of this encyclopedia will take its role in cultivating talented persons of TCM having a very good command of TCM English and in extending, rapidly, comprehensive knowledge of TCM to all corners of the globe.

Chief Editor Xu Xiangcai
Shandong College of TCM
March, 1990

Contents

Notes 8
1 Contribution of Traditional Chinese Proctology 1
   1.1   Disease Name and Its Origin 1
   1.2   Historical Study of the Anorectal Anatomy 2
   1.3   Historical Study of the Anorectal Physiology and
         Pathology 3
   1.4   Understanding of the Etiology of Hemorrhoid 4
   1.5   Differentiation of Syndromes 5
        1.5.1   Classification 5
        1.5.2   Symptoms and Signs, Pulse and the Diseased Meridians ... 7
   1.6   Treatment 8
        1.6.1   Internal Treatment 8
        1.6.2   External Treatment 14
        1.6.3   Acupuncture, Moxibustion and *Daoyin* 18
   1.7   Care and Prevention 19
2 Examination for Anal-Rectum Diseases 21
   2.1   Position of Patients 21
        2.1.1   Lateral Position 21
        2.1.2   Prone Position 21
        2.1.3   Lithotomy Position 21
        2.1.4   Knee-Chest Position or Knee-Elbow Position ... 22
        2.1.5   Flexed-Knee Supine Position 22
        2.1.6   Squatting Position 22
        2.1.7   Standing-Bowing Position 22

2.1.8	Inverted Position	22
2.1.9	Ride-prone Position	23

2.2　Procedure for Examination ······ 23
   2.2.1　Asking ······ 23
   2.2.2　Looking ······ 24
   2.2.3　Finger Diagnosis ······ 24
   2.2.4　Anoscopy ······ 24
   2.2.5　Probing Examination ······ 24
   2.2.6　Localization of the Internal Opening of the Cryptus Hook ······ 25

2.3　Case Writing Record and Examination Record ······ 26
   2.3.1　Special Case History Record form Can Be Used ······ 26
   2.3.2　Requirement for Case History Record ······ 26
   2.3.3　Diagrams Commonly Used for Partial Examination, Code and Its Meaning ······ 29

3　Anesthesia of Anus and Rectum ······ 31

3.1　Acupuncture Anesthesia ······ 31
   3.1.1　Point Selection ······ 31
   3.1.2　Preparation before Acupuncture Anesthesia ······ 31
   3.1.3　Method ······ 31
   3.1.4　Advantage and Drawback ······ 32

3.2　Local Anesthesia ······ 32
   3.2.1　Suitable for Hemorrhoid and Fistula Operation in General ······ 32
   3.2.2.　Method of Anesthesia ······ 32
   3.2.3　Requirements ······ 33
   3.2.4　Advantage and Disadvantage ······ 33

3.3　Yaoshu (DU2) Anesthesia ······ 33
   3.3.1　Indications ······ 33

  3.3.2 Commonly Used Anesthetics ·· 33
  3.3.3 Anesthetic Method ·· 33
  3.3.4 Anesthetic Effect ·· 34
  3.3.5 How to Apply Anesthesia to Yaoshu (DU2) ·················· 35
 3.4 Other Kinds of Anesthesia ·· 41
  3.4.1 Lumbar Anesthesia ·· 41
  3.4.2 Lumbosacral Epidural Anesthesia of Spinal Cord ············ 41
  3.4.3 Refrigeration Anesthesia and General Anesthesia ············ 41
  3.4.4 Intravenous Anesthesia and General Anesthesia ············· 41
4 Pre-and-Post-Operative Management of Anorectal Surgery and Handling of Post-Operative Reaction and Complications ·· 42
 4.1 Pre-and-Post-Operative Management of Anorectal Surgery ·· 42
  4.1.1 Pre-Operative Preparation ·· 42
  4.1.2 Ptst-Operative Management ·· 43
 4.2 Handling the Post-Operative Reaction and Complications ·· 46
  4.2.1 Pain ·· 46
  4.2.2 Bearing-Down Pain ·· 47
  4.2.3 Urinating Disturbance ·· 48
  4.2.4 Hemorrhage ·· 50
  4.2.5 Fever ·· 58
  4.2.6 Local Swelling ·· 59
  4.2.7 Eczema and Dermatitis ··· 59
  4.2.8 Slow Healing of the Wound ··· 59
  4.2.9 Stricture of Anus and Fecal Incontinence ······················ 60
5 Hemorrhoid ·· 61
 5.1 Etiology and Pathogenesis ·· 61

      5.1.1   Integrated Internal Factors 61
      5.1.2   Local External Factors 61
   5.2   Clinical Manifestations 62
      5.2.1   Classification 62
      5.2.2   Symptoms and Signs 65
      5.2.3   The Involved Meridians and Their Relationship 66
   5.3   Diagnosis and Differential Diagnosis 66
   5.4   Clinical Treatment 67
      5.4.1   Internal Treatment 67
      5.4.2   External Treatment 68
      5.4.3   Acupuncture and Magnetic Therapy 99

6 Anorectal Peripheral Abscess 100
   6.1   Etiology and Pathogenesis 100
   6.2   Clinical Manifestations 101
   6.3   Treatment 102
      6.3.1   Internal Treatment 102
      6.3.2   External Treatment 102

7 Anal Fistula 103
   7.1   Etiology and Pathogenesis 103
   7.2   Clinical Manifestations 104
      7.2.1   Classification 104
      7.2.2   Symptoms and Signs 107
   7.3   Diagnosis and Differential Diagnosis 108
      7.3.1   Asking 108
      7.3.2   Looking 108
      7.3.3   Palpation 110
      7.3.4   Probe Examination 112
      7.3.5   Anoscopy and Anal Crypt Hook Examination 112
      7.3.6   Fistulous Pipe Staining Method 114

	7.3.7	Roentgenography	115
	7.3.8	Rules to Know the Relation between the Inner and Outer Openings and the Trend of Fistula	116
	7.3.9	Pathological Section Examination	118
7.4		Clinical Treatment	120
	7.4.1	Internal Treatment	120
	7.4.2	External Treatment	120
8	**Anal Fissure**		**135**
8.1		Etiology and Pathogenesis	135
	8.1.1	Factors of Anatomy	136
	8.1.2	Inflammation	136
	8.1.3	Mechanical Injury	136
	8.1.4	Other Factors	137
8.2		Clinical Manifestations	137
	8.2.1	Stage Classification	137
	8.2.2	Symptoms and Signs	138
8.3		Diagnosis and Differential Diagnosis	139
8.4		Clinical Treatment	140
	8.4.1	Internal Treatment	140
	8.4.2	External Treatment	143
	8.4.3	Acupuncture and Magnetotherapy	150
9	**Proctoptoma**		**151**
9.1		Etiology and Pathogenesis	151
	9.1.1	The Theory of Sliding Hernia	151
	9.1.2	The Theory of Intussusception	152
9.2		Clinical Manifestations	153
	9.2.1	Classification	153
	9.2.2	Symptoms and Signs	156
9.3		Diagnosis and Differential Diagnosis	158

    9.3.1   Diagnosis ································· 158

    9.3.2   Differential Diagnosis ·················· 163

  9.4   Clinical Treatment ······························· 164

    9.4.1   Internal Treatment ······················· 164

    9.4.2   External Treatment ······················ 164

    9.4.3   Acupuncture Therapy ··················· 176

10   Rectal Polyp ······································· 177

  10.1   Etiology and Pathogenesis ····················· 177

  10.2   Clinical Manifestations ························· 177

    10.2.1   Classifications ··························· 177

    10.2.2   Symptoms and Signs ···················· 180

  10.3   Diagnosis and Differential Diagnosis ········ 180

  10.4   Clinical Treatment ······························ 182

    10.4.1   Internal Treatment ······················ 182

    10.4.2   External Treatment ····················· 182

11   Prevention of Anorectal Diseases ············· 185

  11.1   Prevention of Hemorrhoids ···················· 185

    11.1.1.   Physical Exercises ····················· 185

    11.1.2   Keeping off Anger and Worry ········ 185

    11.1.3   Proper Diet ······························ 185

    11.1.4   Having Regular Bowel Movements Every Day ············ 186

    11.1.5   Keep Hygiene of the Anus ············ 186

    11.1.6   Massage and Anus-Lifting Exercise ························ 186

    11.1.7   *Daoyin* ···································· 190

  11.2   Prevention of Anal Fistula ····················· 190

  11.3   Prevention of Anal Fissure ····················· 191

  11.4   Prevention of Prolapse of Rectum ············ 192

  11.5   Prevention of Rectal Polyp ····················· 193

Formula Index ··· 194

The English–Chinese Encyclopedia of Practical TCM
(Booklist) ·· (390)

Notes

Proctology is the fifteenth volume of the English—Chinese Encyclopedia of Practical Traditional Chinese Medicine.

Traditional Chinese medicine has a long history, unique theoretical system and rich clinical esperience in the diagnosia and treatment of anorectal disorders such as hemorrhoids and anal fistula.This volume deals with the etiology, pathogenesis, differentiation of syndromes and treatment of hemorrhoids, perianal abscess , anal fistula, anal fissure, prolapse of rectum and rectal polyp,and the anesthesia, management before and after the surgical operation, and frequently—used prescriptions and herbs.

The compilation and translation of the book have been helped by many specialists .We are especially indebted to Prof. Ding Zemin, Director of the Anorectal Society ,All—China Association of Traditional Chinese Medicine, Prof.Sun Xiangxie of the Shanghai College of Traditional Chinese and Prof. Li Zhenshen of the Henan College of Traditional Chinese Medicine for their valuable suggestions and advices.

The Editor

1 Contribution of Traditional Chinese Proctology

The long-standing traditional Chinese medicine is the accumulation of clinical experience of the Chinese working people in their long period of struggle against diseases.In the past thousands of years the Chinese anorectal medicine gradually developed into a specific branch of traditional medicine with its own theoretical system and rich clinical experience,and it has played an important role in traditional Chinese medicine. Detailed introduction based on documents are going to be made as follows.

1.1 Disease Name and Its Origin

As early as in the Western Zhou Dynasty (11th century B.C.-770 B.C.) the name of hemorrhoid and fistula were recorded. In the period of Warring States abundant record of hemorrhoids was seen.It was listed in *Zhuang Zi. Lie Yu Kou*(770-430 B.C.),in which Zhuang Zi said:"Once the emperor of the Qin State called in practitioners when he fell ill...Those who cured his carbuncle,sore and ulcer were rewarded a cart,and those who took laps at his hemorrhoid were rewarded five carts.The lower the disease treated located,the higher the reward was given..." The word "hemorrhoid" mentioned above was used in a derogatory sense.According to a legend Cao Shang,an envoy of the Song State to the Qin State ingratiated himself with the Qin emperor and was rewarded one hundred carts.He showed off his merits to Zhunag Zi, who was disgusted with Cao and sneered at him by making the above remarks.From this we can see that about two thousand years ago the ancient Chinese had the terms of carbuncle.sore and ulcer.and knew the methods of treatment for hemorrhoids. As for disease names,there used to be "hemorrhoid-disease","five hemorrhoids","hemorrhoid-sore", "hemorrhoid-illness","hemorrhoid-core","hemorrhoid-fistula", " anal fistula" and so on.The term hemorrhoid-core was first found in *Yi Xue Zheng Zhuan*(Oxthodox Medical Problems) compiled around 1515.400 hundred years from now. Some of the names have been introduced to foreign countries where they have been adopted so far.

1.2 Historical Study of the Anorectal Anatomy

The ancient Chinese practitioners had made remarkable contributions to anatomy. As early as the Shang and Zhou Dynasties anatomic investigations into the body was conducted on the spot.It is stated in *Ling Shu. Jing Shui Pian* (Treatise on the Comparison of Meridians to Rivers,Miraculous Pivot) that "A man's skin and flesh can be measured on the surface of the body... Also, when a man is dead,his organs can be observed by autopsy..." *Nan Jing* • *Si Shi Si Nan*(The 44th Problem,Classic on Medical Problems) points out the large and small intestines meet at *Lanmen* or the ileocecal valve,the end is *Pomen* or anus.As early as the Han Dynasty (206 B.C.-220 A.D.) it was known that *Lanmen* was the line of demarcation and it was shaped as a gate, which could stop and pass of contents in the large intestine.The ancient Chinese found that the lower-most end of the digestive tract was *Pomen* or anus. They held that since the lung and large intestine were in pair exteriorly and interiorly and *"Po"* or soul was housed in the lung, the end of the large intestine was called *Pomen* or anus. An illustration of the large intestine was given in *Yi Zong Bi Du* (Reader of Medicine) published in the Ming Dynasty. The large intestine described is similar to the modern illustration of colon. From the medical literature we know that the ancient practitioners made detailed descriptions of the length, size, volume and blood supply of the intestine and their connection with the surrounding organs and tissues. Among the various ancient writings *Ling Shu*(Miraculous Pivot) and *Nan Jing* (Classic on Medical Problems) were two representative works. The ileum was also known as the large intestine in *Ling Shu,* which corresponds to the ileum and most of the colon, while the sigmoidrectum recorded in the book is equal to modern sigmoid, rectum and anus. The term anus was firstly seen in *Nan Jing* (Classic on Medical Problems) and *Tai Ping Sheng Hui Fang* (Peaceful Holy Benevolent Prescriptions) (982-992 A.D.)first listed the term of analrectum. The term rectum was created by Yang Xuancao, an annotator for *Nan Jing* (Classic on Medical Problems) in the Tang Dynasty and commonly known in the Ming and Qing Dynasties.

1.3 Historical Study of the Anorectal Physiology and Pathology

Quite a number of treatises on Chinese medicine focus on the study of the anorectal physiology and pathology. It has been generally held that the large intestine is a *Yang* organ, attributing to metal, governing body fluid and preferring dryness, it is to convey and transform. It discharges without storing and it is continuously cleaned of its contents. Anus is the passage of solid waste. It does not transform anything. *Nei Jin* (Classic of Internal Medicine) points out " *Pomen* is also controlled by the five *Zang*-organs and is unable to contain water and cereals for a long time." The ancient Chinese thought that the function of the large intestine was to transform unusable materials into solid waste. As water is absorbed, these are then expelled from the body. Functional disturbance may lead to constipation, diarrhea, etc.

1.4 Understanding of the Etiology of Hemorrhoid

Detailed description of the etiology of hemorrhoid can be found in the Chinese medical literature. It was more than two thousand years ago that hemorrhoid was thought of as a pathological change of blood vessels. It is stated in *Su Wen • Sheng Qi Tong Tian Lun* (Treatise on Communication of Vitality with Heaven, Plain Questions) (240A.D.) that "Too much food intake causes injury and flaccidity of vessels, leading to hemorrhoid". It is held by *Su Wen* (Plain Questions) that hemorrhoid is due to abnormal swelling and dilation of veins which proposes the initial theory of varicosity. bleeding due to blood heat was advanced by *Tai Ping Sheng Hui Fang*(Peaceful Holy Benevolent Prescriptions). In the Jin and Yuan Dynasties (1127−1168 A.D.) Liu Wansu and Li Dongyuan pointed out that hemorrhoid was caused by functional disturbance of the large intestine, lung, liver and spleen. He advocated the causative factors were pathogenic dampness, heat, wind and dryness. According to *Dan Xi Xin Fa* (Danxi's Experiential Therapy)."Hemorrhoids result from lowered functioning of the *Zang—Fu* organs." *Chuang Yang Jing Yan Quan Shu*(A Complete Manual of Experience in the Treatment of Sores) says:"Hemorrhoid occurring to those who are not good at drinking is brought about by declined functioning of the *Zang—Fu* organs; sometimes,genetic factor plays its part in occurrence of hemorrhoid...",indicating the impact of weakness of the *Zang—Fu* organs and the genetic factors.*Wai Ke Qi Xuan* (Revealing the Mystery of Surgery) advocates the theory of impeded blood flow, saying:"Hemorrhoid is caused by retarded flow of blood." *Wai Ke Zheng Zong* (Orthodox Manual of Surgery) points out that "Accumulation of pathogenic dampness and heat was the cause of hemorrhoid."All of the viewpoints had an influence on the later generations in their medical practice. Much more was discussed about the etiology of hemorrhoid. In short, the causative factors of hemorrhoid are either internal and integratal or external and local. Finally, the mutual affection of the two aspects of factors leads to occurrence of hemorrhoid. These are the clinical summary of the ancient Chinese and has been regarded as the guidance of differentiation of syndromes and treatment through out ages, which has been valued highly and followed by the successors.

1.5 Differentiation of Syndromes

1.5.1 Classification

In the Qin and Han Dynasties hemorrhoids were grouped

under four heads listed in *Wu Shi Er Bing Fang* (Fifty-Two Prescriptions). They were known as "female", "male" vessel and bloody hemorrhoids. In the Sui Dynasty, intestinal hemorrhoid, hemorrhoids due to alcoholism and deficiency were added with vivid descriptions in *Zhu Bing Yuan Hou Lun* (The General Treatise on Etiology and Symptoms)(610 A.D.). The theory of the five kinds of hemorrhoid, i.e. female, male, vessel, intestinal and bloody hemorrhoid, hemorrhoid due to alcoholism and *Qi* stagnation has played an important role in the academic history, which has lasted for several centuries. Based on this theory, the later practitioners developed it into the theory of seven, eight, ten, and eleven hemorrhoids. It should be pointed out that the modern terms of internal and external hemorrhoids were mentioned by practitioners of the Tang Dynasty. *Wai Tai Mi Yao* (Medical Secrets of An Official)(752 A.D.) says: "There are two kinds of hemorrhoids, namely, internal hemorrhoid and external hemorrhoid. Bowel movements with hemorrhage are a sign of the internal hemorrhoid, while the sign of external hemorrhage is different. Blood is often running out from the hole under the external hemorrhoid." Then twenty-five and twenty-four kinds of hemorrhoids were found in the Jin Yuan Dynasties, and the Ming Dynasty respectively. Then the term internal-external hemorrhoid, or "mixed hemorrhoid" appeared. All the descriptions were accompanied by illustrations. In the Qing Dynasty classification of hemorrhoids consisted of five, twenty-four and twenty-five. In 1873 *Ma Shi Zhi Lou Ke Qi Shi Er Zhong*(Ma's Works on Seventy-Two Kinds of Hemorrhoid), the first monography on hemorrhoid in the country, was published, in which anal fissure was mentioned for the first time in history.

From the above we can see that the classification of hemorrhoids was based on rich clinical experience, but there included other rectal disorders owing to the limitation of the time. In *Wu Shi Er Bing Fang* (Fifty—Two Prescriptions) anal fistula was discussed but it was not differentiated from hemorrhoid, and from Qin and Han to Jin, Sui, Tang Dynasties anal fistula was grouped under hemorrhoid. Only in the Song Dynasty hemorrhoid and anal fistula were separated in *Tai Ping Sheng Hui Fang* (Peaceful Holy Benevolent Prescriptions). There was a further discussion of anal fistula in the *Chuang Yang Jing Yan Quan Shu* (A Complete Manual of Experience in the Treatment of Sores) (1569 A.D.),which says:" On either side of the anus,where there is dischage of pus and blood, is known as the single fistula." Nowadays it is called the simple anal fistula. Later different classifications were adopted.

1.5.2 Symptoms and Signs, Pulse and the Diseased Meridians

Ancient Chinese had described all the symptoms of hemorrhoid, such as a swelling and bearing—down pain,proctoptosis, itching, puruloid secretion as the pathological changes. The pulse indicating the condition of the large intestine is felt at *Chi* (on the proximal side from the wrist),according to *Nei Jing* (Classic of Internal Medicine).*Qian Jin Yao Fang* (Prescriptions Worth a Thousand Pieces of Gold) points out that arteria dorsalis pedis is sometimes taken to diagnose the condition of the Meridian of the Large Intestine. In deficiency cases, one may see thready,weak, deep, retarded or hollow pulse,while in excess cases,there may be full pulse, taut or rapid pulse.Disorders of the large intestine is related to Meridians of the Large Intestine,Lung, Liver, Spleen, Kidney, Bladder, *Ren,Du* and

Gallbladder. "In terms of differentiation of syndromes, a swollen end of the large intestine results from pathogenic dampness, pain is caused by pathogenic wind. Constipation is a result of pathogenic fire." *(Lan Shi Mi Cang,* ——A Secret Book Kept in the Chamber, printed in the turn of the Jin and Yuan Dynasties).*Wai Ke Da Cheng*(The Compendium 'of Surgery) makes a further explanation of Li Dongyuan's concept. It says: "Swelling, pain,itching and constipation are brought about by pathogenic dampness, heat, wind and fire respectively." It also describes in detail the condition,development of the disease,which is held for the basis in judgment of the prognosis.

1.6 Treatment

Treatment of the hemorrhoid and anal fistula includes internal, external approaches, acupuncture, moxibustion and *Daoyin,*the necrotizing therapy, ligation method, ligation therapy for anal fistula,surgery, fumigating method,steam and bath method,and catharsis. Besides the internal treatment, there listed other therapies, such as surgery, drug application, madicated bath, fumigating, moxibustion and cupping in *Wu Shi Er Bing Fang* (Fifty—Two Prescriptions).Great importance had been attached to the internal treatment until the Ming Dynasty, when the external treatment was called into practice.

1.6.1 Internal Treatment

The internal treatment is already listed in *Wu Shi Er Bing Fang* (Fifty—Two Prescriptions). It is pointed out in *Jin Kui Yao Lüo*(Synopsis of Prescriptions of the Golden Chamber) that "Bleeding after bowel movements is treated by *Huangtu Tang*

(1), because blood is coming from a distal part of the body." "Bleeding followed by bowel movements is treated by *Chixiaodou Dangui San* (2) because blood comes nearby." The treating principle favored by the four schools of traditional Chinese medicine in the Jin and Yuan Dynasties (represented by Liu Wansu, Zhang Congzheng, Li Dongyuan and Zhu Zhenheng) was to clear off pathogenic heat and cool blood. Li Dongyuan advocated regulating blood and dryness, removing and dispelling. wind to stop pain."For severe cases, herbs bitter in taste and cold in property are administered to remove fire, and herbs pungent in taste and warm in property to regulate blood, eliminate dryness, wind and pain." *(Lan Shi Mi Cang* ——A Secret Book Kept in the Chamber). It is pointed out by Dan Xi Xin Fa (Danxi's Experiential Therapy) that "Blood cooling is the key method for hemorrhoid." "It is effective to treat by cooling blood." *(Chuang Yang Jing Yan Quan Shu*——A Complete Manual of Experiences in the Treatment of Sores). "The general principle of treatment lies in warming and recuperating instead of cooling and purgating. The former may cause blood to travel in the meridians, and blood is controlled by *Qi*." (*Yi Xue Zhen Chuan*——True Experience of Medicine). As for the treatment of anal fistula the treating principle and medication are similar to that for hemorrhoid, but reinforcement is stressed. "The pain and swelling due to hemorrhoid and fistula...are treated by removing dampness." (*Ru Men Shi Qin* ——Confucians' Duties to Their Parents). "In the treatment of anal fistula tonics are given first to produce *Qi* and blood. The tonics include Radix Ginseng, Rhizoma Atractulodis Macrocephalae, Radix Astragali, Rhizoma Ligustici Chuanxiong, Radix Angelicae Sinensis, large dosage of which is given," says

Dan Xi Xin Fa (Danxi's Experiential Therapy)."Herbs to warm and recuperate the internal organs are administered, and myogenic medicines given for the external application."(*Chuang Yang Jing Yan Quan Shu* ——A Complete Manual of Experiences in the Treatment of Sores).*Yi Xue Ru Men* (Elementary Medicine)says "At the initial stage, discharge of pus and blood in anal fistula represents existence of damp—heat,it is suggested to cool blood, eliminate heat and dampness. Presence of damp—cold is seen in persisted cases and it is necessary to remove dampness in the anus and parasites by the warming and recuperating method." "Anal fistula can be described as a crack on a dam,or a leak in the roof.Harm can never be alleviated when there exists fistula. In the treatment of anal fistula,it is advisable to reinforce *Qi* and blood first.Abundant *Qi* and blood can arrest discharge.When body fluid gets more, recuperation can be got...The following six prescriptions are used for persisted anal fistula, which causes hypofunction of the stomach. Herbs sweet in taste and warm in property are used. For cases due to *Yin* deficiency and hyperactivity of *Yang*,herbs to replenish *Yin* and bitter in taste are administered. Semen Nulumbinis, Semen Euryales and Fructus Chebulae can reinforce *Qi* and arrest discharge of blood."(*Wai Zheng Yi An Hui Bian* ——Collected Works on External Diseases).In the treatment of proctoptosis,*Nei Jing* (Classic of Internal Medicine) says:"Tonification is employed in deficiency cases,"and "herbs sour in taste is given to lift the anus." It is said in *Jing Yue Quan Shu* (Complete Works of Zhang Jingyue) that "*Nei Jing* Classic of Internal Medicine points out, prolapse of rectum is treated by lifting. Xu Zhicai says, herbs puckery in taste are good for prolapse of rectum.These are the methods to treat prolapse of rectum."

Medication for hemorrhoid is based on rich clinical experience. Apart from the *Wu Shi Er Bing Fang* Fifty-Two Prescriptions and *Jin Kui Yao Lüe* (Synopsis of Prescriptions of Golden Chamber) over 30 out of 365 herbs listed in the *Shen Nong Ben Cao* (Shen Nong's Herbal Classic) can treat hemorrhoid and anal fistula. There are twenty-six prescriptions for five kinds of hemorrhoid recorded in *Bei Ji Qian Jin Yao Fang* (Prescriptions Worth a Thousand Pieces of Gold for Emergencies),and 213 recipes in *Tai Ping Sheng Hui Fang* (Peaceful Holy Benevolent Prescriptions).If prescriptions for hematochezia are involved, they total 220 prescriptions. *Pu Ji Fang* (Prescriptions for Universal Relief)recorded over 1,200 recipes, among which 136 were for hematochezia due to pathogenic wind in the large intestine, 225 for hematochezia due to toxins in the large intestine, and 800 for all kinds of hemorrhoid and red, swollen anus. There listed about 300 simple and proved recipes and 240 prescriptions in *Gu Jin Tu Shu Ji Cheng Yi Bu Quan Lu* (Collection of Medical Works, Ancient and Contemporary) for hemorrhoids, fistula and proctoptosis. So many recipes, including secret, proved ones, were collected by the ancient physicians in their long-term medical practice.

Yi Xue Zheng Zhuan (Orthodox Medical Problems) points out that "Herbs used to treat hemorrhoid are those such as Radix Scutellariae,Rhizoma Coptidis, Fructus Gardeniae and Flos Sophorae, bitter in taste and cold in property to eliminate fire; or those, for example, Radix Angelicae Sinensis, Rhizoma Ligustici Chuangxiong and Semen Persicae pungent in taste and warm in property to harmonize blood. Radix Gentianae Macrophyllae,

Radix Ledebouriellae and Rhizoma Cimicifugae are given when pathogenic wind stays in the lower part of the body. Fructus Aurantii, Radix Rhei and Semen Cannabis are used for pathogenic dryness and heat. *Ben Cao Gang Mu* (Compendium of Materia Medica)records Li Dongyuan's examples of medication for hemorrhoid.Hematochezia is treated by Radix Sanguisorbae. Rhizoma Atractylodis, Radix Ledebouriellae, Radix Glycyrrhizae and Radix Paeoniae are given with modification for hemorrhoid and anal fistula.*Zheng Zhi Hui Bu* (Diagnosis and Treatment) holds that for hematochezia *Siwu Tang*(3)is the chief recipe. Herba Schizonepelae and Radix Ledebouriellae are added for cases with pathogenic wind; Rhizoma Atractylodis and Radix Gentianae Macrophyllae are added for symptoms due to dampness; Fructus Sophorae, Radix Scutellariae and Rhizoma Coptidis are added for symptoms due to heat; Radix Aucklandia, Rhizoma Zingiberis are added for symptoms due to cold; Rhizoma Ciperi, Fructus Aurantii are added for *Qi* stagnation; Semen Persicae, chive juice are added for stagnation of *Qi* and blood; Radix Ginseng, Radix Astragali, Rhizoma Atractylodis and Radix Glycyrrhizae are added for protracted debility; Radix Aconiti Praeparata and Rhizoma Zingiberis Praeparata are added for debility and cold; Rhizoma Cimicifugae and Radix Bupleuri are added for proctoptosis; Colla Corii Asini and Radix Rehmanniae are added for heat due to deficiency.

For anal fistula, Radix Ginseng and Radix Astragali are usually given. Sometimes *Huanglian Biguan Wan* (4) and *Xiangya Huaguan Wan* (5) are administered. *Chuang Yang Jing Yan Quan Shu* (A Complete Manual of Experience in the Treatment of Sores) usually administered to treat proctoptosis due to deficiency of blood, and for cases due to *Qi* insufficiency, Radix Ginseng, Radix Astragali, Radix Angelicae Sinensis and Rhizoma Atractylodis Macrocephalae are given. For cases due to heat in blood, Cortex Phelloaendri is added to *Siwu Tang*. Proctoptosis due to debility is treated by *Buzhong Yiqi Tang* (6) with modification.*Jing Yue Quan Shu* (Complete Works of Zhang Jingyue) holds that "Proctoptosis was treated by predecessors with Radix Ginseng, Radix Astragali,Radix Angelicae Sinensis, Rhizoma Areactylidis, Rhizoma Ligustici Chuangxiong, Radix Glycyrrhizae and Rhizoma Cimicifugae to lift the anus and improve health, or sometimes, herbs like Fructus Mume are used to exert the astringent function." Among the prescriptions used to treat anal-rectal disorders, *HuaiJiao Wan* and *QinJiu Cangzhu Tang* (7) are often administered. The former is a typical recipe for replenishing *Yin*, removing dampness and heat from blood. It is not only used by practitioners but also is very popular among the people. *Huaizi Wan* (8)and *Xiaohuaishi Wan* (9) are called *Huaizi Yuan and Xiaohuaishi Wan* in *Qian Jin Yi Fang* (A Supplement to the Essential Prescriptions Worth a Thousand Pieces of Gold) with differed ingredients. *Huaij iao Yuan*(10)listed in the *Tai Ping Hui Min He Ji Ju Fang* (Peaceful Holy Belevolent Prescriptions)(1107 A.D.).is the present *Huaij iao Wan*, which is regarded as a traditional prescription. Another *Huaij iao Wan* (11) is recorded in the *Chuang Yang Jing Yan Quan Shu* (A Complete Manual of Experience in the Treatment of Sores).This formula consist of only two herbs——Fructus Sophorae and Fel Bovis, which should be named *Danhuai Wan* or *Huai Dan Dan* in *Yi Xue Ru Men* (The Elementary Medicine).The present prescription contains the same ingredients and dosage as *Danhuai Wan* does, known as

Huaij iao Yuan or the traditional *Huaij iao Wan*. In case of the same ingredients with differen dose it is a supplementary prescription of the traditional *Huaij iao Wan* (12). If the ingredients are not the same, it is not a traditional *Huaij iao Wan* (13). *Qinj iao Cangzhu Tang* was created by Li Dongyuan and from the Jin Dynasty to now it has been praiseworthy of practitioners. In *Lan Shi Mi Cang* (A Secret Book in the Chamber), there are listed seven recipes for hemorrhoid and anal fistula, i.e. *Qinj iao Baizhu Wan* (14), *Qinj iao Cangzhu Tang*, *Qinj iao Fangfeng Tang* (15), *Qinj iao Qianghuo Tang* (16), *Qinj iao Danggui Tang* (17) *Danggui Yuliren Tang* (18) and *Honghua Taoren Tang* (19). Contending that *Qinjiao Cangzhu Tang* can "regulate blood, eliminate dryness and dispel wind and kill pain" because it is pungent in taste and warm in property, which represents Li Dongyuan's ideas in the treatment of hemorrhoid, the author took it as his treating principle for hemorrhoid and anal fistula. It is a typical recipe and *Qinjiao Baizhu Wan* is the second choice. These prescriptions and other similar ones, on which the present prescriptions are based were developed by the predecessor and used for centuries with good results. The modification of the above recipes not only increases the number of similar prescriptions, but also expand the indications. The present prescriptions are widely indicated for other disorders apart from hemorrhoid and anal fistula.

1.6.2 External Treatment

1. Necrotizing Therapy for Hemorrhoid: It is a conventional treatment in traditional Chinese medicine, playing an important role in the treatment of hemorrhoid. It was first applied in the Song Dynasty, and in the Ming and Qing Dynasties it was praised highly. Drugs used in this therapy were *Kuzhi San* (20) and *Kuzhi*

Ding (21). The chief recipe should be *Sanpin Yitiaoqiang* (22) recorded in *Wai Ke Zheng Zong* (Orthodox Manual of External Diseases)(1617 A.D.).Arsenic is the main ingredient, which should go through special preparation before use.Rich experience was accumulated by physicians throughout ages in the external application and inserting of drugs, necrosis of tissues and healing of the wound, side—effect and its management. When *Kuzhi San* is used, the course of treatment is long and patients tend to suffer. Thus this therapy has been given up. However, the *Kuzhi Ding* therapy, including preparation of the drug, clinical application and laboratory experiment has been carried out continuously. The present approach is much improved and it has become one of the important external treatments so far.

2. The Ligation Method for Hemorrhoid and Fistula: The ligation method for hemorrhoid can be traced back to the Song Dynasty or 1,000 years ago and it is the chief and effective approach to have a radical removal of the root of hemorrhoid. The method and apparatus adopted have been discussed in detail. Because of its effectiveness, it has been introduced to other countries.Satisfactory results have been gained on continuous exploration in the treatment of high anal fistula,which is held as one of the modern prominent achievements in traditional Chinese-rectal medicine.

3. Surgery:Surgery of hemorrhoid and anal fistula started as early as the Qin and Han Dynasties. For example, it is recorded in *Wu Shi Er Bing Fang*(Fifty—Two Prescriptions)that " First cupping is applied to the hemorrhoid located beside the anus.A small piece of thread is tied to it and a knife is used to cut it off. When something like a dodder seed or a blood clot is taken out,

the disorder is removed." From the modern point of view it is the thrombosed external hemorrhoidectomy. Another example of fistulectomy is described as follows. "Before the surgery kill a dog and have its urinary bladder. A bamboo stick is put into the bladder and then it is inserted into the rectum. Blow the bladder until the fistula is exposed. Then gradually cut it off with a knife. After the surgical operation, powder of Radix Scutellariae is applied to the wound." Two thousand years ago, the ancient practitioners developed such an advanced unique surgery, after which herbal medicine was applied. *Wai Ke Tu Shuo* (Illustrated Surgery) also describes the surgery of hemorrhoid and anal fistula. It says:" In the treatment of hemorrhoid, pathological conditions should be first observed. For small hemorrhoid, narcotic is applied to the affected part, then cut it with a sharp knife and bleeding is stopped by cotton balls...for persisted anal fistula, insert a filiform silver wire to detect its condition, then make a small opening with a lancet every day. After the operation the wound is covered with cotton balls for half a day. Herbal medicine is applied afterwards. When the anus is involved, a curved knife is used in the operation. Contraindications are as follows: hematopathy, pulmonary tuberculosis in its active stage, anterior and posterior pathological changes of the anus, anal fistula in children and old people." In the Qing Dynasty, apart from surgery of hemorrhoid and fistula, surgery was given to congenital anal atresia and anorectal foreign body. In diagnosis an appropriate body posture was desired then.

For smooth going of the operation, narcotics were used and special surgical apparatus invented. For instance, *Wai Ke Tu Shuo* (Illustrated Surgery) describes about thirty kinds of surgical knives, scissors, forceps, among which the operative appliance includes the rectal detector (anoscope), filiform ballended silver wire, silver needle for anal fistula, rectumcross needle, curved knife, fishhook knife, lancet, etc. Besides, there were other apparatus for dressing change, preparation of herbal medicines, examination and moxibustion. Zhao Lian, the author of *Yi Men Bu Yao* (Supplementary to Medicine) invented a pus cannula to drain pus from sores and ulcers. The book says:" A two *cun* cannula is made of thin copper plate with the size as big as a chopstic. One end is flat and the other is of an inclined plane; when the sharp end is inserted into the affected part, pus soon sprays out." In the Song Dynasty boiling sterilization for the surgical appliance was employed. For example, *Wei Ji Bao Shu* (A Precious Book on Medicine) points out that "...boil a small knife and hook in the decoction of Cortex Mori Radicis and Dalbergia Odorifera for a whole day, and store them in the powder of Dalbergia Odorifera."

4. Catharsis: In the Han Dynasty rectal suppository and enema were used. For Example, Zhang Zhongjing had honey as an enema. He made honey dates, which were inserted into the rectum together with some pig bile and vinegar. A few minutes later, bowel movements began. In the Ming Dynasty drug-spraying catharsis was used. A Bamboo tube loaded with herbal medicines was inserted into the rectum. The other end of the tube was slipped over a pig urinary bladder. When the bladder is pressed, herbal medicines were srayed into the rectum. The Chinese medicines included pig bile, honey, sesame oil, vinegar, onion juice herbal decoction and warm water. *Hui Chun Fang* (Aging Delaying Recipe) illustrates an enema with the head low and feet

high. With this method, half sesame oil and half warm water were given through a bamboo tube.

In addition, for an easy operation cleaning enema was used with mild or drastic purgatives, as *Wai Ke Zheng Zong* (Orthodox Manual of External Diseases)points out :"...in the treatment of internal hemorrhoid, purgatives are given first to clean the intestine and *Huanzhi san* (23) is applied to the anus." *Yi Xue Gang Mu* (Compendium of Medicine) says:"One day before the operation of hemorrhoid purgatives are given to make bowel movements easy, soft stool passing may not rub the hemorrhoids and avoid diarrhea."

1.6.3　Acupuncture, Moxibustion and *Daoyin*

Acupuncture and moxibustion are important methods to treat hemorrhoid and anal fistula, It is stated in *Zhen Jiu Jia Yi Jing* (A−B Classic of Acupuncture and Moxibustion)(282 A.D.)that " For painful hemorrhoids, acupuncture is applied to Cuanzhu (BL2);for hemorrhoids alone, Huiyin(RN1) is needled...;for proctoptosis and disrrhea,acupuncture is given to Qichong (ST30).*Zhen Jiu Zi Sheng Jin* (Experience in Acupuncture and Moxibustion)says:" A Mr. He had hemorrhoids for years,and one treatment of moxibustion given to Qichong (ST30) cured him." Later on,when a book on moxibustion was read and it was found that this point could be used to treat children's proctoptosis and diarrhea, a method developed by *Qi* Bo when he treated children. Then it was used to treat adult hematochezia,for which Changqiang (DU1) was the chief point to select." The commonly used points were Changqiang(DU1), Chengshan (BL57), eight−liao points Zusanli (ST36), Qihai (RN6) and Baihui (DU20). In recent years apart from body acupuncture auriculo-acupuncture is developed, and some new effective points such as Qiheng has been discovered. Acupuncture anesthesia is used in the hemorrhoid surgery. *Daoyin,* an approach for keeping fit and preventing diseases, is described in *Zhu Bing Yuan Hou Lun (General Treatise on the Causes and Symptoms of Diseases)*and *Bao Sheng Mi Yao* (Secrets for Keeping Fit).If one can practise it according to the instructions, disorders such as the five hemorrhoids may be cured.

1.7 Care and Prevention

Great importance has been attached to the nursing of hemorrhoid patients. *Wai Ke Jing Yi* (Essence of External Diseases)of the Yuan Dynasty points out the significance of proper diet, avoiding alcohol,rich food and food purgent and hot in property. Too much sexual activity and worry should be kept off. *Chuang Yang Jing Yan Quan Shu* (A Complete Manual of Experience in the Treatment of Sores) says:"For quick recovery, it is necessary to do less physical labor, keep away from rage and sexual activity and follow diet restraint. It is pointed out by *Yi Xue Zheng Zhuan* (Orthodox of Medical Problems)that "Patients of hemorrhoid or fistula may recover soon if they can follow proper diet,and avoid indulgence of sexual life." Examples will not be illustrated about proper diet,including herbal diet and diet restraint. Many experiences from late practitioners can relieve the sufferings of the patients. *Zhi Zhi Fang* (Most Effective Recipes) points out that patients with swollen hemorrhoid are not able to sit and stand owing to pain. They should be in a supine position and calm-minded, then distending pain may be alleviated. *Yang*

Yi Da Quan (A Complete Book on Sores) introduces a cushion filled with catkins and an opening in the centre. Hemorrhoid patients may sit on it comfortably, Up to now this kind of cushion is frequently adopted by hemorrhoid patients.

Traditional Chinese medicine has attached great significance to the integrated treatment for hemorrhoids and anal fistula. Prevention first is listed in *Nei Jing* (Classic of Internal Medicine). *Zhu Bing Yuan Hou Lun* (General Treatise on the Causes and Symptoms of Diseases) says that continuous practice of *Daoyin* can prevent hemorrhoids. It is recorded in *Ma Shi Zhi Lou Ke Qishierzhong* (Ma's Seventy-Two Kinds of Hemorrhoid and Anal Fistula) that "Very few people can avoid recurrence of hemorrhoid when they get it. It is suggested that boys before sixteen and girls before fourteen take a dose of *Wuxing Huazhi Dan* (Pills for Removing Hemorrhoid) to eliminate congenital and acquired toxins, they may keep away hemorrhoids for the whole life. This drug is a preventive measure to ward off hemorrhoids." From the above we can see preventive methods of hemorrhoids were studied too at that time.

2 Examination for Anal Rectum Diseases

2.1 Position of Patients

2.1.1 Lateral Position

The patient lies on his / her side with his upper limbs slightly bent towards the abdomen while keeping the lower limbs slightly straightened or two legs completely bent thereby completely exposing the anus. According to habit, the patient can lie on the left or right side, depending upon whichever way is more comfortable. It is important to ensure the patient's comfort if and when the operation involves a long time.

2.1.2 Prone Position

The patient is to lie on his / her abdomen with the lower limbs in a slightly elevated position, spreading both legs wide apart. It is a comfortable position, advised to be adopted by weak patients or long duration of the operation. This posture is to ensure adequate exposure of the anus. It is best suited for the examination or operation. During the operation, the buttocks can be separated by applying a wide strip of adhesive plaster.

2.1.3 Lithotomy Position.

The patient is to lie on his / her back with the lower limbs bent laterally. This position ensures sufficient exposure of the anus, but the patient may experience difficult climbing in and out of the operation table .It is best suited for the examination or operation.

For the purpose of demonstration, this posture has its drawback during the operation as there is not much space around.On account of the patient's legs being elevated, this somewhat impedes those assisting during the operation.

2.1.4 Knee-Chest Position or Knee-Elbow Position

The patient is to kneel down with his/her head down and buttocks up. This position is easily achieved with either the patient's chest touching the bed or being supported by both elbows. This posture, though lacking comfort has the advantage of sufficient exposure of the anus for the examination or colonoscope.

2.1.5 Flexed-Knee Supine Position

The patient is to lie on his/her back with the knees flexed acutely held by hands and pressed against the abdomen, thereby exposing the anus for the examination.

2.1.6 Squatting Position

The patient is to assume a squatting position. This is ideal for the examination of prolapse of hemorrhoid or rectum.

2.1.7 Standing-Bowing Position

The patient stands up with the body in a slightly forward inclined position,Both hands can be supported by either the bed or the chair.The chest can be padded with blankets. This position is suitable for the examination. and it does not require any equipment and can be easily implemented. The disadvantage is insufficient exposure.

2.1.8 Inverted Position

The patient is to lie on his/her abdomen with the head well

down, at the same time with both buttocks elevated. With certain adjustment, the patient virtually knees on the edge of the bed. This is to facilitate the easy examination and operation. The patient has the difficulty in climbing up and down the examining table and sometimes experiences great doscomfort if the head is too low down.

2.1.9 Ride-prone Position

The patient is to sit on the top of a specially designed wooden horse bed, with his / her back facing he examiner and the chest on the bed. The patient's head should turn to one side while the body is being supported by two hands holding onto the legs of the bed. This position again renders sufficient exposure of the buttocks for examination and changing of dressings. From the past experience this is an ideal position for examination, change of dressing and operation. However,after a prolonged operation, the patient may collapse as a result of this posture.

The wooden horse is a special design of the hospital and is made of wood. Now,it has been re-designed into an operation table, an all-round improvement on the previous model.

2.2 Procedure for Examination

2.2.1 Asking

The physician should endeavour to patiently listen to the patient's complaints.According to the pattern perception, when questions are asked,there should always be a focal point. Besides paying attention to the complaints, it must be emphasized that special understanding on the wholistic approach as well as the general well-being of the patient are of priority to the physician.In particular, the physician must note if the patient suffers from hypertension, coronary disease, diabetes or other related liver and kidney diseases or tuberculosis, etc.

2.2.2 Looking

The patient should assume a specific posture in order to expose the anus.With the help of good lighting, whether it be natural or artificial, the physician then proceeds with the examination.During the examination, the physician should separate the patient's buttocks in order to closely examine the problem area and the natural appearance of the anus.

2.2.3 Finger Diagnosis

This is for the examination of hemorrhoid and anal fistula. During the examination, first palpate the anus to see if there is any painful spot and any movable or cord—like object. If there is the latter, the next step is to ascertain its pathway. Then cover the index finger with a rubber cap which has been well lubricated and slowly insert the index finger into the anal canal. This is to establish if there is any soft or hard palpable lump on the anal wall. If there is a fistula, feel the inside of the internal orifice by the dentate line and see the condition of the strength of the sphincters and therectal ring.

2.2.4 Anoscopy

First lubricate the anoscope, then slowly insert it into the anus, gradually withdraw the anoscope, observing changes occurring in the rectum and inside the anal passage, such as the color of the mucosa, ulcer, the position of the hemorrhoid, its size and number,etc.

2.2.5 Probing Examination

This is an essential method to examine the anal fistula by the use of differentsized probes with round tips. Insert the probe into the anal fistula in order to examine the length and depth of it,at the same time insert the index finger covered with a lubricated rubber cap into the anus. The index finger should feel the impact of the probe at the rectal wall on the level of the top end of the fistula,if an anal fistula is present and if this occurs in an area parallel to the anal canal.

2.2.6 Localization of the Internal Opening of the Cryptus Hook

This is an important method to locate the inner opening of the anal fistula.Dilate the anus with a procteurysis and use different length of recess hooks for examination.First use a 0.5 cm hook to examine the problem area which has been observed or touched by the finger.Then follow the dentate line to examine the affected area. When coming into contact with the external orifice, easy access is ensured. In the presence of inflammation of the recess, a longer hook can be used (1 cm).If the recess can be reached to some extent by the hook, or the inner orifice easily swallows up the hook and the run of the hook is parallel to that of the anal fistula,it suggests that the hook has gone into it.

Other methods of examination include Methylene blue staining method, local roentgenography, sigmoidoscopy, fibrocolonoscopy, etc. The method involved is entirely dictated by the progress of the disease. Besides partial examination, full examination is also indicated. Generally, it includes blood routine examination, duration of bleeding and coagulation, or white cell count, duration of bleeding and coagulation, When necessary, routine feces and urine examination, E.S.R.,blood type, liver function test, cholesterol test, etc. are conducted. Specific examination like ECG and rhoencephalogram can also be considered.

2.3 Case Writing Record and Examination Record

After examination, detailed records of the patient's case history should be written down (See appendix).

2.3.1 Special Case History Record Form Can Be Used

In the case of inpatient, complete and detailed case history should be recorded for future reference.

2.3.2 Requirement for Case History Record

1. Time:

(1) Date of Admission

(2) It is necessary to record the patient's condition right before the operation. If the general condition is good, the local problem is stable and the hospitalized date is near the operation, the record made on the day of admission may serve as the record before the operation.

(3) No limitation of the number for pages for the post operation record.

(4) It is a routine practice to record the condition of the patient for three successive days. Thereafter twice weekly until the patient recovers. If the patient encounters any obvious discomfort or any deterioration, it is madatory to record everything until the patient's condition is stablized.

2. Content of the Record:

It includes the treatment procedures during the entire period of hospitalization. In another word, it is an entire procedure from the day of admission and progress of recovery or deterioration until death. With the combined traditional Chinese and modern medicine is employed in the treatment of anal fistula and other rectum related problem, it must be emphasized that traditional Chinese four examinations—four diagnostic methods and differentiation of syndromes should be reflected in the record.

(1) Record of the Day of Admission: It is a brief account of the ward admission record. In general, put the date of the record on the top left hand corner before proceeding with the details. The content entails the reason of admission after the full and partial examinations, the method of diagnosis and treatment program. If the condition is serious, important points of the implementation of the treatment and care in particular should be clearly listed.

(2) Pre—Operation Record: Any other systemic disease should also be or recorded .If the patient's condition is contraindicated for undergoing an operation. then treatment must be carried out prior to the actual operation. Once the requirement is fulfilled, the present condition of the patient must be recorded. After the operation, the patient's pre—operative condition can be compared with the post—operative one.If the patient's condition is stablized and immediate operation is indicated, then the admissi on record can also serve as the pre—operative record.

(3) Record of the Operation: It is to record the condition during and after the operation, for instance, if the patient suffers from any discomfort or any related pain anywhere. Any particular reaction should be noted. That operative procedure should be recorded too.

Selection of the body posture, sterilization, anesthetic and details of the operation should all be recorded. After the operation, there is no need to repeat the course of the disease. Upon the return to the ward, it is essential to record the entire condition of the patient. The general condition stems from the operation and anesthetic, such as headache, dizziness, palpitation, sweating, nausea, vomiting, etc. If blood pressure should be taken or serum or blood transfusion are indicaated, they should all be recorded. Other related conditions should also be recorded, such as pain, bearing-down feeling, hemorrhage, dysuria, retention of urine, abdominal distention, etc. Any necessary measure involved to relieve the symptoms should also be kept in the reoord.

(4)Post-Operative Record: After the operation, the condition of the patient and treatment should be recorded: Any related symptoms resulting from the operation should be gradually lessened. However, other symptoms like cold, infection tend to arise after the operation. The content of the record should state if the patient is running a temperature, aversion to cold, bitter taste in the mouth, development of thirst, persperation,sleeping and eating pattern, development of frequent urination and urodynia,color of the urine, bowel movements and its texture, any blood in the feces or internal hemorrhage. Besides recording the above, the incisive wound should be checked to ensure there is no infection.

Any measures adopted for treatment should focus on differentiation of syndromes, This is able to propose a proper prescription and treatment after a thorough analysis of the symptoms. If required, help can be rendered by associated departments. Advice and suggestion given by senior doctors and associated departments should be noted and recorded. During the treatment, if special investigation and treatment are warranted, the reason should be given for doing so. After the examination, results should be recorded. During shift change, the doctor going off duty should ensure that the record be handed over to the doctor coming on duty. The shift change record is similar to a summary. For the seriously ill patient, special notation should be recorded. The record for the doctor coming on duty is relatively simple, it merely records ail the patient's condition. In addition, due to the patient's deterioration, ward transfer is indicated and the reason for the transfer should be elaborated.

Transfer Record: The main thing is to elucidate the reason for the transfer and points to take note, and the doctor in charge's advice. Once transferred in, the record embraces many aspects. The form is identical to the admission record. In addition to the reason for the patient's transfer the patient's condition after the admission, the present condition ,etc should be recorded.

(5) Hospital Discharge Record: This is a systematic detailod record of the patient, including the date of admission,duration of hospitalization, treatment after the admission, and the detailed description of the patient's condition, with special emphasis on the method of the treatment, and things to note after the discharge.

2.3.3 Diagrams Commonly Used for Partial Examination, Code and Its Meaning

1. Lateral Aspect of the Anal Canal Diagram: See Figure 1
2. Anus and Perineum: See Figure 2
3. Commonly Used Code and Its Meaning :See Figure 3

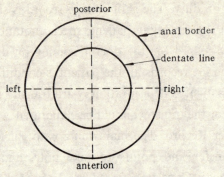

Fig.1 cross section of anal canal

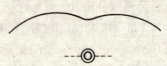

Fig.2 plan of anal canal and perineum

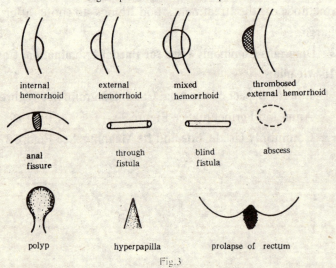

Fig.3

3 Anesthesia of Anus and Rectum

Due to the highly sensitivity of the anus and rectum and the presence of sphincter in the lower part of the rectum, it is important to select suitable anesthetic method in order to satisfy all the requirements, that is complete pain relief, complete relaxation of the sphincter and at the same time full exposure of the operable area, and also to ensure there is no reaction from other organs.

3.1 Acupuncture Anesthesia

3.1.1 Point Selection
1. Auricular Points: Shenmen,Lung, Lower Portion of Rectum, Upper Portion of Rectum, Jisong, etc.
2. Body Points: Chengshan (BL 57), Qiheng (ST30), Changqiang (DU1), Dice, etc.

3.1.2 Preparation before Acupuncture Anesthesia
The advantage of acupuncture anesthesia should be pointed out to the patient, in order to alleviate any worries and build up confidence. Small amount of Dolantin and Promethazine Hydrochloride can be administered accordingly.

3.1.3 Method
Locate the point and insert the needle and manipulate the needle until a distending sensation is experienced. Then connect the needle with electrodes. The intensity of the electric stimulation

can be tolerated by the patient. The duration of stimulation is approximately 30 minutes.

3.1.4 Advantage and Drawback

It is safe and void of any side-effects, but the degree of anesthesia is incomplete with the sphincter not being sufficiently relaxed.

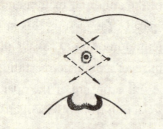 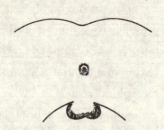

Fig.4 Perianal infiltration anesthesia: stratified anesthesia

Fig.5 Perianal infiltration anesthesia: seven point injection (vertical puncture)

3.2 Local Anesthesia

3.2.1 Suitable for Hemorrhoid and Fistula Operation in General

0.5%–2% Procaine, 1–2% Lidocaine, 0.15–0.5% Bupivacaine.

3.2.2 Method of Anesthesia

1. Peripheral Infiltration Anesthesia: This is generally used for ligation of the mixed hemorrhoid or internal hemorrhoid. See Figs.4 and 5.

2. Infiltration Anesthesia around the Problem Area: This is generally used for the operation on anal fistula and anal fissure.

3. Puncture Infiltration Anesthesia: This method is suitable

for peripheral injection of the rectal area in the case of proctoptosis, about 2 cm from the edge of the rectum.

3.2.3 Requirements

The whole procedure should be conducted in a complete sterile condition, paying attention to the depth of the injection, and the degree of blocking. If after the injection there is a protrusive area, every effort should be adopted to normalize the condition.

3.2.4 Advantage and Disadvantage

Easy implementation, safe, however, this method does not facilitate the easy injection in the high or complicated hemorrhoid fistula cases.

3.3 Yaoshu (DU2) Anesthesia

This is one of the sacral anesthesic methods, i.e. sacral hiatus anesthesia.

3.3.1 Indications

Mixed hemorrhoids, cyclic hemorrhoids, high complicated anal fistula, and ventral tumor.

3.3.2 Commonly Used Anesthetics

2% Lidocaine;2% Procaine.

3.3.3 Anesthetic Method

There is no special posture for this anesthesia.The best position is the prone position in surgery and the anesthic is administered accordingly. When lying in the prone position, the buttocks are to be elevated,giving an ample exposure. Sterilize the area with Iodine or alcohol and then cover the area with a sterile towel. Locate the point by using the midline along the sacrum until the sacrac hiatus. First puncture the point by injecting a little anesthetic solution before the further insertion. Once the resistance disappears, the sacrum is reached and do not insert the needle any further. The sensation of going through without any resistance is indicative that the puncture is accomplished. This means the needle has reached the sacral hiatus.After the successful puncture, the test for absence of blood in the syringe at the same time tells the injection can go in with considerable ease and that there is no protruding area. Proceed slowly in 5 minutes with the 10—20 ml injection. About 10 ml Lidocaine is usually administered. The minimum is 4 ml. About 20 ml Procaine is usually given. On the injection of the anesthetic the needle should touch sacrococcyx and the skin around the anus. Absense of pain shows the success of anesthesia. After the injection of the anesthetic, the operation starts.

3.3.4 Anesthetic Effect

In the past twenty years thousands of cases have undergone such kind of anesthesia and satisfactory result has been seen.The rate of success increases year by year and the rate of failure decreases. The rate of failure was 5.1% in 1966, 2.1% in 1967,and 1.1% in 1968. Since 1969 not a case has failed. The latency of anesthesia shortens year by year. From 1966—1967 it was 5—15 minutes, and half of the cases reached anesthesia within 5 minutes. In 1968 the latency of anesthesia was about 5 minutes, and 80% of the cases had the anesthetic effect within 5 minutes. In 1960 75% immediately had the anesthetic effect.

The effective anesthetic duration is 50—70 minutes when Procaine is administered. The effective duration can be prolonged when 0.1—0.25 ml of 1:1000 Adrenalin is added to or a mixer of 2% Procaine and 0.1% Dicaine is given. In addition, continuous giving of anesthetic in the operation may be adopted.

In the period of anesthesia, patients feel all right, without negative reaction. The blood pressure, pulse rate and respiration are normal. In some cases, mild negative reaction may arise, such as slight dizziness, nausea, palpitation, suffocated chest, and rise of blood pressure, for which no special treatment is necessary because these minor symptoms may disappear after a short rest. However, if spasm and convulsion are present, sedatives such as injections of Dazepam, Luminal Sodium are administered to the case.

3.3.5 How to Apply Anesthesia to Yaoshu (DU2)

1. Point Location

Yaoshu (DU2) is located at the hiatus of the sacrum, in the 21th lumbar vertebra or 3 Cun above Changqiang (DU1) and in the centre of Xialiao (BL34).From the view of modern anatomy, it is located at the 4th sacral vertebra and its hiatus. In other words, it is the lower entry of the sacral canal. The sacral hiatus and sacral canal are not identical,and it has aroused attention at home and abroad. After a careful analysis, it is a long fissure, although different in appearance. It is covered with hard sacral ligaments. The term sacral crest can fundamentally represent its actual appearance.

In medical literature the sacral hiatus of the Chinese is triangle in shape.The upper angle is the bulge of the end of the intermediate sacral crest. The two lower angles are the left and right sacral horns. The center of the triangle is the standard puncturing point for sacral canal anesthesia. Since the appearance of the sacral hiatus is different, the square (trapezoid, or rectangle) between the triangle is the mark of point location too, besides the triangle itself, the square is symbolized by two upper sacral horns and two lower caudal horns. Therefore for point location, when the sense of the body protrusions is found, the point can be easily located.

2. Success of Puncture and Anesthesia

Sudden disappearance of resistance tells the success of the proper puncture,because the sacral fissure is covered with ligaments, through which the needle goes, One end of the sacral fissure connects the sacral canal, and the other communicates with the sacrococcyx. From the bottom to the top, there is a change of depth.In general, the upper end is deeper. The puncture point is between the sacral horns and in front of or behind them. The depth here is about 1.5 cm.If it is relatively long, the sacral fissure can be divided into three parts: upper, middle and lower. The upper part is beneath the bulge of the end of the median sacral crest, where the puncture tends to fail. The middle part is between the sacral horns and in front of or behind them,where the puncture and anesthetic injection is often successful. The lower part is in the sacrococcyx, where the puncture and anesthetic injection only has partial anesthetic effect, that is posterior anesthesia, which cannot meet the clinical demand. In case of short sacral fissure, it is difficult to identify the three parts, the puncture should still be applied between the sacral horns.

Success of the puncture and that of anesthesia are closely related, yet they are the same thing. The successful puncture only implies the needle reaching the sacral fissure, but the anesthetic effect should be observed during the anesthetic injection. There are several puncture points from above to below in the sacral fissure,and not all of them are effective. It is essential to select rigorously the point to exert the anesthetic action. That the past failure of sacral anesthesia attributed to the anatomical change is not right.

3. Regularity of Yaoshu (DU2) Anesthesia

Clinical experiments show that disappearance of the pain sense is felt from above to below, and posterior to anterior in the sacroccoyx and perianal area, which indicates the success of anesthesia. After the anesthetic is given, if disappearance of the pain sense does not go downward, it indicates the punctured point is too low, and an upper one should be used. No presence of anesthesia within this area tells the puncture is too high and the anesthetic goes into the sacral canal. A lower point should be selected and repunctured. Disappearance of the pain sense and timely change of puncture points can ensure the success of anesthesia and absence of anesthetic latency.

4. Analysis of Yaoshu (DU2) Anesthesia

There is no consensus about the Yaoshu anesthesia. Based on keen obser vations in the past years, it has been observed that the Yaoshu anesthesia cannot be considered as the sacral canal anesthesia. Why does anaesthesia lack in some patients when the anesthetic goes into the sacral canal? According to the indication of success of anesthesia, there is no doubt that the anesthetic goes into the sacral fissure. In most of the failed cases, the puncture point is wrongly located at the upper part of the triangle. The upper the puncture is applied, the deeper the needle goes. When the needle goes to the part close to the sacral canal, or to the lower orifice of it, the anesthetic may naturally runs into the sacral canal. Because of the declined penetrating power of the anesthetic, absence of anesthesia would be found with a period of time after the anesthetic goes into the sacral canal. On the contrary, the nerval sheath of the sacral fissure may be thinner than that of the sacral canal, then 2% Procaine can soon exert the blocking action.

It is thought that the Yaoshu anesthesia, in the final analysis, is partial blocking of the sacral fissure with the anesthetic penetration of the lower part of the sacral canal. On the whole, the Yaoshu anesthesia is the area blocking of the sacral fissure and its upper related part (a small part of the lower sacral canal).

When the penetrative action of the anesthetic (e.g. Lidocaine) is strong enough, selection of the puncture point is not so rigorous as above. On puncturing either the upper or lower sacral fissure, block is completed and spread to the sacral canal. The difference of the anesthetic action due to improper puncture point is made up by the penetrative power of the anesthetic. Hence, once Lidocaine is administered the significance of the Yaoshu anesthesia is covered up.

The anesthetic area is identical to the low sacral canal block. It is understandable that an increased dose may expand the block plane. It is because the sacral fissure is located at the lower part of the sacral canal, and there is no obvious separation between them. Extra anesthetic would naturally run into the sacral canal, or the higher part. Although there appears a blocking at the sacral fissure, the sacral canal anesthesia is seen too owing to the strong penetrative action of the anesthetic. It is different from the fact that the anesthetic is directly injected into the sacral canal.

It is generally conceived that the length of latency is related to the selection of the puncture point and the penetrative action of the anesthetic for local anesthesia. With the same dose and concentration limit, different latency would appear if the appropriate puncture point is ont selected. After 2% 20 ml Procaine is given, complete anesthesia will be seen within 5 minutes, and the operation may start without any delay. But in the first several years, the latency was 5-15 minutes, which was associated with the puncture, when the anesthetic was diffused to the main nerves of the anus and perineum, a complete anesthesia was achieved. The longer the time, the more perfect of the blockage. Later on, disappearance of the pain sense as the criterion and timely shift of the puncture point made the absence of latency possible or shortened it. In addition, strong penetrative action of the anesthetic and increased dose made contributions too.

Some people think that it is just the same as the sacral canal anesthesia, because the dose of the anesthetic applied is similar to that in the sacral canal anesthesia. That is not the case. If a large dose of anesthetic is given, aside from the sacral fissure blocking, extra anesthetic may run into the sacral canal or the higher part. Different effect may occur because of differed penetrative action when the anesthetic runs into the sacral canal. No research has shown the volume of the sacral fissure. It is yet unknown whether the sacral fissure is included in the sacral canal.

In short, in vivo, in a broad sense, this kind of anesthesia is a blockage of the specific area in the sacral canal. In terms of anesthesiology and anatomy, it is known as the sacral fissure anesthesia, which is completely different from the sacral canal anesthesia; however, in the past, the sacral fissure was used only as the entry in the sacral canal anesthesia, but not as the blocking area. The new anesthesia takes the sacral fissure as the blocking area, i.e. both the puncture and anesthetic injection are given at this place. It not only simplifies the operation sequence, but also allows lower appearance of the blocking area, suitable to the anal surgery. When one knows the regularity of the superficial disappearance of the pain sense, there will be no or little anesthetic latency. In this sense, the Yaoshu anesthesia enriches the sacral anaesthesia.

5. Point for Attention

The sacral fissure, located beneath the sacral canal is a part of the epidurum, so this kind of anesthesia is also called epidural block anesthesia. Since it is connected with the sacral canal, and the extra anesthetic may enter the sacral canal, points for attention of the Yaoshu anesthesia is similar to those of the sacral canal anesthesia.

(1) Before putting in the anesthetic, the plunger must be drawn back a little to make sure that there is no presence of blood. Otherwise, intoxication may occur when the anesthetic goes into blood.

(2) The anesthetic must be slowly put in to avoid quick absorption and toxic reaction due to a sudden change of the pressure in the sacral fissure.

(3) It is essential to select the puncture point. Pay attention to the changes of the disappearance of the corresponding superficial pain sense, and the successful rate of anesthesia reaches 100 percent, lacking or shortening latency.

(4) Thin and short needle is used, and the needle is not deeply inserted.

3.4 Other Kinds of Anesthesia

3.4.1 Lumbar Anesthesia
It is also known as saddle spinal anesthesia, in which small dose is applied. The ordinary dose of Procaine is 60—70 mg.

3.4.2 Lumbosacral Epidural Anesthesia of Spinal Cord
It has good effect, but skilled techique is required.

3.4.3 Refrigeration Anesthesia and General Anesthesia
They are seldom used.

3.4.4 Intravenous Anesthesia and General Anesthesia
They are seldom used.

4. Pre-and-Post-Operative Management of Anorectal Surgery and Handling of Post-Operative Reaction and Complications

4.1 Pre-and-Post-Operative Management of Anorectal Surgery

It is significant to have proper pre-and-post-operative management, which would lessen the sufferings of patients and ensure a smooth course of treatment.

4.1.1 Pre-Operative Preparation

1. It is important for patients to take a good rest and to be full of optimism and confidence in treatment.

2. It is necessary to have a general check-up and local examination.

3. Diet: In general, normal diet is taken, but some restraints should be carried out when necessary.

4. Preparation for Skin: When conditions are permitted, the patients should take a bath or a hip bath. Local hair should be shaved.

5. Preparation for Intestines:

(1) Enema: In general, enema is not applied. One day before the operation, beginning at 2 o'clock in the afternoon, drink Senna tea (6—9 g Senna contained) to clear the intestines, or take castor oil 2 ml to purgate. Enema is given for asepsis.

(2) Administration of Intestinal Antibiotics: For most anal and fistula operations, it is unnecessary to administer intestinal antibiotics. Antibiotics begin to give three days before the operation.

(3) Sedatives: Point Injection at Zusanli (ST36) is given with 0.1 g Luminal Sodium, 15—30 minutes before the operation.

4.1.2 Post-Operative Management

1. Points for Attention

(1) Patients should be brought to the rest room of the clinic or ward for bed rest after the operation. For outpatients, having half an hour's rest after the operation without hemorrhage, they may go home. But riding bicycle is inhibited.

(2) Ask constantly the patients how they feel and observe the condition keenly.

(3) Measure regularly the body temperature, pulse rate, respiration rate and blood pressure for inpatients.

(4) Promptly handle post-operative pain, dysuria, hemorrhage and complications.

(5) Have appropriate rest and avoid strenuous physical exercise and sexual activity before the wound is healed.

2. Diet: Normal diet is taken or less food on the day of the surgery. Avoid pungent food. Have more vegetables and fruits several days after the operation. According to the previous lessons, dog meat and scaleless fishes should not be taken. But because of individual distinction some felt sharp pain at the wound

owing to eating mutton in the days following the surgery; some had more secretions from the wound owing to eating chicken, but nothing special was found when they ate scaleless fishes and hairtail. It is advisable to have vegetarian diet, more vegetables and fruits in a few days following the surgery.

3. Control of Bowel Movements: Don't pass stools on the day of the surgery. Afterwards regular bowel movements are encouraged. For cases having asepsis, control bowel movements for 3—5 days. Take 5—10 ml 10% Opium tincture, twice a day. For those to control bowel movements, before passage of stools, lubricants are given and enema is applied. After the operation it is essential to ensure free bowel movements and avoid diarrhea.

4. Dressing change : Dressing change is important after the anal and fistula operations.

Procedure of Dressing Change: The patient makes bowel movements first, and then has a hip bath. On dressing change, the patient is in a ride—prone position with the buttocks elevated, while the doctor separates the wound area with the thumb and index finger. The wound is cleaned by cotton balls with alcohol. *Jiuhua Gao*(24) is applied to the hemorrhoid, anal fissure and the interior of the anus, or *Jiuhua Gao* is directly applied to the wound and the interior of the anus by a glycerin enemator. On dressing change for the anal fistula, the opening of the wound should be separated as wide as possible. Wipe out the secretion from inside to outside, then apply *ShengJi Yuhong Gao*(25) to the wound. If the edge of the wound tends to close or there is a sinus, a piece of medicated gauze should be put in, and then fix the dressing.

Points for Attention:

(1) Dressing change should be gentle and careful to lessen pain.

(2) When there is dull-colored granulation or much putrefactive tissue, *Hongfeng Yougao* (26) or *Maoyan Caogao* (27) is applied.

(3) When the granulatin is too long, corrode it with toughened silver Nitrate or Silver Nitrate solution, or cut it.

(4) On dressing change, first have a check to see if there is any branch fistula or other factor impeding the healing. If a branch fistula is found, pus may run out when the edge of the wound is pressed. Clean the pus, and find the sore. Examine it with a probe to see the depth, length and travelling direction of the fistula.

(5) A large and deep wound of the anal fissure should be filled with a piece of medicated gauze to allow the wound to be kept in an opening state. The new granulation may grow gradually from the bottom of it, so as to avoid adhesion of the wound or bridge-shaped pseudohealing.

(6) Treatment should be given when there are ulcer, blister, papular eruption or itching pain around the anus or the wound.Take drugs to relieve he at and toxins or wash the anus with them. Apply medicinal power or ointment to the wound to remove dampness and itching.

(7) Concern about the general condition of the patient. If he is weak or experiences slow healing of the wound, or suffers from much pus and light red blood running, tonics should be given. They include *Buzhong Yiqi Tang* (6), *Shiquan dabu Tang* (28) and *Shengfu Tang* (29).

4.2 Handling the Post-Operative Reaction and Complications

Post-operative bad reactions and complications may be seen in anal and rectal diseases after the operation. These problems must be solved properly. The following is the main bad reactions and complications.

4.2.1 Pain

Post-operative pain to varying degrees is usually found, because the anal skin is most sensitive. Mild pain only brings on a local uneasiness, not affecting the whole body, but severe pain causes great sufferings to the patient. The patient cannot rest well, he groans, and has profuse sweating and no desire to eat. Pains varies from distending pain, burning pain, bearingdown pain and throbbing pain, characterized by persistence. The sharp pain is felt 1-2 days after the operation, then it gradually subsides. But on bowel movements and dressing changes, there occurs severe pain.

Post-operative pain is related to the patient's mental state, tolerance, anesthesia adopted, size of lesion, etc. in addition to the sensitivity of the anal region. Therefore all-round measures should be taken to alleviate pain.

Measures

(1) Proper Anesthesia: Painless and aseptic manipulations are conducted. In the local anesthesia, the narcotics should reach the appropriate site by exerting complete blockade. Long-acting analgesics are used. Good pain-killing effect can be seen when long-acting Methylene Blue analgesics (30) are given, The

analgesic action may last 1-2 weeks.

(2) Set the patient free from worrying before the operation, or give sedatives when necessary.

(3) Operation: Gently change the dressing and ask the patients to keep free bowel movements, and promptly eliminate inflammation.

(4) Giving Analgesics: In accordance with the degree of pain, administer some analgesics to the patients, usually pain-killing tablets are given, but analgesic injections and sedatives are given to severe cases. If there is an extensive lesion, and severe injury is associated with inflammation, herbs are given too. i.e (31)

(5) Acupuncture Analgesia: It can exert a quick action without any side-effect. Strong acupuncture stimulation or electric acupuncture is given until pain subsides or disappears. Points usually used are Chengshan (BL57), Qiheng, Changqiang (DU1), Baliao and Diche. Ear acupuncture is used too. The responsive spots are located at the helix. After acupuncture, small needles are embeded beneath the skin or plant seeds are put on the ear points covered by pieces of tape. Frequently give pressure to the embedded needles or plant seeds to relieve pain.

(6) Magnetic Therapy: A piece of magnet is placed on Yaoshu (DU 2), immobilized with adhesive tape. Carry it for several days when there is no dizziness, nausea and vomiting. Pain tends to be relieved after 5 minutes of the immobilization of the magnet. The stronger the magnetic field, the better the effect. Electric magnet is also used for this purpose.

4.2.2 Bearing-Down Pain

It is usually induced by mechanical stimulation or inflammation. The patient may have a bearing-down sensation of the anus, or a distending feeling, leading to frequent bowel movements, or rectal tenesmus.

Treatment

(1) Elimination of the Irritations: Anal bearing-down sensation is caused by operative irritation or injury. It can be relieved a few days after the operation. Alleviation is felt after removal of the piles in hemorrhoid ligation. For severe cases, *Qinjiu Wan* (32) and *Zhitong Rushen Tang* (31) are given.

(2) Bed Rest: Standing may cause deterioration and bed rest helps to relieve the bearing-down pain.

(3) Acupuncture Therapy: It can be used but the effect is not so obvious as analgesics.

Points for Attention:

Post-operative freqent bowel movements caused by the anal bearing-down sensation can never be considered as enteritis. If there are red, white cells and pus cells in the stool, it does not mean enteritis, rather, it is the result of the wound. Therefore it is unnecessary to have a fecal examination.

4.2.3 Urinating Disturbance

It is usually seen the day after the operaiton. In some cases, it may last a few days with various causes. But it is chiefly brought about by reflex. Reflective urinating disturbance is caused by the operative irritaition, injury and pain, and dressing in the rectum, mental factors and unaccustomed urination in bed also contribute to the disturbance. In mild cases, it is manifested by uneasy urination, but in severe cases, there is retention of urine for a few days. The bladder is full and a distending pain is felt in the lower abdomen. Sometimes, there is urodynia with the lower abdomen involved. Some patients who do not urinate a few hours after the operation should not be considered as urinating disturbance because there is not enough urine in the bladder.

Treatment:

(1) Set the patient free from worries. Drink as much water or tea as he likes. If he is not accustomed to passing water in bed, let him to do it in the toilet.

(2) Hot or Cold Compress: Hot compress is applied to the lower abdomen in difficulty of urination. Half an hour later urination becomes normal. If it fails, continuous hot compress or cold compress is given or first cold compress and then hot compress is applied. The hot or cold stimulation may induce urination. But it is not advisable to use cold compress in winter.

(3) Acupuncture: Points frequently used are as follows. Sanyinjiao (SP6), Yinlingquan (SP9), Guanyuan (RN4), Shuidao (ST28) and others.

(4) *Tuina* and Massage Therapy: Give a up and down massage to the medial part of both thighs until there is a feeling of urination. Finger-pressure is applied to Zhongji (RN3) for 2-5 minutes. The dogskin plaster mixed with 0.25 g Borneol is applied to Guanyuan (RN4) or Zhongji (RN3). Application of hot smashed green Chinese onion to the umbilicus or lower abdomen is also helpful.

(5) When it is assured that there is no possibilty of hemorrhage, take out the dressing from the rectum or put a piece of garlic on the meatus urinatius of the male patients to induce urination. Hip bath is adopted on the same day after the operation when necessary.

(6) Treatment with APC and CNB: Doctor Lu Kijie often administers draught of compound 0.75 g Aspirin (APC) with 0.3 g Caffine

Sodium Benxoate (CNB) for patients with difficult urination. Thirty—forty minutes after medication, urine is passed. Sometimes, 0.8 g APC and 0.75 g CNB are used for injection.Twenty minutes later urine is passed. For patients with difficulty of urination for several days, it is advised to take such drugs as *Wuling San*(33), *Bazheng San* (34) and *Tongpao Tang* (35) (modifications).

4.2.4 Hemorrhage

Among quite a number of reasons causing hemorrhage after the operation, local factors are the chief ones, including hemostatic problems during the operation, too much physical activites after the operation, injury by passing dry stools or inflammation, etc. In a few cases, there exist general hemorrhatic factors. Bleeding condition can be classified into the following groups according to the bleeding time, nature and amount of blood escape.

In terms of time of hemorrhage, it can be divided into immediate hemorrhage and later hemorrhage. The former occurs on the day of the operation caused by hemostatic problems during the operation, while the latter usually occurs within 15 days after the operation. Later massive hemorrhage is a serious complication, happening at the withering period of hemorrhoids and it is difficult to avoid completely where the present surgery of hemorrhoids is adopted.

There are two kinds of hemorrhage: internal and external.

The former refers to blood running to the rectum and colon, caused by obstruction of the anal canal due to anal sphincterismus or pressure brought on by the filling, stopping blood from flowing out. At first the patient may feel nothing wrong because of small amount of hemorrhage. However, when increased blood escape exists, the patient may feel distension of the lower abdomen, desire of bowel movements, or a burning sensation at the anus. On bowel movements, the accumulated dark blood together with clots runs out. Now the patient may have a sense of pulpitation, dizziness, weakened limbs or loss of consciousness in severe cases. There may appear pallor, cold perspiration, thready and weak pulse, and lowered blood pressure. Internal hemorrhage may be neglected, and a mild case would turn to a serious one owing to failure to stop hemorrhage timely. For this reason, it is essential to have prompt discovery and treatment for this condition. External hemorrhage is easy to be found because it can be seen on the dressing, while the patient may have a burning sensation at the anus and feels something running out from it.

There may be massive, moderate and small loss of blood. The first two are considered as serious cases, usually in the form of later hemorrhage or immediate hemorrhage. They must be timely handled. The last one, in the form of later hemorrhage or immediate hemorrhage does not effect the body severely because of small loss of blood.

Symptoms and signs of internal or external hemorrhage vary as mentioned above. In short, on massive acute hemorrhage, there are obvious symptoms and signs, and shock may be present in serious cases; whereas small, slow hemorrhage produces less obvious symptoms and signs.

Management: Among various hemorrhagic factors, local ones are the chief cause. In the prevention and treatment the following should be noted.

(1) Carefully select indications and follow strictly the technique of each therapy. Hemostasis during the operation must be done well.

(2) It is advised to have less physical activity immediately after the operation and ensure free bowel movements.

(3) It is essential to eliminate inflammation.

(4) Avoid hot stimulation to the anus on the withering period of the hemorrhoid. On hip bath, warm medicated water is used for a shorter time.

(5) Take some hemostats in case of small post-operative hemorrhage or no special treatment is given except keen observations. When masive hemorrhage occurs, pay close attention to the condition, blood pressure, pulse rate, and get hemostatic preparation.

Post-operative hemorrhage can be handled in the following ways. prompt stopping hemorrhage, bed rest and control of diet and bowel movements.

(1) Prompt Stopping Hemorrhage: Give hemostats or take measures to check local bleeding.

Hemostats Commonly Used: In general, Vitamin K, Adrenosem Salicylate, Thromboplastin, Dicynone, powder of Notoginseng and other medicinal herbs. The dose, duration of medication and way of administration depend on the case condition.

Proper Local Hemostatic Measures: Different measures are taken according to the condition. For example, small hemorrhage or oozing of blood is handled by change of dressing, pressure bandage or local application of hemostats, such as *Zhixue San*(36) and Alum powder. When there appears fast oozing of blood, forceps hold or ligation is used, or Silver Nitrate is applied to the bleeding part. The hemorrhagic spot must be held with forceps, or ligated, cauterized or eroded.

Massive and moderate hemorrhage, if immediate, is handled by suture of the bleeding wound, or fix the free mucosa and the submucous tissue by means of suture. Ligate the hemorrhoid vessel on the upper part of the wound. It is more difficult to handle later hemorrhage because it often occurs at the withering period of the hemorrhoid, when the fragile tissue is not easy to be sutured. Experience shows that hemostasis by compression has been suitable. The detailed descriptions are as follows. Roller Pressure: Have a 8—10 cm hollow rubber tube wrapped in vaseline gauze to a diameter of 5 cm. The gauze roller is slowly put into the anal canal. Tie a piece of silk thread throught the rubber tube and the gauze roller to the dressing to prevent the roller from moving into the upper rectum.

Ribbon Gauze Pressure: Have a piece of ribbon gauze and make it into strips wrapped in a layer of vaselin gauze. Attach a piece of thick silk thread to its centor and put the ribbon gauze slowly into the rectum, while leave the silk thread outside. Use a finger to feel the gauze and push it to the rectal ampulla. Draw the silk thread and bring the gauze back to the anal canal. At this moment, the gauze is folded and exerts greater pressure. Tie the silk thread to a small gauze roller outside the anus to prevent it from moving upward. The above two methods are called prolonged pressure, usually spplied for 3—5 days.

Baloon Pressure: Put a baloon into the rectum and pump air into it. The opening of the baloon is kept shut by a pair of forceps. The baloon can be replaced by a condom. Cover a short stick with the condom, into which a thin rubber tube is put. Tie the opening of the condom loosely and put it into the rectum. Pump air into the rubber tube. When the condom expands, tie the opening of it tightly. Intermittent pressure can be given by the baloon pressure. In order to avoid sufferings caused by the pressure, air can be released or pumped again.

When the pressure hemostasis is employed, it is necessary to control diet, bowel movements, and to administer hemostatics. Local pressure may produce varied sufferings on patients. Although satisfactory effect can be gained when a sclerosing agent is injected into the mucosa above the hemorrhagic part, patients suffer from anesthesia and injection.

Patients with hematochezia due to internal hemorrhoid or post-operative hemorrhoid hemorrhage have been cured by introducing Alum solution into the anal canal, based on the experience of enema for patients with rectal cancer. Since 1965 application of Alum ointment to the hemorrhagic area has shown desirable effects.

This method is easy to operate with no sufferings and control of diet and bowel movements. In addition, no hemostatic measures are taken at the local hemorrhagic area.

Introducing Alum Solution to the Anal Canal: Dissolve Alum powder in warm water to the required concentration. Put the Alum solution into the anal canal with a glycerine enema syringe, or a urinary catheter. After introduction of the Alum solution, advise the patient to lie in bed for at least half an hour. When it is hard to control bowel movements, pass the solution. If there is no desire of bowel movements, never loose bowels on purpose, and keep the Alum solution as long as possible in the anal canal.

Application of Alum Ointment: Mix *Jiuhua Gao*(24) with much Alum powder (known as the Alum Ointment). Cover a piece of gauze, vaselin gauze or medicated gauze of *ShengJi Yuhong Gao* (25) with the ointment, and put the gauze into the anal canal and cover the whole hemorrhagic area. Digital examination is used first to ensure the bleeding area so as to put the medicated gauze to it. The medicated gauze should be bigger than the bleeding area to make a full cover. In case of later massive hemorrhage, the hemorrhagic area tends to be unsmooth, with protrusion of the edge of the wound and free mucosa. Sometimes, a gap of the free mucosa can be felt. If a large range of free mucosa occurs, digital examination should follow after insertion of the gauze, and the total hemorrhagic area should be covered by the flat gauze. On injection of the Alum ointment into the anus, it is difficult to inject when too much Alum is involved. Adjustment should be done.

Points for Attention for Application of Alum Solution or Alum Ointment:

Concentration, Dose and Number of Application: Concentration and dose are flexible according to different conditions. For example, if only premonitor of hemorrhage is seen, 100–200 ml 1–2% Alum solution is administered. On massive hemorrhage, increase the concentration and dose, 300 ml 2–3% Alum solution is used generally. The maximum concentration and dose are 8% and 500 ml respectively. The number of administration depends on the condition too, once a day for two successive days. Three times are given a day when necessary. In the mixer of *Jiuhua Gao* and Alum Ointment the proportion of the former to the latter is 1 : 1,2 : 1 or 3 : 1. It is applied once a day until cessation of hemorrhage. The drug can be administered again when there are bowel movements after medication on the day of hemorrhage.

Observation and Prediction of Cessation of Hemorrhage: From the stools evacuated after enema one can see if hemorrhage stops or not. Bright red blood mixed with stools indicates fast continuous hemorrhage. It is not easy to determine hemostasis by only one anal enema. Dark brown or dark purple blood mixed with stools refers to slow hemorrhage, for which one anal enema may get the desired result. If oozing of blood remains, hemorrhage can cease by itself. But for safety, anal enema can be applied on the following day. No more anal enema is applied when there is no blood or only brown old blood in the stools. Hemorrhage may cease when there is no more stool passing. 5—8 hours after the first bowel movements. The observation and prediction of hemostatis with the application of Alum Ointment on the hemorrhagic area is almost similar to those of anal enema, But alum ointment application is only in a small area and it can lessen the stimulation of the wound, avoiding or delaying bowel movements. As a result, later massive hemorrhage and shock can be excaped and prevented.

Hemostatic Grounds of Alum Solution or Alum Ointment: Alum, cold in property and acerbic in flavor can remove dampness and phlegm, kill parasites, detoxify, astrict and stop bleeding.

Points for Attention:

a. Too cold or too warm Alum solution is not applied. Abdominal pain may occur in patients with cold due to deficiency when the Alum solution (Alum is of cold property) is too cold. If abdominal pain is present, such treatments as hot compress are given.

b. Gently insert the enemator and inject the Alum solution slowly.

c. Never insert the enemator or urinary catheter deeply. In general, 2 cm in depth is enough.

Determine the hemorrhagic area before the application of the Alum ointment so as to cover the area completely.

Other Measures Taken: Hemostats may be administered sometimes, but it is unnecessary to control diet and bowel movements. Appropriate emergent measures may be taken in case of shock.

Measures for Immediate Post-Operative Hemorrhage: Massive post-operative hemorrhage is often caused by malpractice during the operation. After ligation or suture of the wound, other necessary measures such as Alum enema or application of Alum ointment may be taken. Once massive post-operative hemorrhage due to loose of the ligation was seen in one case on the same day after the internal hemorrhoid ligation. The hemorrhoid was not ligated again. The patient was given anal enema with 200 ml 8% Alum solution, three times a day, and hemorrhage ceased. In addition, on ligation of polyp when it exfoliates soon, the anal enema with Alum solution is used to prevent hemorrhage.

(2) Bed Rest: Bed rest is necessary for cases of massive and moderate hemorrhage. At the same time hemostasis by compression is helpful. After cessation of hemorrhage, bed rest is unnecessary. Have appropriate rest for small bleeding patients.

No special limitations are needed for patients with hematochezia after the prompt management.

(3) Control over Diet and Bowel Movements: Normal diet is taken and it is unnecessary to control bowel movements for small hemorrhage patients after hemostatic measures. But it is significant to control diet and bowel movements in massive and moderate hemorrhage when hemostasis by compression is applied, until the fillings are removed. Usually it takes 3—5 days. If hemorrhage continues after the fillings are removed, Alum Ointment is applied and meanwhile it is unnecessary to control over diet and bowel movements. During this period, liquid or semi—liquid food is given depending on the patient's physical condition. On the control over bowel movements opium tablets may be administered, twice a day, one tablet each time.

Resume normal diet after hemostasis by compression. Lubricants are administered after removal of the fillings to prevent constipation, and on the first bowel movements it is advisable to have enema.

(4) Give fluid infusion and blood transfusion on post—operative hemorrhage, and emergent measures are taken to treat shock.

4.2.5 Fever

Reactive fever due to local irritation is found within three days after the operation, when blood cell count is normal or slightly higher. Sometimes, it is caused by cold—catching due to oversweating during the operation. Low fever without obvious symptoms should not be treated. Medicinal herbs can be administered to high fever based on differentiation of syndromes. If fever is present several days after the operation, and the white blood cell count increases, it is a case of infection. Herbal medicines or antibiotics are given.

4.2.6 Local Swelling

It may be produced by infection, disturbance of venous or lymphatic return, local anesthesia, injury during the operation, poor handling of the wound, etc. The swollen edge of the wound or edema of the skin around the anus causes swelling of the anus. Sometimes an acute attack of prolapse or impaction of internal hemorrhoids may occur, or anal patch ecchymoma is found, and thrombosed external hemorrhoid forms.

Management: Wash the affected part with compound (*Fu fang*) *JingJie Xiyao* (38) 2—3 times a day, 0.5—1 hour for each time.

4.2.7 Eczema and Dermatitis

It is ually produced by allergy, local inflammation, and irritation by secretion. The skin becomes swollen, and ulcerous or papular eruption, blisters and itching occur. In serious cases, there may be general symptoms.

Management: Medicinal herbs that can clear off heat, wind and dampness, and detoxify are administered orally. *Qingge San*(39) and other desensitizers are for the external application.

4.2.8 Slow Healing of the Wound

It may have to reasons: general debility or local factors that hinder the healing.

Management:

(1) Take tonics to reinforce *Qi* and blood, such as *Shiquan Dabu Tang* (28), *Buzhong Yiqi Tang* (6), and *Shengfu Tang* (29).

(2) Use *Hongfeng Yougao* (26), *Maoyan Caogao* (27), etc. for the external application.

(3) Point Injection with Vitamin, B_1: Have point injection at

either Zusanli (ST36) atternatively, once a day or the other day until the healing of the wound. A month makes a course. A new course begins at an interval of 10 days.

(4) Puncture the vicinity of the wound with a health protective needle, 1—2 times a day.

4.2.9 Stricture of Anus and Fecal Incontinence

Stricture of anus is rare. It can be produced by excessive removal of the anal skin during the operation, causing severe damage to the anal canal, or by adhesion of mucosa during the withering stage of the ligated hemorrhoids. For mild cases, the anus can be enlarged or the narrow anus be incised.

Fecal incontinence is ultimately seldom found. There are many causes for this condition, for example, severe damage to sphincters, disturbance of the nervous function, shift of the rectal pressure, etc. Two groups are classified according to the condition.

Complete Fecal Incontinence: There is no or little control over feces, resulting in automatic running of feces, the condition which is difficult to recover to normal itself is known as complete fecal incontinence or incurable fecal incontinence. However, according to clinical observations, partial function may be restored in prolonged cases.

Incomplete Fecal Incontinence: The controlling ability over anus is poor, but it can be gradually restored. It is also called partial fecal incontinence or curable fecal incontinence.

Treating methods are based on particular conditions. For mild cases, no treatment is given, and leave it to restore its function. Medicinal herbs or acupuncture may be used for severe cases. Sphincteroplasty is done when necessary.

5 Hemorrhoid

Any protrusion existing inside or outside the anus is called hemorrhoid in general. The ancient Chinese practitioners held that it was a kind of angiopathy which was commonly found among the people, and a saying goes that "Of ten persons nine have hemorrhoids."

5.1 Etiology and Pathogenesis

Detailed discussi on was recorded in the traditional medical literature. In *Su Wen*. *Sheng Qi Tong Tian Lun* (Treatise on Communication of Vitality with Heaven, Plain Questions) it states:"Too much food intake causes injury and flaccidity of vessels, leading to hemorrhoid. " This is the initial theory of varicosity. It was held that the disease cause was related to integrated internal factors and local external factors.

5.1.1 Integrated Internal Factors

They include disharmony of *Yin* and *Yang*,deficiency in the *Zang-Fu* organs, con-sumption of *Qi* and blood, extreme excitation of emotions and genetic factors.

5.1.2 Local External Factors

1. Interactions of pathogenic dampness, heat, wind and dryness.

2. Injury of *Yin* by pathogenic heat, hemorrhage due to blood-heat, and accumulation of pathogenic heat.

3. Food Influence: Overintake of roast, fatty, raw, cold, pungent and hot food, or drinking of too much alcohol, or improper food intake.

4. Profession and Life Style: Long-time sitting and standing, walking a long way with heavy load or indulgence in sexual activity.

5. Others: Persisted constipation or diarrhea, child delivery, etc.

The above causes were recognized as the etiology of hemorrhoids by the ancient practitioners. Hemorrhoids only occur in human beings because man is an animal of erect standing. Modern medicine usually thinks that hemorrhoids are caused by the increase of the venous internal pressure of the venous plexus and the decrease of the resistance of the venous walls. But through a profound study of hemorrhoids, different ideas have been put forward. Besides the theory of varicose vein, there is added the theory of vessel hyperplasia and that of mucosa slide.

5.2 Clinical Manifestations

5.2.1 Classification

The hemorrhoid area can be classfied into the following according to modern medicine and clinical practice.

1. External Hemorrhoid: It is located below the anal dentate line, covered by skin, and developed by hemorrhoidal venous pleux. Usually it can directly seen. External hemorrhoids are classified into variciform external hemorrhoid, connective tissue external hemorrhoid, thrombosed external hemorrhoid and inflammatory external hemorrhoid.

(1) Variciform External Hemorrhoid: It is often seen, without suffering, On bowel movements and in the squatting position hemorrhoid is obvious. A soft swelling is felt and it attacks with the attack of internal hemorrhoids. In mild cases, a swelling is seen only on bowel movements.

(2) Connective Tissue External Hemorrhoid: It is the proliferous skin tag of the anal margin usually found in different size. It is also called "cockscomb" and "lotus seed ".No obvious sufferings occur when there is no acute attack. Local dampness and itching are felt.

(3) Thrombosed External Hemorrhoid: It is a stagnant spot due to rupture of the subcutaneous small vessels of the anal margin. The elasticity of the subcutaneous vessel walls decreases, resulting from chronic inflammation and other factors, such as bowel movements with strength, excessive drinking of alcohol, etc. that rupture blood vessels. Blood escapes to the subcutaneous layer. Hemorrhage ceases when accumulated blood oppresses the hemorrhagic area. Because of the distinct degree of bleeding, the size of the stagnant spots varies.

Several stagnated spots of different size exist separately or with connection to one another. One to several or a dozen stagnant spots may be seen. Big stagnant spot occupying 1/3, 1/2 or 2/3 anus or even the whole anus exists in some patients. The stagnant hemorrhoid, less hard and movable, is green purple in color. There is tenderness on touching. When it is complicated by inflammation, no obvious green purple is seen, and a hard blood stasis is felt at this moment. It has an acute attack with or without great sufferings and tends to cure spontaneously, i.e. several days later, blood stasis is absorbed naturally and turns to a hard lump.

After an attack, it is advised to wash and steam the anus with warm water to speed up its absorption.

(4) Inflammatory External Hemorrhoid: It is an acute inflammation of the anal margin plica with great sufferings. No hard stagnant lump is felt on palpation.

2. Internal Hemorrhoid: It is located above the anal dentate line, covered by mucose and developed by hemorrhoidal venous plexus. At the initial stage, it is of small size and stays in the anus. It may come out of the anus when it is growing bigger. Three stages are divided, namely the first or initial state, the second or medial stage and the third stage, called the later or advanced stage.

The Initial Stage: It is a small hemorrhoid within the anus and chiefly manifested by hematochezia. Different amount of bright red blood may pour out or drip.

The Second Stage: Hematochezia and prolapse of hemorrhoid are found at the same time. The bleeding is the same as in the initial stage or in large amount. The hemorrhoid becomes bigger and comes out on bowel movements. But it can go back spontaneously.

The third State: It is mainly manifested by prolapse of hemorrhoid. Hematochezia lessens but the hemorrhoid becomes much bigger. It tends to fall down on bowel movements, long-time walking, standing and coughing. It cannot return to normal except with the help of pushing it back or bed rest.

The chief symptoms of internal hemorrhoid are hematochezia and prolapse of hemorrhoid, and the prolapse is the ground for stage classification. In the first stage, no prolapse of hemorrhoid occurs, but in the second stage, it falls down, yet goes back spontaneously. In the third stage, it falls down and fails to go back. Sometimes, four stages are classified and in the last stage, there produces more serious prolapse of internal hemorrhoid.

Three types can be divided according to the pathological changes:

Type of Swollen Blood Vessel:It is as big as a bayberry with thin mucosa,bright red or dark red in color.It tends to bleed and is felt soft on touch.

Type of Venous Aneurysm: The surface of the hemorrhoid appears to be plexiformly or deflectively projected and is green, purple or dark red in color. The thickened mucosa of hemorrhoid is lustrous.It is less bleeding and felt soft.

Type of Fibrous Swelling: It is produced by proliferation of the connective tissues. The hemorrhoid is hard, big, light red or white in color, covered with fibrous membrane, or ulcerous and rough mucosa. No bleeding is seen.

In addition, vascular hemorrhoid and mucosal hemorrhoid are grouped according to the appearance of hemorrhoid and the pathogenic age. The former is often seen in young patients and the latter in aged patients.

3. Mixed Hemorrhoid: It is located above and beneath the dentate line, covered with mucosa and skin, developed by the venous pleux inside and outside of the hemorrhoid. There is no groove between the internal and external hemorrhoids, and they form a united one.

5.2.2 Symptoms and Signs

Hemorrhoid is manifested by hematochezia, prolapse, pain and swelling, bearing—down sensation, itching, etc.

5.2.3 The Involved Meridians and Their Relationship

Hemorrhoids are related to Meridians of the Large Intestine, Lung, *Du, Ren,* Bladder, Liver, Spleen and Kidney.

5.3 Diagnosis and Differential Diagnosis

Diagnosis is quickly made based on inspection, palpation and anoscopy. For instance, the internal hemorrhoid is manifested by a soft prominence above the dentate line, with bright red or dark red color. Multiple hemorrhoids are separated from each other. Anterior right, posterior right and middle left are the primary hemorrhoids or mother hemorrhoids, while those developed at other sites the secondary hemorrhoids or son hemorrhoids, It is essential to tell the duration of hemorrhage, characteristics of hematochezia, color of blood passed and the difference from other he morrhagic disorders.

(1) Time of Bleeding: Bleeding followed by bowel movements is a sign of hemorrhage of the lower part of the large intestine, known as vicinal bleeding, where as bowel movements followed by hemorrhage are a sign of bleeding of the upper part of the large intestine, stomach or small intestine, called remote bleeding.

(2) Characteristics of Hematochezia due to Hemorrhoid: Bloody exudate from the mucosa or bleeding due to mucosal abrasion is called bloody stools. Dripping or spurting of blood on bowel movements is caused by the increase of the abdominal pressure, leading to a sudden rise of the internal pressure of the hemorrhoid vascular group, which occurs in the case of ulcer of the hemorrhoidal mucosa. This is called the pressure hemorrhage,

typical of hemorrhoidal bleeding.

(3) Differentiation of Blood Color: Bright red blood is seen on the internal hemorrhoidal hemorrhage; dark red blood indicates colonic hemorrhage; deep dark red blood shows hemorrhage from the upper digestive system.

5.4 Clinical Treatment

5.4.1 Internal Treatment

It is mostly suitable for the first and second stages of hemorrhoids, prolapse of internal hemorrhoid or aged patients who are debilitating and have other serious diseases. The principle of treatment and prescriptions adopted are as follows based on the information listed in the medical literature and clinical experience.

Treating Principle and Medication

1. Regulating Blood, Dispelling Dryness, Wind and Pain with Medicinal Herbs Pungent in Flavor and Warm in Property: *Qinj iu Cangzhu Tang* (7) or *Zhitong Rushen Tang* (31) is given. This is especially for hemorrhoids due to pathogenic dampness, heat, wind, dryness, leading to swelling, pain, prolapse, hematochezia, local exudate and itching.

2. Replenishing *Yin* and Cooling Blood, Expelling Heat and Dampness:*Liangxue Dihuang Tang* (40) or *Huaijiao Wan* (10) is administered to treat hematochezia due to hemorrhoid, swelling and pain. It is especially indicated for the excess syndrome, or hemorrhoid complicated by hypertensi on and atherosclerosis. It is not suggested for patients with cold and deficiency in the intestine and stomach.

3. **Purging Intense Heat and Detoxicating with Medicinal Herbs Bitter in Flavor and Cold in Property**: *Huanglian Jiedu Tang* (41) or *Xijiao Dihuang Tang* (42) is given to eliminate intense heat toxin.

4. ***Qi* Reinforcing or *Qi* and Blood Reinforcing**: *Buzhong yiqi Tang* (6), *Shiquan Dabu Tang*(28), and *Guipi Tang* (43) are administered, especially for the deficiency syndrome.

Internal treatment is the chief approach for hemorrhoids. It is worthwhile to study how to use drugs to relieve symptoms. Clinical manifestations are handled by the following measures.

(1) Hematochezia: Based on the excess or deficiency syndrome select the above recipes. Hemorrhage in general may be treated by *Heye Wan* (44), *Huaijiao Wan*(10), *Huazhi Wan*(45), *Zanglian Wan* (46)*Xiaozhi Pian* (47) and *Zhining* (48), *Jichang San* (49), *Zangsuan Fang* (50), and Western drugs such as Adrenosem Salicylate, Vitamin K and Vitamin C to check bleeding.

(2) Prolapse of Rectum: Herbs to invigorate *Qi*, e.g. *Buzhong Yiqi Tang* (6) are given.

(3) Swelling, Pain and a Bearing-down Sensation: *Rushen Tang* (31), *Qinj iu Pian* (32) or *Qinjiu Baizhu Wan* (14) are administered.

(4) Constipation or Diarrhea: Catharsis or antidiarrheal is given based on differentiation of pathological conditions.

5.4.2 External Treatment

Multiple approaches are employed, including the necrotizing therapy for hemorrhoids, ligation method, surgery, steaming and washing, fumigation, hot medicated compress, moxibustion and feces inducing, among which some are non-operative therapies and some are operative therapies.They are discussed as follows in terms of clinical practice.

1. Steaming and Washing: It is a conventional approach to treat hemorrhoids,functioning as follows: promotion of blood flow and subsidence of swelling, relieving inflammation and pain, astringency to arrest hemorrhage and stopping itching. After the surgery of the thrombosed external hemorrhoid, inflammatory external hemorrhoid, prolapse and impaction of internal hemorrhoid,local swelling, pain and itching, the steaming and washing method is used in addition to medication. Use steam of hot medicinal decoction or hot water to heat the affected part or after steaming, use the decoction or water to wash the affected part, or dress the affected part with a piece of medicated gauze. It is applied 2−3 times a day, half an hour for each time. Alternative prescriptions are *Fufang Jinjie Xiyao* (38) or *Quedu Tang* (51). For hip bath, the following ingredients are commonly used, i.e. prickly ash peel, argyi leaf, prepared mirabilite, salt, Boric Acid and Potassium Permanganate.

2. Drugs for External Application: It is another effective conventional approach to treat hemorrhage, Apply drugs to the affected part or the anus directly. It functions as the steaming and washing method.

In addition to the similar effect as the steaming and washing method,it is used to remove the necrotic tissues and promote granulation and arrest hemorrhage, which is mostly suitable for an acute attack of hemorrhoid and dressing change. Varied drug forms—ointment, powder, such as *Jiuhua Gao* (24) and Alum Ointment directly cover the affected part or medicated cotton ball and gauze are inserted into the anus. Different—sized ribbon gauze with the ointment can be put on the wound. Drug powder is spread on the affected part or it is mixed with water or vegetable oil to cover the wound. Suppository is a form of medicine to be placed inside the anus and it cannot be used as an ointment spreading on the affected part, because the suppository acts on the local when it is melted. In fact, it is a kind of ointment.

3. Enema: It is used to stop pain, combat inflammation, invigorate blood flow, subside swelling, promote astringency, arrest hemorrhage, and relieve prolapse, indicated for thrombosed internal hemorrhoids, hemorrhoid bleeding, inflammation of the anal canal, and later hemorrhage after the operation. Medicated suspension or solution is introduced into the anus with a glycerin enema syringe, producing a marked effect on the lower part of the rectum. For example, Alum solution is injected to arrest bleeding.

4. Reposition: It is suitable for prolapse and impaction of hemorrhoid, Have a piece of gauze covered with a lubricating agent or *Jiuhua Gao*. Push the hemorrhoid with the piece of gauze gripped between the gloved middle finger and index finger. First pressure is exerted to one side of the hemorrhoid. Then even strength is given continuously. When the hemorrhoid is felt smaller, push it with an increasing force. More strength is given to the fingers on pushing the hemorrhoid in, and the fingers should not move. Prop the hemorrhoid with the gauze for some time to cause blood return and reduction of the hemorrhoid, so as to easily push it into the anus.

If the hemorrhoid pushed in falls again, re—push it in and prop it for several minutes. Then push the second hemorrhoid in with the other hand. When it is pushed to the orifice of the anus, draw back the finger from the anus and the second hemorrhoid is continuously pushed with other fingers, to support the first one which will not fall. Usually, push in bigger ones first, and small ones next. When all the hemorrhoids go back to their right places, support them with a wedge-shaped gauze pad. The focal point of this method lies in pushing the hemorrhoid with unmoved fingers. Two hands can be alternately used to reposit the hemorrhoid. The author usually does it with facility. Ask the patients to breathe naturally when the method is applied. For this reason, patients and operators often feel at ease. It is really a desirable approach to reposit hemorrhoids because the operator is never in a muddle.

After anesthesia, it is easier to return the hemorrhoid, but it is not so simple as this one and it is essential to have aseptic manipulation. Prolapse and impaction of hemorrhoids for a few days without withering can be tried to put back to their original positions although they have turned to dark color. Withered hemorrhoids may be treated by steaming-washing or medical application.

5. Necrotizing Therapy for Hemorrhoids: It may be subgrouped under the *Kuzhi San* therapy, *Kuzhi Ding* therapy, *Kuzhi Ye* therapy because of different drug forms and medications. *Kuzhi Ye* in fact, is a kind of injection the rapy, which will be dealt with in the section of the injection therapy.

(1) *Kuzhi San* Therapy: Mix *Kuzhi San* with water or vegetable oil, and apply the mixer to the hemorrhoid, to let it wither, necrotize and drop off. The application of the drug is similar to other methods when drugs are spread over the affected part. But the action of the former is different from the latter. When the

hemorrhoid prolapses, it is easy to put *Kuzhi San* on it. Otherwise, first put a cotton ball with *Huanzhi San* (23) into the anus to stimulate the internal hemorrhoid to become larger and prolapse. Before the application of *Kuzhi San,* cover the vicinity of the hemorrhoid with *Kuzhi Gao* (52) or a strip of vaselin gauze to prevent corrosion of the healthy tissues. The duration of the application depends on the quality of the drug, once, twice or several times a day, for a few days or every other day, until the hemorrhoid withers and turns to black. After it drops off other herbs are applied to regenerate tissues and heal the wound.

This therapy has been rarely employed since it needs a long course of treatment and patients suffer greatly. But for prolonged necrotic hemorrhoids or patients with other disorders who cannot be operated on the therapy is still available.

(2) *Kuzhi Ding* Therapy: It is also known as the medicinal strip insertion therapy adopted in the internal hemorrhoids of different stages and the internal hemorrhoid of mixed hemorrhoids. The orange red drug containing arsenic is made by Fujian Institute of Traditional Chinese Medicine and Pharmacy. The drug—needle is 3 cm long with two sharp ends and either of the ends can be inserted into the hemorrhoid. In view of the arrangement of the *Kuzhi Ding*(21), there are sparse, dense and basal inserting methods. In the first two methods, the *Kuzhi Ding* is inserted obliquely into the hemorrhoid and in the last one it is straightly inserted into the root of the hemorrhoid. Several *Kuzhi Ding* are lineally arranged to cause necrosis of the hemorrhoid from its root and drop—off. It is usually inserted by hands. The drug—needle is gripped between the thumb and index finger and inserted into the hemorrhoid. It can be inserted into the

hemorrhoid by a gun which forces out a drug—needle by pressure. But it is only used in sparse inserting or when the drug—needle is not so sharp. The following is a description of the dense inserting method.

Techinqie: The patient is in a ride—prone position or lateral recumbent position. After routine anesthesia, draw out and fix the internal hemorrhoid with hand or a pair of tissue forceps. The *Kuzhi Ding* is inserted into the hemorrhoid at an angle of 15—45 ° with the rectal wall. Hold the *Kuzhi Ding* and whirl it in or directly insert it into the hemorrhoid to a proper depth. When it goes half way or less, cut the rest of it with 1—2 mm left. 4—5 pieces of the *Kuzhi Ding* are inserted into a hemorrhoid as big as the tip of a little finger. In the treatment of multiple hemorrhoids, 20—30 are usually applied. Then push the hemorrhoid back to the anus and apply *Jiuhua Gao* (24) or *Xiaoyan Zhitong Gao* (53)to it. Give dressing change once a day until healing.

Points for Attention: Have the hemorrhoid exposed totally and insert the *Kuzhi Ding* properly. The following should be concerned with, i.e.the depth of the insertion, amount and the arrangement of the drug.

6. Injection Therapy: It is a way to Inject drug into the internal hemorrhoid to cause it to atrophy and wither. Two kinds of drug are adopted—sclerosing agents and withering solutions, indicated for the internal hemorrhoid.According to the action of the drug, the injection therapy may be divided into two.

(1) Sclerosing—Atrophying Therapy: It is also known as the sclerosing agent injection therapy or withering solution injection therapy. The hemorrhoid becomes sclerosed and atrophied after the drug injection. The concentration of the drug solution is

weaker than that of other solutions for this purpose. A small dose is applied for superficial injection, after which the hemorrhoid becomes bigger without color change of the hemorrhoidal mucosa or sometimes it turns to pale white. The injection is given every day or at an interval of several days until sclerosis and atrophy of the hemorrhoid. The commonly used drugs include 5% Sodium Morrhuate, 5% Phenol Glycerite or Phenol vegetable oil, and 1-5% Alum injection (54). The injection is done with the aid of an anoscope or the injection is given to the prolapsed hemorrhoid. The sclerosing therapy for the primary hemorrhoidal root has been developed by *Jishan* Hemorrhoid-Fistula Hospital, Shanxi province. Here is a brief introduction.

Technique: After routine anesthesia, put the gloved finger into the anus and feel if there is any arteriopalmus at the primary hemorrhoidal area in the right anterior, right posterior and left middle. The place where arteriopalmus is felt is used as the injecting spot. A fan-shaped injection of 4-7 cm anesthetic (1-2 ml for each) is applied to the upper root of the hemorrhoid along the anal canal from the border of the anus. The syringe needle goes 3-4 cm in depth. This is the first step of the operation, known as the injection on the primary hemorrhoidal root. Then the injection is given to the hemorrhoid itself, which is similar to the sclerosing therapy, but more drug is administered. The injection is also applied to the upper root of the hemorrhoid if there is no arteriopalmus, 4-6 ml anesthetic is given to the hemorrhoids, first to small ones, then to bigger ones. After the injection the internal hemorrhoid dilates a little. The total dose amounts to 8-15 ml.

Points for Attention:

The drug must be injected to the hemorrhoidal arterial area in the primary hemorrhoidal root injection. The drug injected to the sphincter may produce pain, edema and necrosis of it. On the hemorrhoidal injection the drug must be injected to the vascular plexus instead of to the muscular layer and the skin area beneath the dentate line.

In recent years an injection (55)(56) containing Tannic Acid and Citric Acid—active agents extracted from Galla Chinensis and Fructus Mume, has been developed according to the concept that "Sourness serves to astringe" and "Puckery arrests discharge" in traditional Chinese medicine, by the Guang An Men Hospital, China Academy of Traditional Chinese Medicine, Beijing, and the Affiliated Hospital of Nanjing College of Traditional Chinese Medicine to treat internal hemorrhoids and mixed hemorrhoids with good effect.

The following is a description of *Xiaozhi Ling* (55) made in Beijing.

Indications: Internal hemorrhoids and internal hemorrhoid of mixed hemorrhoids.

Injecting Method: The patient is in a ride-prone position, or a prone position, or lateral recumbent position. After routine sterilization and anesthesia, a cotton ball covered with Bromogeramine is put into the anus to enlarge it. Don't take the sterilized cotton ball out because when pushed upward by the anoscope it can prevent sewage running down. Slowly insert a widemouth simple stem inclind anoscope into the anus and observe the mucosa of the lower rectum, the site, number and size of the hemorrhoids. After the second insertion of the anoscope, inject the drug to the upper part or root of the hemorrhoids. It is called high or high plane injection. Shi Zaoqi named it the superior hemorrhoidal arterial area, or the first area to be injected in the four procedures of the injection. The procedure is as follows: Sterilize and clean the mucosa for the injection. Inject 1—3 ml *Xiaozhi Ling* and diluent (1∶1) with a No.5 syringe needle to the mucosa of the hemorrhoid in a depth of 3—5 mm. Turn the direction of the anoscope and apply the injection to the right posterior, left middle and right anterior parts. After that draw back the anoscope. Then apply the injection to the lower part of the mucosa, muscular layer of mucosa and the place slightly above the dentate line with *Xiaozhi Ling* and diluent (2∶1 or 1∶1). It is called the low or low plane injection. Shi Zaoqi divided a hamorrhoid into three parts for the injection: submucous layer, muscular layer of the mucosa and superior dentate line. Insert the syringe needle to a depth of 5 mm into the center and middle part of the hemorrhoidal mucosa above the dentate line.

Usually the dose of the drug is 3—10 ml and the hemorrhoid becomes swollen. On the surface of the hemorrhoidal mucosa criscross minute vessels are seen, which is known as a sign of red stria, which is not obvious when there is severe proliferation of the hemorrhoidal fibrous tissue or inadequacy of the injected drug. When there appears a sign of red stria, and the hemorrhoid is seen as a blister, it indicates full injection of the drug. White spots like papular eruptions by the skin test appearing on the mucosa, show the drug has been injected into the mucosa, cease the injection and change the injecting site because it is possible to cause necrosis of the superficial layer. If the dose is not enough and the color of the hemorrhoid does not change or change a bit, a new injecting site should be chosen to cause change of the color.

Not any of the injecting site above the dentate line be left out. Inject the drug to the three primary hemorrhoids first, and to the small hemorrhoids. On the injection of the hemorrhoid itself, it should be done one by one according to the divided injecting site. Each time the anoscope should be inserted and withdrawn, but on the injection of the submucosa of the hemorrhoid, the anoscope is only inserted once and the visual field is changed. The total dose is about 15-25 ml. The maximum dose for bigger ones is 30-40 ml. After the drug injection, apply either a cotton ball covered with *Jiuhua Gao* (24) or *Jiuhua San* only to the affected part or a dressing. Dressing change is done each day or every other day. If the hemorrhoids are not completely withered, give the injection again 7-10 days later. For small hemorrhoids the injection is given with the aid of an anoscope without anesthesia.

Points for Attention: Aseptic manipulation is guaranteed. Avoid deep puncture of the needle and insertion into the mucosa. On drawing back the plunger, no blood is found, then inject the drug. After the injection the hemorrhoids must be fully puffy. Don,t leave out any part above the dentate line, and do not make bowel movements on the day of treatment.

Because large dose is used in this therapy, it is necessary to dilute *Xiaozhi Ling*. The 1 : 1 diluent is made of one portion of *Xiaozhi Ling* and one portion of 1% Procaine. The diluent may be about 2 : 1. After the injection, the hemorrhoid becomes puffy, several times larger than the original one. At the same time, a bearing-down sensation is present because of the irritation of the rectum. The curative effect obviously improves owing to the increase of the dose. Big hemorrhoids of the advanced stage as well as the small ones can be removed, therefore, it is different from the commonly-applied sclerosing agent injecting therapy, and it can be called hemorrhoid-removing injecting therapy. The sclerosing agent injecting therapy is only for the internal hemorrhoid at the first and second stages. As for the third stage hemorrhoid, there is increased proliferation and dilatation of the vascular plexus and different conditions of fibrous hyperplasia. The drug of a large dose and low concentration can have successful result by completely filling the hemorrhoid with the drug.

(2) *Kuzhi Ye* Therapy: It causes necrosis and drop-off of the hemorrhoid after the drug injection. The concentration of the drug is higher than that of the sclerosing agent of the same kind, which may be called a strong solution. A large dose is used and the drug reaches the deeper site. After the injection of the drug, the hemorrhoid becomes bigger and the color of the mucosa turns to dark grey and black. One injection is usually applied to a hemorrhoid. The commonly-used drugs are *Neizhi Kutuo You* (57), 10% Calcium Chloride Injection (58) and *Lusha* Injection (59).After anesthesia, have the hemorrhoid pulled out and inject the drug under an anoscope. This therapy follows the mechanism of the necrotizing therapy of hemorrhoids in traditional Chinese medicine. A high concentrative strong solution is prepared for the injection, indicated for the internal hemorrhoid at various stages with a better result. In form it is similar to the sclerosing agent injecting therapy, but in nature, they are different.Thus, a new approach has been developed.

Technique: Full expose the internal hemorrhoid after routine sterilization and anesthesia. Draw the hemorrhoid out and fix it. A proper dose of the drug is injected into the hemorrhoid until swelling of it and change of the color of the mucosa. Push back the hemorrhoid and apply *Jiuhua Gao* (24)to it. Dressing change is done daily.

Points for Attention: Don't inject the drug too deep.

7. Ligation Method: Ligation method has experienced a thousand years, being the chief conventional therapy for hemorrhoids. There is a record about it in *Tai Ping Sheng Hui Fang* (Peaceful Holy Benevolent Prescriptions).It says: " A hemorrhoid falls after it has been tied tightly with spider's silk threads"This approach was widely adopted in the Ming Dynasty. The earliest practice was very simple, known as "tying", indicated only for the small-rooted hemorrhoids, i.e."a piece of medicated thread is tied to the hemorrhoid." In ancient times materials used for ligation were cobweb, hair from horse tail, natural silk thread and medicated thread. Now medical silk thread and rubber ring are employed. The detailed methods are as follows.

(1) Simple Ligation: It is completed only by medicated thread. In practice there are two methods.

Non-Penetrative Ligation: It is indicated for hemorrhoids at the second and advanced stages, known also as the simple ligation because of the easy technique.

Technique: After routine sterilization and anesthesia, have hemorrhoid pulled out and grip the root of it with a pair of all-tooth blood vessel forceps. Tie a piece of thick medical silk thread to the root of the hemorrhoid. Tighten it up while the forceps is loosened. The root of the hemorrhoid must be gripped and deformed. Then the ligation can be completed.

Penetrating Ligation: It is indicated for the internal hemorrhoids at the second and the third stages and the mixed hemorrhoids. Single or double thread is tied to hemorrhoids. In terms of the shape of ligation, it can be divided into the "8" ligation, petal ligation and emulsive ring ligation.

Technique: The patient is in a ride-prone position, or in a prone position with a raised hip or lateral recumbent position. After routine sterilization, the local anesthesia or Yaoshu anesthesia, grip the hemorrhoid with a pair of tissue forceps. A needle with a piece of thread goes through the root of the hemorrhoid and ligate it with the thread. Ligate the hemorrhoid shaped in "8" with double thread or ligate it ring by ring with single thread. The actual operation is the same to that employed in the external stripping and internal ligating therapy. Dressing change is done daily until healing.

Points for Attention: Tie the hemorrhoid tightly and retain the healthy mucosa between hemorrhoids when the multiple hemorrhoids are ligated at a time.

(2) Other Measures Taken: They include the drug injection and incision aside from the ligation method as the chief approach. Ligation associated with the drug injection is called the "injecting-ligating therapy", i.e. the drug injection follows ligation. The drug injection may speed up necrosis of the hemorrhoid. The ligation accompanied by compression is known as the "ligation-compression therapy", i.e. the drug injection follows ligation. After that the hemorrhoid is gripped flat with a pair of all-tooth vessel forceps. Ligation with incision is called the cut-ligation or external stripping and internal ligation, external cut and internal ligation. It is used for the ring-shaped mixed hemorrhoids.

Technique: The patient is in a ride-prone position or in a prone position with a raised hip. After routine sterilization, the local anesthesia or Yaoshu anesthesia put a cotton ball covered with Bromogeramine into the anal canal. Expose the hemorrhoids with an anal rectracor and see the number and site of the hemorrhoids. Separate the opposite tissue to the hemorrhoid to have a full vision. Pull out the hemorrhoid with two pairs of tissue forceps one after another. Tie the medicated thread to the upper root of the hemorrhoid. If the ligation is shaped in "8",double thread is used. If the emultion ring ligation is adopted, single thread is used.Tie the internal hemorrhoids tightly, and cut the edge of the external hemorrhoid open to the margin of the upper part of the dentate line.The wound of the external hemorrhoid is shped in a shuttle or " V ". If there are hemorrhagic spots, pressure is given to stop bleeding. In general,no ligation is applied to the external hemorrhoid, and when necessary,long thread is left out for easy taking off. Afterwards, ligate the lower part of the internal hemorrhoid. Then tie the upper and lower parts together.When the "8"-shaped ligation is performed, tie the upper and lower parts together. The two pairs of tissue forceps used to lift the hemorrhoid may be loosened alternately to make the hemorrhoid tied tightly. Push the hemorrhoids or their remains into the anus after cutting off part of the ligated hemorrhoids and trimming the edge of the wound. For cases of the big ring-shaped mixed hemorrhoids, remove the varicose vascular group which is higher in position than the wound. When the internal hemorrhoids are too big to be separated, handle them one by one. The operation is completed by dressing and fixing. Dressing change is done daily until healing of the wound.

  Points for Attention: Healthy skin should be retained between the wounds of the external hemorrhoids.

(3) Elastic Ring Ligation Therapy: It was developed in 1960's and since then it has been widely adopted in the world. Dr.Barron in the U.S.A. described this therapy in 1963 and the research on it started in 1964 in our country, based on the traditional Chinese conventional ligation therapy. This therapeutic method should be encouraged for its simple operation, good curative effect, less suffering and medical cost.

Historical Development: According to the report of Holley, the hemorrhoid surgery has undergone several centuries. Ligation, incision and cauterization were employed by Hippocrates, but there is no written record about ligation. The ligation therapy initiate at the beginning of the 19th century. In 1829 Salmon reported the withering and drop-off of hemorrhoids. In 1873 Allingham performed and described the internal hemorrhoid ligation associated with incision, and in 1926 Hirschman reported his ligation of internal hemorrhoids and incision of external hemorrhoids in mixed hemorrhoids.

In 1950's the ligation therapy developed to a new phase. Blaisdell invented a small and exquisite apparatus, known as the first hemorrhoid ligator in the world. He ligated the internal hemorrhoids with silk thread or catgut suture. But the ligation thread tended to loosen too early, occasionally leading to massive hemorrhage. Later, Blaisdell improved the method and ligated hemorrhoids with rubber rings. In 1960's, Barron first adopted the rubber ring ligation therapy. Based on the principle of Gravlee's umbilical ligator he slipped an emulsive ring over a ligature casing for ligation of the internal hemorrhoids. This ligator has been improved on the model of Blaisdell's. Afterwards Mcgivney developed a new ligator, which has been very popular among the medical circles.

In the past 20 years the therapy has been adopted in the U.S.A., Japan, Britain, Canada, Germany, Australia and Southeast Asian countries. Besides the rubber ring ligation, drug injection, incision or refrigeration are added. It was reported that thousands of cases had been cured and there are monographs on the late result.

Domestic Report: The hemorrhoidal ligation therapy is one of the chief conventional therapies in China with a history of a thousand years. For example, there is a record in *Tai Ping Sheng Hui Fang* (Peaceful Holy Belevolent Prescriptions) describing "the technique to remove a hemorrhoid by tying it with a spider's silk thread." The approach was widely adopted in the Ming and Qing Dynasties. According to the principle guiding the ligation in traditional Chinese medicine the rubber band ligation therapy has been used since 1964 by the Affiliated Hospital of Shandong College of Traditional Chinese Medicine. Model 7, a popular ligator for the internal hemorrhoid was put on show on the national scientific conference in 1972. In 1974 Lu Qi from Zhejiang province developed a suction ligator, based on which an electric-powered cupping ligator was turned out by Deng Zhengming from Fujian province. The suction ligator became popular. Later on, different kinds of ligators were available. In 1977 Yu Dehong et al from Shanghai developed the suction or traction ligator. Du Keli from Tianjin and Rui Hengxiang from Hebei made suction ligators of different structure. Li Runting from Liaoning province turned out a simpler blood vessel forceps-emulsive ring ligation therapy, which did not need any specific apparatus. The suction ligation therapy used by the Harbin 3rd Hospital was very simple too. The suction process was done by a ready syringe. In recent years Han Houji has developed a new model of ligator to treat rectal polyp and sigmoid colon with better result. Since 1964 the rubber band ligation therapy has been popular in China and 4300 cases were treated by this therapy in 1976 in four hospitals. Now there are several factories producing the ring ligators for the internal hemorrhoids in our country, and the ring ligator therapy is widely employed.

Mechanism: A special ligator slips a rubber ring over the root of a hemorrhoid, blocking blood circulation by the contraction of the rubber ring, leading to ischemic necrosis and drop-off of the hemorrhoid eventually.

Application Methods:

Apparatus and Other Materials: At present there are two kinds of ligators—traction ligator and suction ligator. The front casing are different, including the visual type, incline type and lateral type.

Traction Ligator: It uses a pair of forceps to draw a hemorrhoid into the ligator, which slips a rubber ring over the root of a hemorrhoid.

Blaisdell ligator has two types—hospital type and clinical type. The handle casing is connected to the outer casing and the inner casing is longer than the outer one. The emulsive ring is placed on the front end and the back end is connected to the axle center, over the end of which a distal cap is put. On the operation a pair of tissue forceps is used to lift the hemorrhoid and a common cylindrical anoscope is employed.

Barron Ligator: It is a knee-shaped improved model based

on the Blaisdell's ligator. All the structure is the same to that of the Blaisdell's ligator. It cannot be dismantled and cleaned, but the handle casing can be replaced by different-length handles with casings. The inner casing is of 11 cm in diameter and the handle looks impressive. Its gripping forceps is knee-shaped too. Maurice named it ternaculum forceps. Flat black emulsive rings are used. The central hole is of $\frac{1}{12}$ inch in diameter. On the operation, a cone is used to expand the ring and a common cylindrical anoscope is adopted.

Rudd Ligator: It is a slightly improved model based on the Blaisdell ligator. There are no caps on the handle casing and the distal end of the axle center. At the end of the handle there are two parallel rings in which the index and middle fingers can put when the handle is held. At the end of the axle center there is a ring in which the thumb is put. It is shaped like the vessel forceps and the handle is slightly bent. A cone is used to expand the emulsive ring.

Mcgivney Ligator: It is an improved knee-shaped model based on the Blaisdell ligator and Barron ligator. The structure of it is nearly the same as that of the latter two, only with different connection of the handle casing to the handle. The joining partcan turn 360° for easy ligation of the hemorrhoid. The ligator is liable to be dismantled and cleaned. New improvement has been made in recent years and the handle looks more impressive. The join of the handle and the handle casing has been newly designed. When the handle is held, the inner casing retreats to the outer casing and in this way the emulsive ring is pulled out. The tissue forceps is used to pull out the hemorrhoid, but the head of the tissue forces is knee-shaped. A cone is employed to expand the emulsive ring.

    The Author's Ligator: It is a knee-shaped ligator of Model 7, designed for popularization, consisting of the casing, handle casing, axle center and hand. The direct vision casing connected to the handle casing is called the hand head, which is not long. The whole device is small and equisite.The inner casing is tightly connected to the handle casing by a screw.The axle center controls the outer casing by going through the handle casing and the long hole on the lateral wall of the inner casing to connect with the round hole on the lateral wall of the outer casing. The join between the handle casing and axle center and the handle is newly devised. Handle casings with a casing can be quickly replaced. The ligator has three handle casings of various size, i.e. three heads on one handle. The diameter of the inner casing is 12,14 and 16 mm.Therefore different-sized hemorrhoids can be ligated. The casing and handle casing can be dismantled and cleaned.On the operation, the tissue forceps is used to pull out the hemorrhoid. There is no visible central hole on the emulsive ring. Because of more prestressing force the ligature can never be loosened. The hemorrhoid is fully seen when a big-mouthed simple stem inclined anoscope is used. If the hemorrhoid prolapses naturally, an anal retractor is used in ligation. A cone with a cone protrusion at the front end of it, shaping of a small neck, is used to dilate the emulsive ring. The cone protrusion is named the second cone by the author. It means there are two cones to expand the emulsive ring. It is designed for easy placing of the emulsive ring on the cone. A nice emulsive ring dilator has been produced to replace the expansion of the ring by hand.

The new Model 8 ligator is operated by one person, to complete the whole process of ligation, i.e. gripping the hemorrhoid by forceps, moving the casing forward and backward, and pulling out the emulsive ring.It is a ligator which has one handle and three handle casings, easy to use but still the structure has to be improved.

Furthermore, Li Ruanting uses a pair of vessel forces and emulsive ring instead of a ligator to complete the ligation.

Suction Ligator: A suction device is used to suck the internal hemorrhoid into the casing, then an emulsive ring is pushed to the root of the hemorrhoid by the ligator.

Lu Qi's Ligator: It is a knee-shaped ligator of direct vision.After the join of the inner and outer casings with the axle center and handle casing, the end of the casing is sealed by a piece of glass to form a negative pressure in the casing and observe the suction process. A sealed hollow handle is attached to the rear handle casing. At the end of the handle another tube is joined for easy connection with the suction device. The axile center is connected with a lever and an emulsive ring can be readily pushed out. Because of a spring the outer casing can be retreated automatically after the ring is pushed out by it. The suction ligator is powered by electricity. An emulsive ring is expanded by a cone and an inclined anoscope is adopted. Deng Zhengming does not use electric suction ligators but a cupping device to form a negative pressure.

Stille Company's Ligator: It is made of metal, knee-shaped. The handle is in a "T" shape and the holding part is round and solid. The hollow part is small tubular-shaped, the end of which is attached to a suction apparatus.The handle casing axle center is joined by the handle. A lever is on the holding part. The inner and outer casings connect the handle casing axle center vertically. It uses Barron's emulsive ring with a central hole. There are two kinds of cone which pushes out the ring. It is a more advanced model.

Auxiliary Instruments and Other Materials: They include tissue forceps, rubber ring, anoscope, anal retrator, suction apparatus, anal retractor, cones for expanding the rubber rings and dilator, suction apparatus for suction ligation, sterilized cotton balls, lubricates, *Jiahua Gao* (24), and dressings.

Indications

The traction ligator therapy is indicated for internal hemorrhoids at various stages, internal hemorrhoids of the mixed hemorrhoids, prolapse of the rectal mucosa, eversion of the remaining mucosa after hemorrhoidal circumsision, low rectal polyp and papillary fibroma. The suction ligation is indicated for small internal hemorrhoids at the first and second stages. For the aged and debilitated patients and patients with such chronic diseases as anemia, pulmonary tuberculosis, heart diseases and hypertension, the therapy is adopted when condition permits. On inflammation, edema of hemorrhoids or thrombosed hemorrhoids delay the healing process.

Operating Methods

Emulsive rings are slipped over the root of the internal hemorrhoids under an anoscope and it can be done with an anal retractor when the internal hemorrhoid falls. Anesthesia is unnecessary. The hemorrhoid is pulled or sucked into the ligator. In terms of the pull ligation therapy, an internal hemorrhoid is gripped by a pair of tissue forceps and the hemorrhoid can be pulled out easily. Some of the handle casing can be changed as desired for ligation of various-sized hemorrhoids. On doing the external incision and internal ligation, after the external hemorrhoids are incised and stripped, the internal hemorrhoids are dealt with by the ligator. It is easy to operate. For the suction ligation, the suction apparatus, suction cylinder and hollow needles are adopted. On the suction, a negative pressure is formed in the casing and the hemorrhoid enters the casing gradually. When the suction force is inadequate, the hemorrhoid cannot or cannot completely enter the casing. Sometimes the hemorrhoid cannot enter the casing because of the suction force which causes peripheral enlargement of the hemorrhoid. On performing the incision of the external hemorrhoids and ligation of the internal hemorrhoids the suction ligation therapy cannot be adopted because the internal hemorrhoids are not in good order and the field of the operation is stained with blood.

Detailed Description of the Traction Ligation Therapy: The patient is in a ride-prone position with the buttocks elevated without anesthesia. After sterilization of the anus, insert an anoscope and see the site and number of hemorrhoids (Fig.6). Sterilize the hemorrhoids and anal canal, put a pair of tissue forceps into a ligator with the same diameter as the hemorrhoid and insert it into the anoscope. Open the tissue forceps (Fig.7) and grip the upper part of the hemorrhoid into the ligator (Fig.8). At the same time, push upward the ligator and when the inner casing reaches the root of the hemorrhoid, tighten the forceps, and the rubber ring is slipped over the hemorrhoid (Figs.9,10). Open the forceps and draw back the ligator. The ligation is completed (Fig.11). For naturally falling of the internal hemorrhoids, if they are fully exposed, the ligation is done with an anal retractor. After the ligation, apply *Jiuhua Gao* (24) and dressing to the wound. It is a simple approach, usually takes 3—5 minutes. As for the mixed hemorrhoids (Fig.12), after the incision and stripping of the external hemorrhoids, the internal hemorrhoids are handled in the same way (see Figs.13,14).

Points for Attention: Expose the hemorrhoid completely. Grip the upper part of it for easy drawing out the whole hemorrhoid. Don't exert too much force to pull the hemorrhoid to avoid rupture of it. On the ligation of one hemorrhoid, don't touch other hemorrhoids. The outside edge of the emulsive ring should be above the dentate line to lessen sufferings. Make sure that the emulsive ring is at the root of the hemorrhoid, otherwise, the hemorrhoid cannot be totally removed. No matter how many hemorrhoids there are, and how big they are, the ligation can be completed in one operation. When necessary no more than three sites are given ligation. If there are more than three hemorrhoids, the neighboring hemorrhoids can be tied together.

Treatment before and after the Ligation: Explain to the patients the therapy to relieve his worries. Before the ligation, ask the patient to loose his bowels and pass urine. After the ligation don't make bowel movements on the same day. Keep bowels open. Take some Ecphractics when necessary. Have regular digital examinations to see if the ring has dropped and to avoid mucosal adhesion. The condition should be keenly observed to prevent hemorrhage. It is unnecessary to have dressing change daily. After the therapy, give digital examinations and anoscopy to assess the curative effect.

Points for Attention: On giving the traction ligation therapy, two important steps must be taken. The first one is to slip the emulsive ring right over the root of the hemorrhoid. It is the key in the operation, which is completed by the correct use of the ligator and other auxiliary instruments. The second importance is the good quality of the emulsive ring, which ensures complete withering of the ligated hemorrhoids. This is the key to the cure. What we have used are those produced by the Shanghai Emulsive Product Plant. It is a quality product. After the ligation the hemorrhoid may gradually wither and drop. No natural slip of the hemorrhoid has happened, once tied up, even if it is a small hemorrhoid.

Ligation at a Time or for Several Times: In abroad one hemorrhoid is ligated at a time at an interval of a week. Usually three times are maximum. Barron only reported one hemorrhoid was ligated once, he did not mention the intervals. Engene reported 490 cases who had undergone 1625 time of ligation, 3.3 times for each patient on average. Most of them had undergone only once, but the maximum was 9 times. More than one hemorrhoid ligated at a time amounted to 1.5%, 8% of which suffered great pain. One at a time produces no sufferings, which permits normal working as usual, or only a short rest is needed, but the course of treatment prolongs. The author has ligated hemorrhoids in a patient once forever since 1970, no matter how many ones there are and how big they are. But the ligation is usually applied to three sites at most. For example, the ligation was applied to 6 sites in a patient having 8 hemorrhoids with good result. According to the clinical observation, the ligation once forever may keep off the sufferings when the anoscope is again put into the anus. Seven-ten days after the first ligation, although the hemorrhoid is withered and drops, the wound has not been healed. Insersion of the anoscope again for the second ligation may produce pains and the possibility of later hemorrhage. Long intervals delay the course of treatment. Prolonging course of treatment is indicated for the aged and debilitated patients and those who have chronic diseases.

The emulsive ring must slip over the root of the hemorrhoid, if it falls, religation is necessary.

The emulsive ring must be put 2–3 mm above the dentate line. If it should be very close to the dentate line, analgesia is applied.

Duration for Dropping of the Emulsive Ring: The emulsive rings dropped between 5–19 days in 694 cases observed at the Affiliated Hospital of the Shandong College of Traditional Chinese Medicine from 1970–1973. The emulsive rings dropped on the 7th day were seen in 36 cases, among which 3 suffered from profuse hemorrhage. Two hundred and seven cases saw the drop of the emulsive rings in 8–10 days, 327 cases in 11–13 days, only one case of massive bleeding was found, and 56 cases in 14–15 days. In 3 cases, individual rings dropped on the 16th day, 17th day and 19th day. Besides, two cases single ligated part came out of the anus on the 13th day and 15th day and the emulsive ring tended to drop. The withered tissue was only 3–4 mm in width, and it was incised. These two cases were included in the group whose emulsive rings dropped on the 13th day and 15th day.

Course of Treatment: Among the 694 cases, two were completely cured in 14 days—the shortest course of treatment, and ten were cured in 37 days—the longest course of treatment. Three hundred and thirty-eight cases were cured in 15–20 days,

225 cases in 21—25 days, 90 in 26—30 days, and 9 in over thirty days. The course of treatment is related to the number and size of hemorrhoids,and the general condition of the patient. In general, those who had small wound and strong physique were cured soon. But most of them had several ligations at a time, as a result, the healing was delayed.

Observation of the Curative Effect: This therapy is similar to the medicated silk thread ligation therapy, i.e. the whole hemorrhoid was ligated and withered, ensuring a complete cure. On examination the ligated spot was smooth. Before 1976 470 cases were treated by the Harbin 3rd Hospital.Out of them 466 were cured, amounting to 99% of the total. Three hundred and eight cases (93.9%) and 13 cases (4%)out of 328 were cured by the First Affiliated Hospital of the Zhejiang Medical University. Two thousand five hundred and seventeen cases treated at the Shenyang Hemorrhoid—Fistula Hospital from 1970—1973 and 694 cases at the Affiliated Hospital of the Shandong College of Traditional Chinese Medicine were completely cured in view of the short— term effect. David reported that he made a follow—up for 125 cases in 3.5—6 years, 4.8 years on average, and found 89% late result was satisfactory. Forty—four percent of the cases was without any remaining symptoms.

Reaction and Complication: Cases treated by this therapy have fewer or no sufferings. Routine treatment is given in case of pain, a bearing—down sensation, hematochezia and dysuria. If there is later hemorrhage, Alum enema is given or Alum Ointment applied to the hemorrhagic area.

Merits: It is a simple approach, easy to learn and to be popularized among the grass—root hospitals. Since it is effective, curable with less sufferings and complications, most of the cases can be handled at clinics. Cost is much lower than in the hospitalized treatment.

Defects: There still exist possibilities of pain, a bearing—down sensation, dysuria and later hemorrhage. For this reason, anlgesics or Alum Ointment are used when necessary.

From the above, we can see the ligation therapy may after all be accepted as an important method for treatment of the internal hemorrhoids when there is no breakthrough in the prevention of hemorrhoids.

8. Surgical Operation

Surgical operation has been adopted widely to treat hemorrhoids in modern medicine. In the country specialists of anorectum have accumulated much experience. There are various kinds of surgical operation. According to the condition of the wound, whether it is sutured or not, there are sutured and unsutured wounds. Here is a brief account of the surgical operations done.

(1) Thrombosed External Hemorrhoidectomy: It is done when the steaming and washing treatment fails.

Technique:After routine sterilization and anesthesia,cut a radial incision on the surface of a hemorrhoid.Blood stasis covered by fibrous membrane is all stripped and removed. The clots of blood stasis must be all eliminated.If the blood stasis is ruptured on stripping, clean the spot. Trim the edge of the wound and apply hemostasis by a compression.Afterwards the wound is pushed to close or given a suture. Dressing change is unnecessary. Sometimes squeezable technique is used,i.e. after anesthesia, squeeze the thrombosed hemorrhoid slowly to allow stagnated blood to flow in tissues. Steam and wash the affected part with warm herbal solutions to promote absorption of blood.

(2) Excision of the Varicose External Hemorrhoids and Connective Tissue Hemorrhoids:

Technique: A shuttle incision is made for varicose external hemorrhoids.Strip and cut the venous plexus.Trim the edge of the wound and retain the healthy skin between the wounds. Cut a V-shaped incision of the connective tissue hemorrhoid and remove the hemorrhoid. Don't suture the wound.Dressing is changed daily until a complete recovery.

(3) Extirpation of the Hemorrhoidal Vascular Plexus:It is indicated for the bigger separate internal hemorrhoids and mixed hemorrhoids,by removing all the varicose vessel groups.

Technique:After routine sterilization,the local anesthesia or Yaoshu anesthesia,open the anus with an anal retractor to expose the hemorrhoid.Make incisions on either side of the root of the hemorrhoid.Connect the incisions at the dentate line and trim them inwardly.Strip the varicose vessel plexus upwardly until a small part is left. Grip it with a pair of forceps,then tie a piece of thread to the root of it, and cut the remaining part off. For the mixed hemorrhoids,the incisions at the root of the hemorrhoid must be extended to the dermatome,1-2 cm beyond the external hemorrhoid.The wound of the mucosa is partially open and the wound of the dermatome is totally open.Dressing change is done daily until recovery.

Howard and Turner's hemorrhoidal extirpation is similar to the above operation. The technique is as follows.

After sterilization and anesthesia,dilate the anal canal to the width of four fingers,which is a step to fully expose the hemorrhoid and lessen the post-operative cramp of the sphincter.Explore the three-grouped hemorrhoids and grip each group of the internal and external hemorrhoids with a pair of forceps. Tie a piece of catgut suture to the hemorrhoidal vessels above the internal hemorrhoid together with the mucosa. Cut a V-shaped incision at the root of the external hemorrhoid and cut it continuously straightly upward until a thin stem.Grip the root of the hemorrhoid and remove the internal and external hemorrhoids.Suture the remaining skin and mucosa and leave some space for drainage. Dressing is changed daily until recovery.

(4) Separate Hemorrhoid Incision and Hemorrhoidal Ligation:

Indications:The internal hemorrhoid and mixed hemorrhoids at the first and second stages.

Technique:The patient is in a ride-prone position. After routine sterilization and anesthesia,or the Yaoshu anesthesia dilate the anus with the two index fingers.Separate the anus with the two thumbs.Then tell the patient to increase his abdominal pressure or squat down to make the hemorrhoid prolapse.

Sterilization is applied again.Grip and lift the hemorrhoid with a pair of tissue forceps. For mixed hemorrhoids,cut a V-shaped incision,extending to the dentate line and grip the hemorrhoid with a pair of forceps.But for a simple internal hemorrhoid,grip the upper or lower part of the hemorrhoid with a pair of curved or straight all-tooth blood vessel forceps,with or without minor space between the two pairs of forceps.The head of them are in parallel,but their other two ends are in opposite directions.Grip the root of the hemorrhoid,and do not injure too much mucosa.Cut off part of the hemorrhoidal tissue above the all-tooth forceps,which is removed after that process.With the blood vessel forceps,grip the part which has been held flat by the all-tooth forceps.Remove the blood vessel forceps,clean the affected part with a piece of Saline gauze and see if there occurs bleeding. If any, change the gripping part until there is no hemorrhage.Ligate the hemorrhoids from outside to inside. Special attention should be paid to 2-3 gripping spots.Ligate them again.Make sure there is no obvious hemorrhage,fill the incision with *Zhixue San*(36) and a piece of vaselin gauze. Change dressings daily until recovery.

Points for Attention

The all-tooth forceps must grip the hemorrhoid along its original direction.Because of different locations of hemorrhoids,the angle between the all-tooth blood vessel forceps and the anal groove must vary.

When the hemorrhoid is at the middle from the left and right the forceps meets the anal groove at the right angles.When the hemorrhoid is at the middle from the anterior and posterior,the forceps should be in parallel with the anal groove. When the hemorrhoid is at the right anterior or posterior,left anterior or posterior,the forceps should be approximately in parallel with the anal groove or meets the anal groove at an angle.No matter where the hemorrhoid locates,the gripping must be along the original direction of the hemorrhoid to avoid much injury of the mucosa.

On section ligation,special care is given to the inside end of the wound.After removal of the hemorrhoid,only the mucosa of the corresponding area and the hemorrhagic spots of the submucosal layer are ligated.The deep hemorrhagic spots are often easy to be ligated.The biginners tend to grip the part higher than required. Then on the post-operative examination,it is often found that the ligation site is far above the rectal ring.It must be pointed out that there is abundant blood flowing in the rectal mucosa,wide injury of which,in addition to the loose ligation,may cause profuse hemorrhage due to free movement of the mucosa and continuous oozing of blood.Therefore the inside end or the upper part of the wound must be handled carefully.The two-three gripping spots must be ligated again.

When several mixed hemorrhoids are incised at a time,the healthy skin must be retained between the wounds, which can promote healing and avoid stricture of the anus due to the large-area scars.

(5) Internal Hemorrhoid Suture:It is indicated for the internal hemorrhoid at the second and third stages.It is a simple approach with little hemorrhage.

Technique:After routine sterilization and anesthesia,separate the anus with an anal retractor to expose the hemorrhoids.Grip and lift a hemorrhoid,and grip the root of it with a pair of blood vessel forceps.Tie the hemorrhoid together with the forceps with a non-traumatic suture needle. Remove the forceps and tighten the suture.The hemorrhoid is sutured at its original spot. Dressing change is unnecessary.

(6) Incision and Suture of Hemorrhoids:It is indicated for the internal and mixed hemorrhoids at the advanced stage.

Technique:After routine sterilization and anesthesia,grip and lift the hemorrhoid with a pair of tissue forceps and then grip the root of the hemorrhoid with a pair of blood vessel forceps.Cut off the hemorrhoidal tissue above the blood vessel and suture the wound with No. 0-1 catgut suture or silk thread.Remove the forceps and the suture is tigthened naturally.For the mixed hemorrhoids,keep the wound open.

5.4.3 Acupuncture and Magnetic Therapy

1. Acupuncture Therapy:It is indicated for an acute attack of hemorrhoids,such as pain and swelling.Points selected are the same as in the treatment of the post-operative pain.Zusanli (ST36) is added in the presence of hematochezia and prolapse of hemorrhoids.

2. Pricking Therapy: It is indicated for hemorrhoidal pain,swelling, hematochezia and prolapse of hemorrhoids.

Technique:Find out the "hemorrhoidal spots" on the back of the low back.After routine sterilization,prick them with a three-edged needle and pick out white fiber-like substances from the subcutaneous tissue.Apply Iodine tincture to the spots and cover them with a piece of adhesive tape.

3. Moxibustion:It is often indicated for hematochezia. Moxibustion is applied to Zusanli (ST36),Zhongwan (RN12),Qihai (RN6) and Changqiang(DU1).

4. Magnetic Therapy:It is indicated for an acute attack of hemorrhoids,such as pain and swelling.Treatment is the same as that of post-operative pain.

6 Anorectal Penipheral Abscess

Any suppurative conditions around the anus and rectum are grouped under anorectal peripheral abscess in traditional Chinese medicine.

According to modern medicine and clinical practice,anal abscess must be differentiated from boils.Anal carbuncles and boils held by traditional Chinese medicine include anal peripheral abscess,and other swellings or fistula abscess and non-fistula abscess in modern medicine.

6.1　Etiology and Pathogenesis

In general ,anal peripheral abscess is caused by pouring-down of damp-heat and accumulation of noxious heat. The excess syndrome is mainly due to alcoholism,taking too much rich food, leading to accumulation of dampness,whereas the deficiency syndrome results from weak function of the lung,spleen and kidney and pouring-down of damp-heat.Modern medicine holds it is caused by an infection of the anal crypt,extending to the peripheral tissues of the anus.The onset is from inside to outside and the anal crypt is the gate for pathogens to enter. There are three stages of infection: infection of the anal crypt, the reaction stage of the anorectal peripheral tissues and local lesion,or formation of abscess.During the three stages,there appears anal cryptitis first, then inflammation of the circumanal glands and anal peripheral tissues and finally abscess. Most of the infection results mainly from bacillus coli, although there exist many kinds of germs in the intestines.

6.2 Clinical Manifestations

Anal peripheral abscess may occur at various parts. The superficial abscesses include subcutaneous abscess, posterior anal abscess, while the deep ones, ischiorectal abscess, when the abscess spreads to the part of the pelvis and diaphragm, pelvi-rectal space abscess and posterior anal space abscess. Pelvic diaphragm abscess affecting a wide and deep area, is not easy to be diagnosed. One side of pelvic and rectal space abscess and ischiorectal abscess may extend to the other side. Rectal submucosa abscess, though it is near the surface of the intestinal cavity, is within the intestine, and is a deep affection. The syndromes can be divided into deficiency and excess ones.

Excess Syndrome: It is manifested by pain, red and hot skin, tenderness, thick foul pus on ulcer. For deep affection, there may be extended swelling, hot sensation of the skin, with its normal color sometimes, and fever.

Deficiency Syndrome: It is manifested by moderate pain, flat affected area, dark red or normal skin color, absence of hot sensation, thin and slightly foul pus on ulcer.

In both excess and deficiency syndromes, anal digital examination shows a swollen crypit, that is the inside end of the anal peripheral abscess, which is different from anal peripheral boils.

6.3 Treatment

6.3.1 Internal Treatment

For the excess syndrome it is advised to clear away heat and toxic materials,administering *Sanhuang Tang*(60) and *Sanmiao San* (modification) (61).or *Huangliang Chishi Tang* (62). For the deficiency syndrome,it is suggested to replenish *Yin* and remove dampness,taking *Zhiyin Chyshi Tang* (63)(modification).For both syndromes antibiotics or antiphlogistics can be administered.

6.3.2 External Treatment

1. Local steaming and washing or hot compress are applied.On steaming and washing *Jingjie* Solution (38) or Detoxication Solution(64) are used,2–3 times a day, half an hour once. The hot-water bag,etc.is used for hot compress.It can be given continuously.

2. Local Application of Drugs: Alternatively use *Suanxiao Huji*(65) and *Huangcu Huji*(66) or anti-inflammatory and pain-killing ointment.

3. Surgery: Cut the affected part open and remove pus; after the operation, the steaming,washing therapy and external application of drugs are given too.On subsidence of inflammation and swelling,handle it as an anal fistula or incise the anal peripheral abscess.The incision is wider than other common abscesses,i.e. the incision extends from the fluctuating area of the abscess to the posterior anal border. The ligation therapy can be partially applied to the inside of the anus. After the operation change dressings regularly until healing. No remaining fistula is found after the operation,but care must be given to infection.

7 Anal Fistula

Anal fistula is a common long pipe-like ulcer with continous oozing of exudate from the anus or rectum.

7.1 Etiology and Pathogenesis

It is held by traditional Chinese medicine that the etiology of anal fistula is similar to that of hemorrhoids, caused by pouring-down of damp-heat and accumulation of noxious heat in case of deficiency in the *Zang-Fu* organs.Clinical practice tells us that anal fistula is a sequela of the anal peripheral abscess, which is actually the acute primary stage of anal fistula.Anal fistula is the chronic stage of anal peripheral abscess i.e. subsidence of the inflammatory swelling and formation of fistula.In this sense, anal peripheral abscess and anal fistula are two different phases of the same problem.The cause of the former is the cause of the latter.It is difficult to have a spontaneous cure of anal fistula, the reasons of which are as follows

1. On rupture of incision, pus is drained outward, and the inner orifice is continuously infected.

2. Fecal pollution.

3. A small caliber of frequent closing and opening of the outer orifice of the fistula affects free drainage of pus.

4. Curved of deep fistula affects free drainage of pus.

7.2 Clinical Manifestations

7.2.1 Classification: Modern medicine classifies anal fistula under various groups. In light of the clinical practice and on the basis of medical literature anal fistula is grouped as follows

1. Classification Based on the Number of Orifices of Fistula and the Anal Fistulous Canal

(1) Simple Anal Fistula: One fistulous pipe and one outer orifice.

(2) Complicated Anal Fistula: Two fistulous pipes and two outer orifices and one inner orifice.

2. Classification on the Depth of the Fistula

(1) Low or superficial anal fistula, felt on touch.

(2) High or Deep Anal Fistula: It is usually judged by the fistula passing the sphincter. The judgment is believed to be not completely suitable for practice. According to the author's experience, the characteristics of the high anal fistula can be summarized as follows. a. The anal fistulous pipe is paralleled or almost paralleled to the anal canal. b. The fistulous pipe is located deeply and on the examination, only a local hard mass at the ulceraous orifice can be felt. c. Probe examination can make sure of the trend of the above fistulous pipe, which is of over 4 cm. d. On probe and digital examinations, the finger in the anus can feel an impact by the probe at the rectal wall. e. Fibrosis of the rectal ring.

3. Classification Based on the Inner and Outer Open Orifices of the Anal Fistula

(1) Through Anal Fistula: It consists of the inner and outer

orifices and fistulous pipe, which is also called complete, or inner-outer fistula.

(2) Partial Open Anal Fistula: It consists of an open inner orifice and an open outer orifice of the anal fistula. The open inner orifice fistula is one in which the skin is not broken through and the open the outer orifice fistula is produced by infection due to the puncture.

4. Classification Based on the Trend of the Anal Fistulous Pipe

(1) Straight Anal Fistula: Usually at the prezone of the anus.

(2) Curved Anal Fistula: Usually at the posterior position of the anus. For the long curved anal fistula the outer orifice is at the prezone of the anus and the curved part at the posterior position of the anus. The inner orifice is at the posterior middle. The curved pipe may be shaped as a sickle or a hook. And the curved pipe can be in the form of a horse's hoof, the one in which bilateral pipes meet in the posterior position.

5. Classification Based on the Number of the Inner Orifice

(1) Single Anal Fistula: It consists of an inner orifice and a pipes.

(2) Multiple Anal Fistula: It is a typical one consisting of over two inner orifices and pipes without a branch fistula.

6. Classification Based on the Relation between the Pipe and the Sphincter

(1) Low Anal Fistula: The fistulous pipe passes through the inner sphincters with one outer orifice near the margin of the anus.

(2) Sphincter Anal Fistula: The fistulous pipe passes through the space between the inner and outer sphincters with several out-

er orifices and branch pipes.

(3) Anal Fistula above the Sphincter: The fistulous pipe passes through the lavator ani muscles to the ischiorectal fossa, having an opening at the skin.

(4) Anal Fistula outside the Sphincter: The fistulous pipe passes through the lavator ani muscles and meets the rectum, rarely seen clinically.

7. Classification Based on Pathology

(1) Non-Specific Anal Fistula: It is a kind of inflammatory anal fistula, most commonly seen.

(2) Specific Anal Fistula: It often refers to tuberculous anal fistula, and other specific infectious ones such as syphilitic anal fistula are rarely found.

Although there are various classifications of the anal fistula, it is difficult to tell the condition only based on one particular classification. Several classifications should be combined to explain a condition. The classification should be as concise as possible for easy clinical application. In consensus with the institution concerned, according to the number and the depth of the fistula the anal fistula is divided into four groups.

(1) Low Simple Anal Fistula: It has one pipe, passing through the superficial layer of the external sphincter with one inner orifice, located at the anal crypt.

(2) Low Complex Anal Fistula: It has more than two pipes and outer orifices. The pipes with one or more inner orifices pass through the superficial layer of the external sphincter. The inner orifices are located at the anal crypt.

(3) High Simple Anal Fistula: It has one pipe and an inner orifice, passing through the part above the deep layer of the external

sphincter. The inner orifice is located at the anal crypt.

(4) High Complex Anal Fistula: It has two or more pipes or branch pipes. The main pipes go through the deep layer of the external sphincters. There are two or more outer orifices, one and more inner orifices locate at the anal crypt (including the multiple hemorrhoids).

7.2.2 Symptoms and Signs

It is marked by pus and exudate. Profuse thick pus runs out of the newly-formed fistula, but little, thin pus runs out of the old fistula. The outer orifice may be sealed for some time and it seems to heal, but soon pus runs out again. If pus does not run from the original fistula, it runs from a new fistula. The condition tends to repeat. The patient suffers no pain in general, but on difficulty in pus running due to a sealed orifice, there appears pain and swelling. In addition, itching of the anus due to irritation of the exudate is felt. Signs vary according to the number and depth of the pipe. Simple anal fistula has one outer orifice, a straight or curved pipe. In the complex case, there are several outer orifices and winding fistulous pipes. Hard cord extending to the anus is felt in the low anal fistula. The clinical features of the high anal fistula have been described as above. In terms of differentiation of the deficiency and excess syndromes, the outer orifice is raised, the pus thickene and the complexion normal with a hard cord felt. In the deficiency syndrome, the outer orifice with an invisible edge is depressed, the pus thin and the complexion dark brown with or without any cord felt.

7.3 Diagnosis and Differential Diagnosis

In a narrow sense it is not difficult to make a diagnosis of the anal fistula by inquiry of the case history and local observation.But further definite diagnosis,that is the classification of the fistula,depends on the careful examination of the position of the inner orifice,trend and depth of the fistulous pipe,existence of any branches,their relation with the sphincter fibrosis of the rectal ring and the nature of the anal fistula.These are the focal points of diagnosis for the anal fistula.A careful examination must be conducted. The diagnostic approaches are as follows.

7.3.1 Asking

Patients tend to have a history of the rectal peripheral abscess.The first step of inquiry is to know the time of the first attack, main symptoms, such as pain,swelling, ulcer or incision, pus running from the anus or from the outer orifice, amount, color, viscosity, smell of the pus discharged, continuous or intermittent running of pus, etc. When profuse pus runs out, it shows a deteriorated condition.Besides,ask the patient whether there is any pass of gas or feces from the fistulous opening,and whether there is any hard mass or pipe beside the anal canal,and ask about their occurrence of sequence,if there are some masses or pipes.

7.3.2 Looking

Inspect the look of the anus, its size of the lesion area,number of the outer orifice,its location,shape and change of the peripheral tissues.

1. Look of the Anus and the Size of Lesion:See if there is any displacement,excavation or defect of the anus.Make sure of

the size of the lesion.

2. The Number of the Outer Orifice,Its Location and Appearance: Simple anal fistula has one outer orifice.When two outer orifices are at both sides of the posterior anus,and there is a raised cord between the orifices,it is a horse—hoof—shaped fistula.But in most cases,the straight prominence between the two orifices is not obvious and the fistulous pipe has two orifices.In some cases,there is an evident prominence,but no pipe exists. If on both sides of the anterior outer orifice there exist fistulous pipes,it is the horse—hoof—shaped fistula.When the outer orifice is at a distance from the anus in the anterior anal fistula,the fistula may affect the subcutaneous scrotum,a manifestation of tuberculous anal fistula.It is then essential to inspect the change of the skin at the scrotum and the bottom of the hip, and to see if there is any straight prominence or nodular swelling.

When multiple outer orifices are present at one or either side of the anus,there are complex fistulous pipes,and extensive multiple anal fistula is marked by unsmooth skin surface, varied outer orifices and appearance. It is significant to measure the distance between the anus and the outer orifice,which is helpful to observing the depth of the pipes.

In general,when the outer orifice is near the anus,the fistulous pipe is shallow; when the outer orifice is at a distance from the anus, the fistulous pipe is deep.But the contrary condition may be found in some patients.The shallow fistulous pipe only extends subcutaneously instead of going deeply.

The examination of the outer orifice of the anal fistula can help to understand the nature of it and its course.A new fistula does not have proliferative nodes;in a prolonged case, there may be granulation of tissues, a fibrous node or cicatricial pitting in the center, of which an fistulous orifice is found. Sometimes, the outer orifice is at one side of the root of the node or it is closed.Sometimes,there exists the anal fistula and connective tissue external hemorrhoids. The anal fistula may be neglected because it does not have an outer orifice.

Varied size and appearance of nodes can be seen in the outer orifice of an inflammatory anal fistula.The tuberculous anal fistula has irregular outer orifices without nodes. The edge of the outer orifice inwardly rolls up and the granulation is grey.

3. Skin Color Change of the Lesion:A brown halo around the outer orifice is found in the complex anal fistula,esp. in a tuberculous one. When the skin where the fistula is located is in diffuse dark brown color or normal color is seen among the color changed areas of the skin or there is an evident brown halo,a subcutaneous pipe often exists and there is one or several lacunae, or areolar lacunae.

7.3.3 Palpation

Palpation is an important method which can directly dicide the sign of an anal fistula,straight or curved,horse-hoof-shaped or hooked,one fistula or multiple ones, location and number of the inner orifice,the condition of the rectal ring,the relation between the fistulous canal and the sphincters,and the function of the sphincters.

1. Palpating Outside the Anus:A cord from the outer orifice to the anus may be felt in a chronic inflammatory anal fistula.A new and short tuberculous anal fistula tends to have no cord.

If several outer orifices are close to the edge of the anus, feel the tissues of the outer orifices to tell the difference between the fistulous pipe and the fibrous sphincters and the latter is not so hard as the former.When several orifices are located at one side or either side of the anus,branches may be found and should be felt carefully. But in the complex anal fistula where the lesion is often hard and unsmooth,it is difficult to feel the branches and their trend.

In the low anal fistula,it is easy to feel the fistula because there is an obvious boundary between the hard cord and the anal fistula, The fistulous pipe runs in parallel or almost parallel to the anal canal, and feeling at the anus only finds a hard cord at the outer orifice,no separate hard cord is found.

On diagnosis by feeling,the author first uses the pressure-moving feeling method and complex feeling method.The pressure-moving feeling method is done by vertically touch of the fistulous pipe. It can help to feel the depth of the pipe because the pipe is harder in comparison with the surrounding tissue.Repeated feeling of the fistulous pipe and the lateral tissues help to differentiate the condition of the pipe.This method is not indicated for the complex anal fistula.

2. Palpating Inside the Anus: Insert a finger into the anus and feel it from outside to inside,finding out the lump and hard cord in the presence of the submucosal abscess and fistulous pipe.Feel the dentate line area to search for the inner orifice.A process or pitting node can be felt. But it is difficult to find the inner orifice when it is sealed and has no obvious node. Care should be given to the rectal ring,the extent of the fibrosis and its area, the relation of the fibrosis with the pipe and the inner orifice. Shape the finger as a hook to feel the upper part of the rectal ring.On a combined examination by a probe and a finger

for the high anal fistula, the finger at the top of the fistulous pipe may feel the impact of the probe on the corresponding rectal wall, which may be seen as a significant sign. In addition, see the contractility of the sphincters.

3. Complex Palpation: Apply the finger examination to the inside or the outside of the rectum with force to see the condition of the fistulous pipe.

7.3.4 Probe Examination

Patients are often not ready to accept this examination because of pains.But it is an important examination,therefore,it is necessary to persuade patients to accept it willingly.

On examination first insert the index finger into the anus, and find the inner orifice of the fistula. A probe is thrusted into the fistulous pipe gently.The index finger and the probe go together to the end of the fistulous pipe.If the inner orifice is closed and the fistulous pipe runs in parallel to the anal canal,this examination may predict the distance between the fistulous pipe and anal canal.An impact of the probe can be felt at the inner orifice and the top of the anal canal.Gently move the probe, otherwise an artificial pipe would be made. On the examination of the complex anal fistula,several probes can be used to see if the fistulous pipes are connected and the inner orifices are at the same position.If the probes meet in a place,it indicates a branch is formed at this place.The finger inserted into the anus can tell the positions of the probes.

7.3.5 Anoscopy and Anal Crypt Hook Examination

It is an effective way to see the position and appearance of the inner orifice,closed or open, and the difference between the inner orifice and crypt.

1. Anoscopy: Before the examination lubricate the anoscope completely and keep it moving in the posterior anal groove. When the patient is distracted, strongly press the posterior anus, which makes the posterior anus move backward, and makes it easy to insert the anoscope, then slowly insert the anoscope into the anal canal. This method may avoid unnecessary nervousness due to sudden insertion of the anoscope and spasm of the sphincters.

After the insertion of the anoscope, draw out the cylinder to observe in good light. While drawing it back slowly, observe the change of the mucosa. Usually there may be found congestion and swelling at the dentate line, inflammatory crypt and nodes. Because of the dilation of the anal canal which exerts pressure to the fistulous wall, sometimes pus runs from the inner orifice to the rectal cavity. If stain is injected into the fistula, one may see the pigmentary area of the inner orifice.

2. Location of the Inner Orifice by a Cryptic Hook: It is an important way to determine the existence of the inner orifice. Dilate the anus with a two-winged anoscope and explore it with the cryptic hook of different size. There are two kinds of the commonly used cryptic hook (0.5 cm and 1 cm of the hook head). First a 0.5 cm hook is used to examine the evident lesion. Along the dentate line find the inner orifice and insert the hook directly into it. But when the inner orifice is closed, the hook is not easy to enter. For a deep anal crypt due to inflammation, the one with a long hook head is used. If it is only a crypt, it only swallows a part of the hook, but if it is an inner orifice, the whole hook is put in it. The running direction of the hook is the same as that of the fistula felt outside of the anus. This is because the cryptic hook has entered the fistulous pipe via the inner orifice. For a low anal

fistula,insert a probe from the outer orifice,and the hook and probe may meet.

7.3.6 Fistulous Pipe Staining Method

1. Methylene Blue—Eosin Staining Method:

(1) Filling of a Gauze Roll: Insert an anoscope into the anus,and pull out the cylinder. Put a lubricated gause roll into it, or have a two—winged anoscope to dilate the anus and put the gauze roll into it.Withdraw the anoscope and leave the gauze roll there,or insert a gauze roll directly into the anus. If this method is not adopted,a harder gauze roll is fully lubricated and inserted into the anus.

(2) Injection of Methylene Blue—Eosin: Inject a certain amount of 1—5% Methylene Blue—Eosin solution from the outer orifice into the fistula. A blunt point needle is used for the injection.If the orifice is big, the injection without a needle is given.When the patient has a distending pain,withdraw the needle soon and block the orifice with hand.Gently rub it for 1—3 minutes and take the gauze roll out.

(3) Examination of the Stained Area :Direct and indirect examinations are given. The former is done by examining the stained area when the stain is being injected. The examination of the stained gauze roll is called indirectly examination.When the gauze roll is pulled out, first see if it is stained. If there is a round blue or irregular stained part on the gauze roll,it indicates the presence of the inner orifice.From the stained part and its distance from the outer end of the gauze roll one may know the location of the inner orifice.Big stained area often causes difficulties in determination of the inner orifice. On condition of a sealed inner orifice or a curved fistulous pipe or sphincterismus,the stain

tends not to pass through the inner orifice and the gauze roll cannot be stained. For this reason,if the gauze roll is unstained,it does not necessarily mean the absence of the inner orifice.

2%Gentian can be used as the coloring agent because it is strong without any side-effect.

2. Injection of Procaine Solution:It is easily condcted and suitable to the direct examination. Before the injection,insert an anoscope into the anus,0.25% Procaine Solution in a certain amount is injected from the outer orifice, and where Procaine runs out is the very position of the inner orifice.

7.3.7 Roentgenography

Roentgenography helps to confirm the depth,trend, branch of the fistula,the size of the fistulous pipe and its relationship to the surrounding tissues. Iodized oil is commonly used as a contrast medium. Because the high concentration of it causes pain,irrigation of the anus is necessary after the contrast examination. Image of high density is produced with the application of the paste of Bismuth Nitrate or Bismuth Subnitrate (one portion of Bismoth Nitrate or Bismuth Subnitrate,two portions of Vaselin mixed on heating and used on cooling),or the paste of Barium Sulfate.

The process is as follows:First put a metal chain (1 cm for each ring) into the anal canal.Inject the contrast medium from the outer orifice into the fistula.When it runs out from the inner orifice or a higher pressure is felt in the anal canal, stop the injection.X-ray examination is made to ensure that the fistula is full of the contrast medium,and then roentgenogram is done.But this is not a routine examination.

7.3.8 Rules to Know the Relation between the Inner and Outer Openings and the Trend of Fistula

1. Salmon's Law: Draw a horizontal line across the center of the anus. If the outer orifice of the fistula is located at the anterior part of the line and 5 cm from the anus, it indicates a straight fistula, the inner and outer orifices are on the same dentate line, facing each other. If the outer orifice is located at the posterior part, it shows a curved fistula and the inner orifice is above the dentate line of the mid-posterior anus, not facing the outer orifice.

2. Goodsall's Law: Draw a horizontal line across the anus. When the outer orifice is located at the anterior of the line or above it with a distance of 2.54-3.81 cm from the anal margin, it is a straight fistula, and the inner orifice is located at the same dentate line. If the outer orifice is located at the posterior part of the line, it is a curved fistula and the inner orifice is at the mid-posterior dentate line. If the outer orifice is at a distance over 2.54-3.81 cm from the anal margin, whether the outer orifice is located at the anterior or posterior part of the line, the fistulous pipe curves to the mid-posterior part.

The above two laws are similar to each other, and they are named Salmon-Goodsall's law. But they cannot solve the problem of how to measure the long curved fistula. Based on his clinical experience, the author has modified the above law. The central horizontal line and the space between the outer orifice and the anal edge are taken as the basis. If the outer orifice is located at the anterior part of the line, and the fistulous pipe is shorter than 5 cm or the outer orifice is less than 5 cm from the edge of the anus, it is a straight fistula, the inner and outer orifices facing each other. When the outer orifice is located at the posterior part of the line, it is a curved fistula, and the inner and outer orifices do not face each other. If the posterior fistulous pipe is located at the anterior part of the line, although the outer orifice is less than 5 cm from the edge of the anus, it is still a curved fistula and the inner and outer orifices do not face each other (Fig. 15).

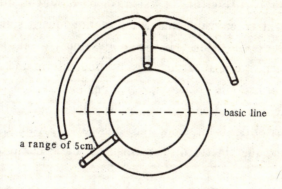

Fig.15 Revised Salmon Goodsall's law

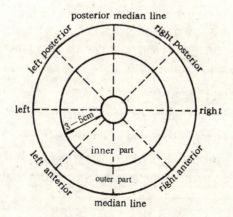

Fig.16 Park's division

3. Park's Classification:

In terms of the marks of the natural anatomy, Park's divided the anal-perineum into eight parts with the anus as the center, namely, anterior median line part, left anterior part, left part, left posterior part, posterior median line part, right posterior part, right part and right anterior part. The place 3-5 cm from the anal plica is called the inner part, while the place 3-5 cm beyond the anal plica and other related parts to the anus are known as the outer part (Fig.16). The lesion is named in light of its position, e.g. right outer fistula, and left posterior inner fistula. If the outer orifice of the fistula is located at the inner part, the fistulous pipe is usually vertical to the anus in a radiatiform and most of the inner orifices are at the corresponding anal crypt. The fistula of the inner part is often confined to the anterior part of the anus. If the outer orifice is located at the outer part, the fistulous pipe is curved, and the inner orifice is usually at the posterior median line.

7.3.9 Pathological Section Examination

It is the most reliable examination to determine the nature of a fistula. But it is essential to get a good specimen, which should include the anal fistulous wall and the tissues related to it, and the specific changing tissues.

Differential Diagnosis:

The differential diagnosis of the anal fistula is quite complicated. The following is the main differentiation.

1. Sinus Formed by the Anal Peripheral Boils: It is rarely seen. There is no fistulous pipe connecting with the anal canal and no inner orifice.

2. Post-Ulceration of the Bursitis of Ischiatic Tuberosity: The wound is closely at both sides of the ischiatic tuberosity, and at a distance from the edge of the anus. The pipe is

deep without the inner orifice and the rectal ring is not fiberized.

3. The Sinus of the Sacrococcyx: The orifice of the sinus is at the sacrococcyx, quite far from the edge of the anus. The sinus is shallow without an inner orifice.

4. Post—Ulceration of the Teratoma of the Sacrococcyx:

The lesion is at the posterior part and the wound at the sacrococcyx or peripheral anus. The pipe is extremely deep without an inner orifice and the rectal ring is not fiberized. The Roentgen examination shows the local occupying lesion. Sometimes there is hair, substance of bone, glands in it, which can be confirmed by pathological sections.

5. The Sinus Formed by Damage of the Substance of Bone at the Sacrococcyx: In case of bone tuberculosis or osteomyelitis, roentengenography can prove that the substance of the bone of the sacrococcyx is damaged or that there is sequestrum. Sometimes hard substances discharge from the wound or sometimes the bone chip is stuck in the sinus.

6. A Fistula Developed from Inflammation of the Abdominal—pelvic Cavity: Abdominal—pelvic abscess is complicated by an internal fistula, which ulcerates at the peripheral anus and hip, e.g. a combination of Clone's diseases and anal fistula. Such patients have a poor general condition.

7. A Fistula Formed by the Low—Back Abscess due to Cold: For example, it is caused by the lumbar tuberculosis complicated by an abscess due to pathogenic cold with the hip involved. Roentgenography of the lumbar vertebrae may help to make correct diagnosis.

7.4 Clinical Treatment
7.4.1 Internal Treatment

Practitioners throughout ages paid special attention to internal treatment, which can make inflammation subside and heal the wound after medication.The treating principle and medication are similar to that for hemorrhoids, but tonification is more stressed.They have accumulated rich experience and cured many cases,but relapse is still found.Thus it is necessary to have a further study of the internal treatment. Prescriptions that can heal the wound, include *Hulian Zhuidu Wan*(67),*Huangliang Biguan Wan* or *Hulian Biguan Wan*(4),*Xianya Huaguan Wan*(5),and their healing action should further be investigated.At present,the internal treatment is mainly indicated for the debilitated patients to improve their health and get them ready to be operated on,or for checking inflammation,pain and swelling in an acute attack,or for free bowel movements.

7.4.2 External Treatment

1. General Treatment:Keep local hygiene, external application is combined with intake of medicine,the steaming and washing therapy.

2. Fistula—Removing Therapy:An erosive agent is applied to the fistula,causing necrosis of the fistulous wall.New granulations are grown to heal the fistula. It is a very simple approach without surgery.suitable only to the low straight anal fistula. But it is not indicated for the curved fistulous pipe, deeper fistulous pipe or fistulous pipe with bigger cavity.

Technique: First remove the fistula and then seal the inner orifice. In the former first put a probe into the fistulous pipe to see if it can get through.Measure the length of it at the same time. Douche the pipe when there is too much pus. Put a piece of erosive medicated thread into the fistula within a short distance from the inner orifice for fear of eroding it. Another end of the medicated thread should be out of the outer orifice.Apply a dressing to it and fix it with a piece of adhesive tape. The erosive agent is called *Hongsheng Tiao* (68).On the second day take out the medicated thread and the necrotic tissue,then douche the fistula and put in another medicated thread. After 3—5 times, put in a piece of medicated thread for growth of new tissues. The next step is to seal the inner orifice. On growth of the new tissue in the fistulous pipe, seal the inner orifice by injection of a sclerosing agent around it. The procedure is as follows.First find the inner orifice with an anoscope,sterilize it and inject a small dose of low concentrated Alum solution or Sodium Morrhuate to the peripheral mucosa.One injection is enough.The injection may turn the inner orifice smaller,but it cannot seal it. The conventional approach to remove the fistula does not have such an operative step.This therapy can also be applied to the complex anal fistula when the branch fistula is intended to remove.

3. Surgical Operation:Fistula surgical treatment has long been mentioned in traditional Chinese medical literature.For example,incision of the anal fistula was recorded in *Wu Shi Er Bing Fang* (The Fifty—Two Prescriptions)and *Wai Ke Tu Shuo* (Illustrated Surgery).In the latter illustrations of instrument were listed. Reports on the recent research point out that this therapy is of higher curative effect with less suffering and short course of treatment.Similar to the ligation therapy,it has its own characteristic advantage,which plays an important role in the treatment of

the problem.It was held that the surgical operation was not indicated for the high anal fistula.If necessary,the operation should be performed several times.But the author has got successful result only by following his own techniques.The condition was cured without any side—effect.The techniques are described as follows based on the depth and number of the fistulous pipes.

(1) Low Anal Fistula Incision

Technique:The patient is in a ride—prone position with the buttocks elevated.After routine sterilization,and the local or Yaoshu anesthesia,a probe is put into the fistulous pipe from the outer orifice and gets through the inner orifice guided by a finger put in the anus. Then the probe is pulled out.According to the trend of the pipe cut it open. If it is a curved pipe, incise it during the probe exploration. Cut it totally open after finding the inner orifice.On the free passage of the pipe incise it with a probe—knife. Put the probe—knife to the front part where the probe is. Then insert it into the anal cavity via the inner orifice.The finger in the anus gets the front part of the probe—knife and brings it out of the anus.The probe—knife is pushed inward by the other hand. The fistulous pipe is cut open with two hands,or the fistulous pipe is cut open when the probe—knife is pushed and pulled. When there is no outer orifice or it is sealed but a hard cord can be felt, an incision is made at the hard cord and the closed outer orifice.Insert a probe into the pipe through the incision and cut the fistula open. Sometimes,enlarge the anal canal with an anal retractor and put a hooked probe into the inner orifice,under the guide of cryptic hook the fistula is cut open from inside to outside.The branch pipes must be cut open one by one. Trim the edge of the wound and remove slough. Do not cut off the fistulous wall, but it is necessary to partially trim it. The incision is "V" shaped for easy healing. When there is no hemorrhagic spots or a little blood oozing, apply a piece of gauze with *Zhixue San* (36) to the wound, dress and fix it. Dressing changes daily until healing.

Points for Attention: Careful exploration is conducted with a probe in order to avoid an artificial pipe. Cut the pipe open along its trend. Vertically cut the sphincters. The incision is as small as possible. Control bleeding.

(2) Incision of the High Anal Fistula

Technique: The patient is in a prone position with a raised hip or in a ride-prone position with the buttocks elevated. After routine sterilization, and the Yaoshu or saddle spinal anesthesia, explore the depth of the fistulous pipe with a probe, and feel the rectal ring's hardening degree with a finger to design a reasonable incision. For a simple high anal fistula, the fistulous pipes exist ssparately. When the incision reaches the inner orifice, vertically cut the rectal wall open. The incision is in a "△" or "Γ" form for easy drainage. But the "△" or "Γ" form wound varies greatly because of differed depth of the fistulous pipes, and varied parallel of the fistulous pipe to the anal cavity. As for a high complex anal fistula, while cut all the branches open, the corrsponding rectal wall to the main pipe must be cut open too. The size of incision of the rectal wall is based on the condition of fibrosis of the rectal ring. Usually, the incision of the anus should extend to the dentate line or above it, and the rectal ring is not totally cut. Along the main pipe slowly cut the main fistulous pipe open from inside with a pair of blunt point scissor, cut the rectal circular muscular bundle. During the surgical operation, an index finger is put into the anal canal and it reaches the medial side of the operated area.The finger may feel the impact of the probe.The fiberized rectal ring should be cut open,making a pitting defect,which will never cause fecal incontinence.On the contrary condition,it should not be cut open.Slough in the anal canal must be removed before the incision of the anal canal wall.Partially cut the fistulous pipe wall off.Trim the wound to make its edge meet neatly.Try the best to make the skin edge and the wound well meet.Pay attention to hemostasis.After the operation apply *Zhixue San*(36)to the wound and dress it. Dressing changes daily until healing.Care is given to keeping regular diet and bowel movements as usual.

Points for Attention:

a.Cirrhosis of the rectal ring area is an important precondition for the surgery of the high anal fistula. How to incise a high anal fistula has been one of the research topics.Formerly,the operation failed because a wide range of the anal canal wall and the entire rectal ring were cut.According to his clinical observation,the author found the cirrhosis of the rectal ring area due to an extended abscess in the high anal fistula.A report which dealt with the treatment of 1250 cases of superficial or deep anal fistulas made by the author revealed that out of 360 cases 330 had rectal ring cirrhosis of various degrees,amounting to 91.6%. The extent of cirrhosis can be divided into three types—mild,moderate and severe,and the posterior is more obvious than the anterior.Cirrhosis takes place in the corresponding area of the inner orifice,the minor semi–circular,semi–circular,major semi–circular ring or the whole circular.The extent of fibrosis and range is related to the simple or complex fistulous pipes,the distance between the fistulous pipes and anal canal and the disease course.In general,if there are several pipes and the main pipe is close to the anal canal in a protracted case, wide range of severe cirrhosis is seen.

Cirrhosis of the rectal ring weakens the function of its sphincters,but cirrhosis itself is a favorable factor for the operation.Incision of it will not cause retraction of the muscular fibers without a fecal incontinence.Thus in management of the inner orifice and the inner part of the fistulous pipe there is not much difficulty,and success of the surgery is possible.Two points about the impact of the cirrhosis of the rectal ring area on the surgery and complications must be clarified.

(a) The Extent of Fibrosis and the Range of Incision of the Rectal Ring Area:The range of the incision of the rectal ring area depends on the extent of fibrosis of it.When there is severe cirrhosis,cut most or total of the area open. On mild cirrhosis,part is cut open. In case of complete cirrhosis with an extensive area,it should be cut entirely open. However,if there is a large area defect, fecal incontinence never occurs. Where there is no cirrhosis,do not cut it open. The ligation therapy or incisions one by one is applied.

(b) Extensive Incision of the Anal Canal Wall and Severe Complications:In the high anal fistula it is necessary to incise the anal canal wall corresponding to the inner end of the fistulous pipe,which is considered one of the key points for the success of the treatment.In general, the incision should extend to the dentate line or above. In cases of severe cirrhosis of the rectal ring area,the incision is made from the edge of the anus to the rectal ring area corresponding to the inner end of the fistulous pipe. The wide incision of the anal fistulous wall can avoid recal incontinence.Where there is no fibrosis of the rectal ring area and the fistula is far from the anus, the incision is performed only from the wound base to the proximal anus where the probe goes through.No incision of the anal canal is made for the time being or for good, or partially incise it when necessary.Otherwise there may occur fecal incontinence, profuse hemorrhage due to large scale mucosa free movement and persisting blood oozing. Then, the ligation therapy or incisions one by one are applied to the rectal ring corresponding to the inner orifice of the fistula.In short,cirrhosis of the rectal ring should be first taken into consideration in the treatment of the high anal fistula,and the occurrence of cirrhosis must be carefully noticed.

b. Incision of the Important or Unimportant Areas :The unimportant areas refer to the lesion far from the anus, e.g.the outer orifice of the fistula,the majority of the outer part of the fistula,branch fistulous pipes,etc. The important areas indicate lesion close to the anus,e.g.the inner part of the fistula and inner orifice. The former less markedly affects the success of the surgery so that the management is flexible,but the latter fully does because the inner orifice and the inner part of the fistula must be incised,which is worth handling carefully.

In a high anal fistula,sometimes the anal canal wall should be cut open,then it is significant to make the wound of the outer end connect the anal canal.Fibrosis of the rectal ring is a precondition for this operation.

c. Importance of the Inner Orifice and Inner Part of the Fistula in the Treatment of the Shallow Deep Anal Fistula: Removal of the inner orifice and the inner part of the fistula is the key to success in the treatment of the anal fistula. The inner orifice and inner part of the fistula are at the same position in the low simple anal fistula. But in most cases the high anal fistula is not at the same position.In the treatment of all the cases of the low anal fistula and several cases of the high anal fistula,removal of the inner orifice determines the success of the treatment.If the inner orifice is not cut off, the anal fistula cannot be healed,or relapse often happens.In a high anal fistula when the inner orifice and inner part of the fistula are separated,it is important to remove both of them practically.The incision of the inner orifice in a simple anal fistula is more important to a successful treatment.In the whole process of the operation,removal of the inner part of the fistula necessarily includes that of the inner orifice,because,in fact, they are at the same position. It means two unfavorable factors affecting healing are eliminated simultaneously,which ensures the success of the treatment.

In the treatment of the high anal fistula,because the inner orifice and inner part of the fistula are not at the same position the management is not so easy.

Clinical experience tells us it is significant to remove the unsealed inner orifice and inner part of a high anal fistula.Never incise the inner orifice only and the inner part of the fistula is left behind and vise versa.Therefore, on the operation of the posterior horse—hoof—shaped or lateral curved anal fistula,incision is made from the outer orifice to the inner part of the anal fistula and then to the inner orifice. It is not desirable to make a straight incision at the inner and outer orifice and cut them off together with the partial fistulous pipe, and leave the inner part of the pipe unremoved.If the inner orifice is losed, the inner part of the pipe is at a distance, and there is no direct connection between them, it is necessary to remove the inner part. What is important is to make a rational surface of wound, eliminate the dead space and slough for free drainage and easy healing. Removal of the inner orifice means no access of the waste contents of the intestine to the fistula, preventing pollution of the fistula, which is regarded important in the treatment. But the author does not agree to the argument that recovery cannot be attained when the inner orifice is not removed.

d. Treating Principles for the High Anal Fistula

(a) Carefully make sure of the extent and range of fibrosis of the rectal ring area and its relation to the fistulous pipe.

(b) Incision of the Rectal Ring Area Once for All of the Fiberized Rectal Ring or One by One: Incision once for all is made for the fibrized rectal ring area. But the range of incision depends on the intensity and size of cirrhosis. In case of necessary section in the absence of fibrosis, incisions are made one by one or once together with the ligation therapy.

(c) The Range of the Anal Canal Wall Incised and Extent of Tissue Injury: It is not necessary to remove all of the anal fistulous wall, only the part affecting healing is cut off. But for tuberculous anal fistula, the slough of the fistulous wall must be eliminated thoroughly to help healing. Cut off the healthy skin as less as possible, otherwise it may cause deformity or stricture of the anus, or weakened its control function.

(d) Care must be given to the extent of incision of the inner orifice and inner part of the fistula. Special care should be attached to the degree of the incision of the anal canal wall.

(e) The incision of the fistulous pipe must be as thorough as possible to help free drainage.

(f) Dressing Change: Keep free drainage, a smaller surface of the wound and bigger space inside to allow growth of the granulations from the base and prevent a bridge—shaped pseudo—healing.

(3) Incision of the Inner Orifice: It is adopted to shorten the course of the treatment and decrease sufferings. On the basis of the general incision therapy,the incision of the inner orifice and inner part of the fistulous pipe,also known as the incision of the inner orifice or root—removal therapy for short,has a satisfactory effect on the low anal fistula. The following is a brief account of it.

Indications: The low simple anal fistula,esp. the low horse—hoof—shaped and long—curved anal fistula.

Technique: The patient is in a ride—prone position or in a prone position with a raised hip, or lateral recumbent position.After routine sterilization and anesthesia,dilate the anus with an anal extractor to expose the inner part of the fistula.Determine the position of the inner orifice with a cryptic hook,guided by which cut the inner orifice and inner pipe open to about 1 cm.If the cavity is bigger, a longer incision is made.Remove the slough and trim the edge of the wound. If there are long fistulous pipes of the posterior horse—hoof—shaped fistula,after the incision of the postero—medial inner orifice,a 1 cm incision is made at both curved parts of the fistula. Separate the subcutaneous tissues and prick the fistulous pipe.Remove more decayed tissues from the wound of the anus to the distal part of the anal fistula with a curet, which is inserted into the wound.No suture is applied to the wound and no drainage—gauze is fixed at the incisions of the left,right posterior part to accelerate the healing.For the long-curved anal fistulas,the incision of the pipe follows the above example except for that of the outer and inner orifices.When the ligation therapy is applied to a high anal fistula the inner orifice and most of the outer pipe are not cut open.A curet is put into the outer orifice to remove part of the decayed tissues,then insert a pair of curved blood vessel forceps to the curved part,press the handles of the forceps,the head of which raises the skin, where a 1-2 cm incision is made.Use another blood vessel forceps to separate the tissue and finally prick the fistula.Now the two forceps meet. A probe is put from the incision to the inner part of the fistulous pipe,prick the pipe and the rectal wall to pull out a rubber band to complete the ligation.Because the inner orifice is not cut open, the incision is smaller than the usual cut, reducing the damage to tissues.It is easy to heal. Dressing is changed daily until recovery.

Mechanism of Treatment: Removal of the inner orifice is a decisive factor in the treatment of the low anal fistula.When the inner orifice and inner part of the fistula are cut open,a new surface of wound is made to accelerate the healing process because the original inner orifice and the fabrized inner part hinder the healing. After the healing of the wound,there is no access of infection and when the distant fistulous pipe is closed,no ulceration will occur.

Merits and Defects: It is more easily done than the general incision and incision with suture,with better curative effect and shorter course of treatment.For the complex anal fistula and high anal fistula,the above technique can be conducted flexibly according to the condition if the incision of the inner orifice cannot help the closure of all the fistulous pipes, some of the pipes can be cut open. When the ligation therapy is applied because of the deep pipe, the outer part needs not to be cut open. On the acute inflammation of the anal fistula or presence of a cavity in the inner part of the pipe this approach is not adopted. Relapse has been found in the high anal fistula.

(4) The Ligation Therapy: This is a conventional therapy in the treatment of the anal fistula in China beginning in the Ming Dynasty. Since then, it has been highly valued and improved. The device for the therapy, such as medicated thread, probe, etc. has been improved too. In recent years, the medicated rubber band, medicated thread and silk thread are used, but the rubber band is more commonly employed. The fistulous pipe can be slowly broken by force and gets a healing. It can be termed the slow incision therapy. In light of the kind of the thread used, the therapy can be divided into the weight ligation therapy and elasticity ligation therapy. The former usually employs medicated thread or silk thread, which has no self-reduction pulling force. If we want to accelerate the breaking process, a plummet is attached to the thread, thus named the weight ligation therapy. The latter uses the rubber band or emulsive ring, making advantage of its own pulling force to break the fistulous pipe, without any help from outside, thus named the elasticity ligation therapy, indicated mainly for the simple anal fistula.

Technique: The patient is in a ride-prone position with his buttocks elevated. After routine sterilization and local anesthesia, a probe with a rubber band is inserted into the outer orifice, and drawn out from the inner orifice to the outside of the anus, the band being also outside. An incision is made at the area where the rubber band is planned to put. Tighten the rubber band and tie it with a piece of silk thread to make the band inlay in the incision.As to the ligation for the high anal fistula, please refer to the incision with the ligation therapy.There are two ways to get the rubber band or medicated thread into the fistulous pipe,i.e. from outside to inside and vise versa. For example,the thread gets access to the fistula pipe via the outer orifice and comes out from the rectum,or the thread goes through the rectum, via the fistulous pipe and comes out from the outer orifice.The author prefers to the former.In terms of the tightening of the thread or band, if a rubber band is used,tighten it once for all in the operation in general,known as once tightening.Ten—fifteen days later the fistula drops. If a piece of medicated thread is used or condition permits,the fistula is to be cut off slowly after the operation,the thread must be tightened again. Dressing is changed daily until healing. If a medicated rubber band is used, tighten it during the operation only. Ten—fifteen days later the fistula drops. If a piece of medicated thread is used or condition permits, the fistula to be cut out slowly, After the operation, the thread must be tightened again.Dressing is changed daily until healing.

(5) Incision with the Ligation Therapy:It is indicated for the high anal fistula,e.g. the high simple anal fistula and the high complex anal fistula.

Technique:The patient is in a prone position with a raised hip, a ride—prone position with the buttocks elevated or lateral recumbent position.After routine sterilization, the Yaoshu anesthesia or saddle block anesthesia, incise the outer orifice,most of the main pipe,branch pipes and cavities one after another.Trim the wound and remove the slough and make the wound open. Put a probe with a rubber band into the pipe. Prick the fistulous pipe wall and the rectal wall (if there exists a secondary inner orifice,through which the probe gets access to the rectum) and finally draw the probe and a part of the rubber band out of the anus. Cut the skin on either side of the anus and tighten the rubber band along the incision,then ligate it.According to the range of the tissue involved,the rubber band and medicated thread or silk thread can be used together.The probe and rubber band cannot be easily come out from the rectum when they go starting from the outside because the high anal fistulous pipe is far away from the anus. If it is performed in the opposite way, other aid should be ready.Because the rectal wall is slowly tightened,a fecal incontinence can be prevented in the treatment of the inner end of the main pipe of the high anal fistula.Treatment for the high complex anal fistula is expected to be successful in one operation.When the main fistulous pipes of the horse-hoof-shaped fistula are deep,at the deepest place cut the majority of the main pipe open.In order to prevent deformity of the anus and too big a wound, a 1 cm skin or cutaneous muscle bridge is kept between the wound and anus, apply the ligation therapy to the inner of the main pipe, and slowly tighten the rubber band to make the wound open. At the deeper place,cut the majority of the main pipe open and dig a tunnel stretching from the posteriormedial anococcygeal ligament,connecting the opposite ligated wound.After the operation fill a piece of gauze in the tunnel and remove it 2-3 days later to make a cavity.Prevent hemorrhage during the operation.Dressing changes daily until healing.

(6) Removing Therapy: It is indicated for the shallow and short anal fistula.

Technique: After routine sterilization and anesthesia put a probe into the fistulous pipe and draw it out from the anus. Remove the whole fistula and the surrounding hardened tissues. Trim the edge of the wound to make it flat.Dressing changes daily until healing.Removal and suture can be used together,i.e. incise the whole or partial fistula and suture it. It is undesirable to have the suture to go through the wound, but the base of the wound.Sutures are removed 7 days later.

Points for Attention: Enema is given before the operation.Asepsis is conducted.After the operation, control diet and bowel movements.

8 Anal Fissure

Anal fissure often occurs between the edge of the anus and the dentate line manifested by pain. It is usually found at the posterior and anterior parts of the anus. According to case analysis, the author finds that solitary anal fissure of the posterior part of the anus is mostly seen in man and woman, young and adult, seldom see in children and the aged. In addition to the type of the posterior fissure there are two types: that of the antero-posterior medial single fissure and that of the antero-posterior medial multiple fissure. These three types are believed to be the main ones. The incidence of an anal fissure is high and the suffering great. Thus the anal fissure is one of the three chief anal disorders.

8.1 Etiology and Pathogenesis

It is caused by constipation due to excessive heat and dryness in the intestines, and by over-exertion on bowel movements. As *Yi Zong Jin Jian* (The Golden Mirror of Medicine) says: "Constipation, pathogenic fire and dryness are the cause of the anal fissure." According to modern medicine and clinical experience the etiology of the anal fissure has a certain relation to the anorectal anatomy, but is chiefly related to the local inflammation and mechanical injury, and both of them are cause and result. The etiology will be discussed as follows.

8.1.1 Factors of Anatomy

1. Small Elastic Force of the Anus and Poor Blood Circulation: Due to distribution of the external sphincters, a triangle area is formed. The superficial part of the anterior and posterior anus has small elastic force and poor blood circulation.It is held that the anal posterior internal sphincters do not have enough support from the external sphincters,but on both sides of the anus the external and internal sphincters are tightly related to each other.

2. Heavy Pressure on the Posterior Anus: The natural angle formed by the anal canal (from the antero-lower to the postero-upper) and the rectum increases the pressure on the posterior anus on bowel movements.

The above two factors illustrate the reason of the occurrence of the anal fissure frequently at the front-back position,especially at the back position.

8.1.2 Inflammation

Inflammation decreases the tissue's elasticity and increases its fragility.When mechanical injury is added,anal fissure easily takes place.

8.1.3 Mechanical Injury

Mechanical injury is the direct pathogenic factor and anal fissure is considered an initial stage lesion.Chronic anal fissure may develop on continuous inflammation,Constipation is the main cause,but other causes,for example,injury by foreign body,anal and rectal examination and operation exist.From the above,we know that the chief cause is injury and inflammation.Inflammation makes the tissue become brittle and brittle tissues are easily ruptured.Mechanical injury further make the brittle or healthy tissues be damaged by inflammation,either of the factors, mechanical injury and inflammation, being both a cause and effect. The affected part cannot heal or relapse is frequently seen.

8.1.4 Other Factors

It is held that the anal fissure is related to conjunctival belt, or the fibromembranous tissues, short or elasticity, between the dentate line and the white line under the distortional skin. Because of this condition, the anal canal is constantly in a strained condition and the sphincters cannot easily relax.

Some people think that the anal fissure is closely related to the internal sphincters, and point out it usually takes place at the internal sphincters. At the base of the edge of the fissure in chronic anal fissure patients, the internal sphincter fibrosis can be seen, but in the acute anal fissure patients there is no such condition. On measurement of the pressure and motility of the anus, it has been found that the anal pressure in anal fissure patients markedly increases and there are present very slow undulate forms caused by dysfunction of the internal sphincters. It seems that the internal sphincters are chronic over-exerting. But it is not clear which is the primary or secondary result.

Special chapping or ulcer due to tuberculosis is rarely seen clinically.

8.2 Clinical Manifestations

8.2.1 Stage Classification

It is necessary to mention the clinical stage classification for better treatment.

Anal fissure can be divided into the acute and chronic

stages. The acute or initial stage is manifested by inflammation, swollen, congestive edge of the fissure, and severe pain. Inflammation gives rise to hyperplasia of the connective tissues at the edge of the fissure. The chronic or late stage called the old stage lesion is marked by relapse, hyperplasia of the affected connective tissues, causing its edge swollen and forming typical skin vegetation—a skin tag at the end of the fissure, called formerly *Shao zhi, Shao bing zhi*.

Based on the author's observation the acute attack does not necessarily occur at the initial stage and the early fissure develops to the chronic stage without a process of inflammation. Therefore anal fissure can be grouped under the initial stage, chronic stage and a special acute attack. The early anal injury is produced by a mechanical injury. Some people maintain that it is an injury of the anus due to rubbing, which is different from the anal fissure. No matter what it is called and how serious it is, it is exactly the anal fissure, a precondition of inflammation. The early anal fissure is easily to heal. The chronic stage has been described as above. An acute attack may deteriorate the condition, which occurs at any time between the initial stage and chronic stage. The acute attack can be termed as the inflammatory state of the anal fissure. It indicates only the condition of the acute inflammation, not the time of attack. Sometimes the anal fissure is divided into the first, second and third stages.

8.2.2 Symptoms and Signs

1. Main Symptoms

(1) Specific Pain: Anal fissure is manifested by severe pain, although it is a local limited lesion. Therefore the main suffering is a characteristic pain. Pain is present on bowel movements. A radia-

tion pain is felt, esp. on passing hard feces.Typical cases are marked by moderate pain on bowel movements and severe pain after that,with an interval between these pains,forming a specific pain cycle.The severe pain after an interval is brought about by sphincterismus,while the moderate pain on bowel movements is the result of the direct injury or irritation.Sphincterismus due to pain exerts strong pressure on the fissure and makes the anus in a state of constant tension.

(2) Hematochezia: Anal pain and hematochezia of different extent occur simultaneously on bowel movements in some patients. This bleeding is different from that caused by the internal hemorrhoids marked by the absence of pain.An examination may tell the coexistence of hemorrhoid and fissure.

(3) Constipation:Passing of dry stools may cause the anal fissure.Patients are afraid of pain on bowel movements so that they dare not to make bowel movements,which produces severe constipation,resulting in a vicious circle,and habitual constipation easily leads to anal fissure.

2. Local Signs

In general,the early anal fissure looks red in color with orderly border and has no skin vegetation.Prolonged anal fissure is dark red in color,and there is fibrous tissue hyperplasia at the edge and base of the fissure.A skin tag produces outside the fissure.The skin tag at the anterior, posterior and middle positions is the typical mark of the chronic anal fissure.

8.3 Diagnosis and Differential Diagnosis

It is easy to make a diagnosis of the anal fissure,determined by the case history and local physical signs. Patients often suffer from constant constipation, pain, and it is easy to tell hematochezia due to internal hemorrhoids from that due to the anal fissure.On examination it is easy to find the fissure occurring at the anterior or posterior anus only by expanding the anus. Local signs should be under careful consideration. For individual patients the anal fissure cannot be discovered naturally, then anesthesia is followed by examination.

8.4 Clinical Treatment

The treating principle is to keep one's bowels open and heal the fissure.The anal fissure is a mild condition with a severe pain.It can be cured but recurs frequently.It is significant to know this point,because it is helpful in differentiation of syndromes.At the initial stage treatment is focused on moistening the intestines and make free bowel movements,kill pain and stop bleeding. Operation, in general, is unnecessary.In protracted cases when there is a skin tag or other complications,surgery is applied.

8.4.1 Internal Treatment

It is essential to moisten the intestines and make free bowel movements,and then give other therapies. So the internal treatment is significant in cure and prevention of the anal fissure. Clinically,it is most important to keep bowels open instead of dealing only with the fissure itself.Comprehensive measures can be adopted to keep bowels open.Here is a detail account.

1. Proper Diet :It is a main link. Intake of less food,lack of water and food with less cellurose may cause constipation.It is advisable to take more vegetables and fruits,water and beverages

helpful to keeping bowels open. The following is recommended. The stuff suggested is carrot, radish, celery, chive, spinach, Chinese cabbage, banana, pear, honey, sesame oil, sweet potato, yam, water chestnut, raw or cooked peanut, walnut, sesame, pine nut, white and black edible fungus,pear juice,jujube juice, hawthorn juice and orange juice.

Banana: It helps bowel movements. At any time you can take it, or take it on an empty stomach in the morning until free bowel movements take place.For those who suffer from deficiency and cold in the spleen and stomach,heat bannanas with its skin in hot water and then take them hot to avoid abdominal pain.

Pear: It helps bowel movements,moistens the lung and stops coughing. Have it mixed in hot water and take it. Good effect is seen when it is taken on an empty stomach in the morning.

Sesame Oil: It functions to eliminate heat and make free bowel movements.Mix some in boiling water and take it on an empty stomach.

Sweet Potato,Yam: Both function to make free bowel movements. Take cooked sweet patoto or yam as much as you like.

Waternut: It functions to eliminate heat,and makes free bowel movements.Take it raw or cooked as much as you like.The powder of waternuts can be mixed in water or prepared into porridge and take it on an empty stomach in the morning or several times a day.

Peanut: Take it raw or cooked.The roasted or fried peanuts cannot make free bowel movements.

Walnut: It functions to strengthen the kidney,moisten the lung and makes free bowel movements. Take it raw.

Sesame, Black Sesame: They function to strengthen the liver and kidney, and moisten the intestines. Take it raw or roast it and grind it into powder, then take it with honey.

Pine Nut Kernel: It contains rich Vitamin E, functioning to moisten the intestines. Appropriate amount is taken each time.

White, Black Edible Fungus: It helps to make bowels open, replenish *Yin* and moistens the lung. It can be taken as a single ingredient or cooked.

Fruit Juice Helping Bowel Movements: Appropriate amount of pear juice, jujube juice, hawthorn juice mixed with water can be taken several times a day. Orange juice is good for regulation of *Qi* flow, free bowel movements and whetting appetite.

In the treatment of constipation, in light of individual constitution, it is advised to eat one kind of vegetable or fruit or several kinds of vegetables and fruits a day. When the diet therapy fails, take some purgatives, cessation of which follows if bowel movements turn to normal. But the diet therapy should go on.

2. Medication

It is advisable to take drugs keeping bowels open. They include Tab Phenolphthaleinum, Isaphenin, *Tongbian Ling*, Liqiid Paraffin, *Runchang Wan* (69), *Maren Wan* (70), *Maren Zipi Wan* (71) *Runchang Pian* (72) fried Semen Cassiae and Folium Cassiae tea. Oleumricini has a strong action to relax the bowels, so it is only used for constipation. Suppositories like glycerin suppository, *Daobian* suppository and *Kai Sai Lu* can also make free movements of the bowels. In addition, acupuncture, moxibustion and massage are helpful to keeping bowels open.

In the morning after getting up it is high time for defecation because peristalsis of the stomach and bowels is accelerating, which may promote defecation. Although time of defecation varies in different individuals,keeping the regular time is important.For habitual constipation,give drugs according to differentiation of syndromes. Timely treatment must be given to severe cases of constipation.

Analgesics are administered for severe pain of the anal fissure.Take hemostats if there is much bleeding. No treatment is needed for a little hemorrhage.

8.4.2 External Treatment

1. Steaming, Washing and Application of Drugs: The drugs used are compound *Jingjie Xiyao*(38),Pericarpium Zanthoxyli, Folium Artemisae Argyi, Potassium Permanganate and salt, once or twice a day.*Jiuhua Gao* (24)and other anti-inflammation herbal medicines are used.Anal suppository of similar action is given to speed up the healing.

2. Erodent Therapy:It is indicated for persisting anal fissure without a skin tag. *Hongsheng Dan* (68),Hydrargyri Oxydum Rubrum (red mercuric oxice)and Silver Nitrate are used to erode the rotten surface and discard the necrotic tissues,and then apply *Shengji Yuhong Gao*(25),*Niuhuang San* (73),*Zhushe San*(74)and *Shoukou San*(75)to promote growth of granulations.

3. Radiation Therapy:Ultraviolet ray is used to radiate the anal fissure with success.Ultraviolet ray not only kills bacteria,but also promotes cell metabolism and growth of the epithelial cells to heal the wound.It is simple and has no side-effect,indicated for fresh anal fissure.

Technique:Ask the patient to have a proper posture to expose the lesion completely. Apply a sterilized ultraviolet crook pipe directly to the fissure.In general,the first time of radiation is

6 seconds and 3 seconds increase progressively each time. The treatment is given once a day and four times make a course. For cases complicated with infection the first radiation lasts 11 seconds,and 4 seconds increase progressively each time,once a day.

4. Cauterization: It is to burn the fissure with a very hot iron or heated wire.After that an eschar falls and a fresh wound is present.Then heal the wound. Now an electric cautery is often used instead.Anesthesia is given before the treatment.

5. Block Therapy:Procaine is injected around the lesion to block irritation of vicious circle, and relieve pain and spasm of the sphincters, promoting the recovery. Usually 5—10 ml 0.5—1% Procaine is injected into the two edges of the fissure respectively. Maintain bowels open during the treatment.

It is recommended to inject Procaine and alcohol to block the nervous tissues, alleviate pain and spasm of the sphincters. Nutrition of the tissues is improved and granulation promoted. The result is good.

Because 10—96% alcohol can give rise to obvious retrograde degeneration in morphology of the nervous fibres, this method is considered as a perfect chemical"nervous apocope".

Technique: Sterilize the lesion with 5% Iodine tincture and then inject 10 ml 1—2% Procaine into the skin at a distance of 0.5—0.7 cm from the lateral portion of the fissure. The drug penetrates the anal subcutaneous tissue and some of the sphincters. The needle is not drawn out, then inject 1 ml 70—96% alcohol into the place beneath the fissure, at a depth of 0.8—1 cm.

After the injection keep bowels open. This is most effective to the early anal fissure.In recent years Methylene Blue, a long—acting analgesic is used with satisfactory results. Other long-acting local analgesics, or nacrotics, astringing agents or medicines promoting blood circulation can be used too with the same result.

6. Dilation of Anus: Simple and effective, the therapy also called anus-dilating approach is used to dilate the anal sphincters.

Technique: After routine sterilization and anesthesia, put the gloved index fingers into the anal pit and push the anal canal open, i. e. the right index finger pushes the left lateral anal pit wall while the left index finger pushes the right lateral anal pit. After that insert the middle fingers into the anal pit and push the anal canal open again. With the index and middle fingers, dilate the anus again. Now four fingers are in the anal pit. Exert strength evenly, or dilate the anal pit with the left index and middle fingers by pulling the anal pit wall on either side. The anal pit can be dilated anteriorly and posteriorly. In general, the anal pit is enlarged to house four fingers. But the Cord's process suggests that 6-8 fingers be housed. Someone advocates rupture of partial submucous tissues. Probably he refers to the inner sphincters and breaking the mucous annular tissues at some point. The dilation only lasts a few minutes and the therapy can alleviate or remove sphincterismus.

An enlarged fissure may speed up the healing. Dressing change is done daily.

7. Surgery

But there are various operations and different results for the anal fissure. Surgery for the anal fissure has early been recommended. The author thinks satisfactory results often false to get because the etiology and pathogenesis of the anal fissure are not comprehensively understood. The author advocates different therapies should be given to differed conditions. For example, surgery is indicated for the chronic anal fissure with or without a skin tag, or protracted cases. The frequently used surgery includes épluchage of the anal fissure, lysis of the sphincters and incision of fibromembranous tissues.

(1) Épluchage of the Anal Fissure: It is to remove the proliferous edges of the fissure, skin tag, inflammatory crypt and hypertropic mammilliform. Trim the base of the anal fissure, and no suture is applied to the wound. Some people advocate resection and suture. There are vertical suture on the vertical cut, and herizontal suture on the vertical cut, horizontal suture of mucosa on the vertical cut and leaving the skin wound open. But the vertical suture on the vertical cut may lead to a narrow anus so that the anal fissure may recur.

(2) Lysis of the Sphincters: It is to cut some of the sphincter bundles to alleviate or remove the sphincterismus.

Technique; After simple épluchage separate and cut vertically some of the sphincter bundles at the posterior middle position with a pair of blood vessel forceps or directly cut the sphincter bundles without separation. No suture is done on the wound. After the operation, the wound is applied with *Zhixue San*(36). Dressing is changed daily until healing.

Points for Attention:

a. Before cutting the sphincters, remove the necrotic tissues of the anal fissure first, and do the simple épluchage.

b. This operation is only indicated for the posterior anal fissure. It is not indicated for anterior anal fissure. On the operation special care is given to female cases who have the anterior anal fissure.

c. The Size of the Incision and the Size of Sphincters to Be Removed: Too small incision may result to relapse. Too big incision may delay the healing. In general, the length of the incision is 2 cm and the depth 1 cm. Only partial sphincters are cut. If there is a bigger skin tag and the fissure is fairly deep, the incision can be extended and deepened.

d. Leave the incision open without suture.

(3) Incision of the Fibromembranous Tissues: Make a V—shaped incision at the base of the anal fissure after the simple épluchage, cutting the fibrous membrane and some sphincters. Suture the wound or leave it open, or only suture the skin and mucosa. A bridge space is to remain for full filling of the connective tissues.

(4) Posterior or Lateral Incision: Treatment is given to the fissure itself. Make an incision at the posterior or lateral portion of the anus and cut the tissue beneath the fissure to speed up the healing.

Technique: After routine sterilization and anesthesia, make a 0.5 cm long radial incision at the place 1—2 cm from the posterior middle of the anus or one side of the anus. The incision is deep to beneath the skin. A pair of blood vessel forces is put into the incision. Take a part of the sphincters with a pair of blood vessel forceps and cut it. One suture is made in the wound.

If the incision is made at the opposition of the anal fissue, the incision should be 1—2 cm from the anal fissure's outer edge. While cutting the deeper layers the incision must not meet the fissure.

Trim the anal fissure edge slightly in chronic cases. Dressing change is not done daily.

(5) Apocope of the Lateral Subcutaneous Internal Sphincters: In 1969 Notaras first adopted this therapy, and the fissure was healed in three weeks. In this therapy only the internal sphincters was cut, so the ruptured sphincters were still covered by skin and external sphincters. A bridge was formed at the ruptured position. There was no umbilicate scar left and the anus could close properly. Even moderate failure of the anal control was seldom seen. For this reason he considered it as a new approach to treat the anal fissure.

Technique: The patient is in a lateral recumbent position or lithotomy position. Give local anesthesia or general anesthesia. After local anesthesia and disappearance of the local projection caused by it the operation begins. Insert a twowinged anoscope into the anal canal and dilate slightly the anus. One feels that the wings of the anoscope are surrounded by the inner sphincters, the lower part of which can be touched. Insert upward a pair of forceps into the spincter groove. The thickened lower part of the sphincters are exposed. When the inner sphincters are recognized, a blade is inserted into the medial part of the left and right (point 3 or point 9) through the perianal skin. The blade goes until the dentate line along the inner sphincters and anal skin, then the sharp point of the blade turns to the sphincters and makes an incision of 0.5 cm laterally. The inner sphincters are cut open and when the inner sphincters are thoroughly cut open, the blade meets a little resistance and the two−winged anoscpe's tense decreases. Withdraw the blade from the original access and tighten the handle of the anoscope to dilate the anus slightly. Some bloody exudate runs out of the wound. But after withdrawing the anoscope and stop of the action of anesthesia, the running of bloody exudate ceases. The surface wound is less than 1 cm and it is not sutured so as to allow drainage of blood.

The anal fissure itself is not handled. The hypertrophic papilla or big skin tag must be incised with a pair of sharp-headed scissor. A small wound is seen without injury of the deep layer of the sphincters. No dressing is put in the anus after the operation. A piece of gauze is placed on the perineum to absorb bloody exudate.

In order to simplify the process, the author uses an anal extracter instead of a two-winged anoscope to dilate the anus. When the internal sphincters are cut, dilate the sphincters with fingers. Feel the ruptured part and find a groove there, which extends to the submucosa and deepens on dilation of the anus by fingers This groove is just the wound of the internal sphincters. When it is healed the groove disappears and only something hard is felt there. During the operation. it is easier to dilate the anus with fingers than an anoscope. If it is an old anal fissure, besides the above treatment, cut the external sphincters at the posterior position and a better result is found.

(6) Ligation Therapy: After routine sterilization and anesthesia, the simple épluchage is used. Then make a small incision slightly outwards at the upper edge of the wound. Insert a probe into it and pull it out from the anus in order to form an artificial fistula under the anal fissure for the ligation. Tighten the silk thread to block blood circulation and cause necrosis of the local tissue, forming an open wound. Dressing changes daily. The silk yarn or rubber band can be used to ligate because of the small area of the tissue involved.

8.4.3 Acupuncture and Magnetotherapy

Treatment given is the same as that of hemorrhoids. In addition, a three—edged needle is used to puncture the fissure directly after anesthesia. In general, puncture in several lines and dressing changes daily.

9 Proctoptoma

Protoptoma is the anorectal prolapse or even the prolapse of a part of sigmoid colon frequently seen in children, old people, pluriparas and young people of weak physique.

9.1 Etiology and Pathogenesis

The cause of the disease has been detailedly described by traditional Chinese medicine, but the main cause believed is insufficient *Qi* and blood, declining function of the *Zang-Fu* organs, leading to sinking of *Qi* and failure of *Qi* to lift the rectum. The local functional disturbance is due to failure of control, lifting and contraction. Modern medicine considers that functional declining of the whole body, especially the nervous system is the chief cause of proctoptoma. But the local factors such as defects of anatomie structure and dysfunction, the enterogenous disease, and increased abdominal pressure, and the cause too. There are two theories depicting the complete proctoptoma of adults.

9.9.1 The Theory of sliding Hernia

It is held by some people that proctoptoma is the sliding hernia of the rectovesical pouch or rectouterine excavation of peritoneum. The rectouterine excavation is also known as peritoneal recess. Under the pressure of the organs in the abdomen, the wall of the peritoneal recess gradually goes down and the anterior wall of the rectum is pushed into the rectal ampulla and finally there occurs prolapse of the rectum. The author thinks that it is similar to the sliding hernia because the small intestine or omentum sinks into the peritoneal recess when the abdominal pressure is getting higher, resulting in a pressure on the wall of the rectum, and proplapse of rectum. If the anus is considered as a hernia foramen or a hernia ring, from which the rectum prolapes, the prolapse of the peritoneal recess and its content is viewed as a big hernia containing a small hernia. The former is the prolapsed rectum and the latter the hernia sac. The vertical procident plane is on the point where the anterior rectal wall turns back. Because the peritoneal recess can move downward, so does the prolapse plane. But they are all above the rectal ring.

9.1.2 The Theory of Intussusception

Some people think that proctoptoma is an invagination of the sigmoid colon and the rectum, and they find that the invagination begins at the boundary between the sigmoid colon and rectum. The procident plane is higher. When the invagination is formed and moves down the rectum is pushed far ahead. Because of repeated invagination, the sigmoid colon moves further down. Meanwhile because of lowered functioning of the lateral ligament of the rectum, there occurs prolapse of the rectum. The author contends that in terms of invagination, the more active upper part of the intestine often goes into the fixed lower part of the intestine, i.e. the sigmoid colon invaginates into the rectum. For protracted cases, proctoptoma is, in fact, the prolapse of the sigmoid colon with the rectum involved. Now prolapse of the rectum is not the chief problem. On diagnosis, when there is no prolapse of the rectum, the reflected pit does not touch the upper border. But sometimes, it is found that there is the prolapse of the rectum, and the reflected pit touches the upper border. In this case it is assumed that the condition of the prolapse of sigmoid colon is viewed as the prolapse of the rectum which involves the falling of the higher intestine. Some of the reports from abroad advocate the view, but it should not be readily accepted. Into the bargain some think there is no fundamental difference between these two views because what they are talking about is only the extensity of prolapse.

Some people think that the above two theories have no difference in nature, they only indicate the extent of prolapse.

9.2 Clinical Manifestations

9.2.1 Classification

There are several ways of classification, but so far they are not totally agreed. The commonly used classification is as follows.

1. Complete and Partial Prolapse of Rectum and Sigmoid Colon: The classification is based on the difference of the prolapsed tissues. Prolapse of the whole rectal wall is called true prolapse or complete prolapse while only mucosa coming out is known as partial prolapse or mucosa prolapse. But some consider either rectal muscosa prolapse of prolapse of the whole rectal, in which the prolapse involves the perineal wall, the complete prolapse, and prolapse confined to one aspect of the rectum, not involving the total perianal wall, the partial prolapse. Classification of this kind indicates a narrow sense, for falling of the inversedly turned rectal wall may happen in one aspect of the rectum, and then falling of the other aspect follows. They come out of the anus simultaneously or one after another.

Prolapse of a single aspect is rarely seen clinically because the author has only seen one case in the past 30 years. It is true that there are complete prolapse or partial prolapse of the perianal mucosa. If they are divided into prolapse of complete mucosa and partial mucosa, it only suggests the range of the mucosa prolapse. Some regard the prolapse of mucosa as an anal turnover and prolapse of the total rectal wall as the prolapse of anus, and others call the total prolapse of rectum, or rectal falling and mucosa prolapse, the prolapse of anus or rectal mucosa falling.

2. Internal and External Prolapse: The classification is based on the condition whether the prolapsed rectum is visible or not.

(1) Internal Prolapse: The rectum moves downward, but it cannot be seen from the outside of the anus. This condition is caused by two possibilities, the first is that it is a mild case, in which short downward moving of the rectum results in an unseen prolapse, and the second is that the upper part of the sigmoid colon moves into the rectal ampulla, but not coming out of the anus. In fact these are the initial phenomena of prolapse of rectum. However, in some protracted cases, the internal prolapse does not deteriorate, the condition is called the rectal invagination.

(2) External Prolapse: Prolapse of rectum can be naturally seen, commonly found clinically. Furthermore, some of the classifications are based on whether the prolapse of rectum is visible or invisible.

3. Classification of Three Grades: It is based on the condition of prolapse and, the reflected pit, existence of the annular concavity between the prolapsed rectum and the anal canal and rectum.

Grade I: Separate prolapse of the rectal mucosa and muscular layer is classified under this group. It is a mild case, in which the rectal mucosa separates from the muscular layer and moves out of the anus. Some people do not agree to this classification, because they consider that the complete prolapse of the rectal wall and prolapse of mucosa are different in cause, and they cannot be viewed as the extent of severeness. They say that it is not proper to label the prolapse of mucosa as the 1st grade and the complete prolapse of the rectal wall as the 2nd or 3rd grade.

Grade II: The rectal wall completely moves out of the anus, and the reflected pit or most of the pit can be seen.

Grade III: The rectal wall completely moves out of the anus, and no reflected pit or a little can be seen, indicating prolapse of both the rectum and rectal canal or majority of the canal, and sometimes, the sigmoid colon is involved. Patients often have loosened anus.

4. Classification based on Three Types:

Prolapse of Anus: There only exists prolapse of the rectal canal. Prolapse of mucosa is called the anal canal mucosa falling, and the prolapsed mucosa involves the perianus or is confined only to one aspect. The total prolapse is known as the complete falling. In case of complete prolapse of the rectal wall, the reflected pit cannot be completely or mostly seen.

Prolapse of Rectum: The prolapse starts from the rectal ring, and the total rectal wall moves out, the reflected pit is still seen.

Mixed Type: The rectal canal and rectum completely move out and the reflected pit cannot be seen.

Classification by Altemir:

(1) Prolapse of Mucosa: It is a pseudo-prolapse. Internal

hemorrhoids or mixed hemorrhoids are often seen in adults in this case.

(2) Invagination: Prolapse of the rectal canal and sliding hernia are not complicated.

(3) Sliding Hernia: Complete prolapse of rectum and rectal canal, a commonly seen true rectal prolapse.

5. Single Prolapse and Non—Single Prolapse: Single prolapse means there is no perineal median hernia, on the contrary, it is called non—single prolapse. Rectal prolapse associated with hemorrhoid prolapse is also included in this group.

9.2.2 Symptoms and Signs

1. Main Symptoms: The disorder comes slowly and no obvious discomfort is found at the initial stage. A bearing—down sensation is felt accompanied by tenesmus in protracted cases.

2. Irritative Symptoms: At the initial stage, they are not obvious, but in protracted cases pathological changes occur because of persisting prolapse and forced return by fingers, as a result, there is congestion, swelling, erosion and ulcer on the rectal mucosa, and hematochezia with red or brown blood. If there is no complications of the internal hemorrhoids or polyp, hematochezi a is seldom found. Mucus is often seen, and it is mixed with stools or on the surface of stools passed. Mucus is either thick or thin, and the amount varies. Sometimes mucus may escape automatically, wetting the anus and underpants. Because the skin around the anus is irritated by mucus, it is constantly wet and the plica becomes thicker, eventually eczema occurs.

Patients may suffer from diarrhea or constipation due to functional disorders of the intestines. Sometimes there is present no diarrhea, but bowel movements increase daily because of the bearing-down sensation. There may occur slight incontenence of feces and a few cases may have pain in the lower abdomen and frequency of urination. No pain occurs without incarceration.

3. Prolapse of Rectal Canal.

(1) Prolapse Sequence: Clinical observations vary as to which part of the rectal canal prolapsing first. In the sliding prolapse, because of the abdominal pressure, or the downward moving of the small intestine and omentum, the anterior rectal wall moves down first followed by the rest of the wall. However, in the invagination prolapse, all of the rectal wall moves out at a time.

(2) Size of Prolapse: The prolapsed rectum varies in size and width. At the early stage, small part of the rectum prolapses, but in protracted cases, large part of it prolapses. The prolapsed part looks bigger when it is accompanied by a perineal median hernia.

(3) Time and Frequency of Prolapse: Prolapse of the rectum usually occurs on bowel movements. Some patients have no sooner sat on the toilet than when they make bowel movements the rectal canal prolapses. For some patients, passing stools, and prolapsing rectal wall happens simultaneously; but for a few patients prolapse of rectal wall immediately follows the ending of defecation. Higher frequency prolapse is seen in protracted cases, for which besides prolapse occurring on bowel movements, it may be caused by physical labour, walking long distance or squatting, or passing urine and coughing.

(4) Reposition: The prolapsed rectum may go back by itself or by short bed rest in mild cases. But in severe cases, reposition must be done by hand or by longer bed rest. Some patients may feel uncomfortable at the anus after reposition of the prolapsed rectal canal and a short rest is necessary. The size of the prolapsed

rectum decides its easy or difficult reposition. If a bigger part of the rectal canal prolapses, it is difficult to reposit it. If a small part of the rectal canal prolapse, it is easy to reposit it.

(5)Incarceration: Incarceration may occur if the prolapsed rectum is not reposited timely. It may become swollen due to stasis and the anus hurts. A strangulated necrosis should be timely handled.

4. Loosened Anus: It is frequently seen in protracted cases. In mild cases it is only found on digital examination, but the anus can open and close naturally. In severe cases the anus is loosened, forming a hole and watery stools may run out.

5. Influence of Prolapse of the Rectum on the Body: Because it is a protracted illness, it may affect the mental state besides the local suffering, and it may cause other diseases and dysfunction of the vegetative nervous system. In recent years, it has been observed abroad that mental disorders often occur simultaneously with prolapse of the rectum. Statistics shows that nearly half of the cases is accompanied by psychosis. It also leads to general debility or prolapse of uterus.

9.3 Diagnosis and Differential Diagnosis

9.3.1 Diagnosis

It is not difficult to make an accurate diagnosis, but it is essential to examine carefully to know the types.

1. Case History: Prolonged diarrhea is often seen. In some cases there is constipation or alternation of constipation and diarrhea. Detailed inquiry should be made about the time of the first onset, possible causes and typical symptoms.

2. Inspection: Observation of the prolapsed part can tell the type, severeness and loosened condition of the anus. Before the examination, ask the patient to exert force on the anus, or squat down to defecate and attract the anus with an anal sucker to make the anal canal fall out of the anus. Observe the following points on examination.

(1) Appearance: The prolapsed part is short or turnover of the anus if it is only prolapse of mucosa. Long part is seen when all the rectal wall prolapses. If a part of the small intestine or omentum moves down ward, the prolapsed part looks bigger. The anterior part is far bigger and the prolapsed anal canal curves backward, shaped as a curved horn. Red smooth mucosa is present in the initial cases, but in protracted cases, because of repeated prolapse and reposition, there is rough dark red mucosa or with ulcer. If the prolapse of the rectum has lasted for some time before examination, the mucosa may become dark red due to circulative disturbance, and it is not the real color. Therefore, the prolapsed rectum should be handled timely.

(2) Appearance of Plica: Obvious or unobvious radiative plicae indicate prolapse of mucosa. Typically, the radiative sunken pit is chrysanthemum-shaped extending from the peripheral anal wall to the center of the prolapsed part. Obvious or unobvious round plicae are found in the complete prolapse of the rectum. If there are proliferative nodes we can see eminences of different size and congestion on the surface of the plicae.

(3) Loosened Condition of the Anus: In mild cases, the anus can close naturally. Inspection cannot tell the difference. But in severe cases, the anus would naturally open to a hole on the knee-chest position and ride-prone position. The more loose the

anus, the bigger the hole.

3. Palpation and Measurement: It is to examine the reflected pit, length and size of the prolapsed part, the power of the sphincters and other pathological changes of the rectum, anus and other related organs.

(1) Digital Examination outside the Anus: First feel the prolapsed part to see whether it is soft or hard. Elasticity is seen on the complete prolapse of the rectum, measure it carefully and make notes. On examination, observe the following points.

a. Existence of the Reflected Pit: Disappearance of the reflected pit indicates the complete prolapse of the rectal canal. Careful touch is given to see if it disappears completely or partially. If it does not completely disappear, measure the height of the reflected pit, i.e. the distance between the edge of the anus and the reflected point.

b. Measurement of the Length and Size of the Prolapsed Part: The length of the prolapsed part should be measured from the reflected pit to the top of the prolapsed part. On disappearance of the reflected pit, the measurement begins at the edge of the anus, and measure all of the surrounding walls. For most patients, the anterior wall is longer than the posterior wall, and the walls on both sides are nearly the same in length. The length is within 15 cm in general. The length of the prolapse of the rectum is decided by the part outside of the anus, but the prolapse of the rectum is a fallingdown of the double rectal walls. The outside wall is the lower anal canal, and the inner wall is the upper anal canal, so that the real length should be doubled. For example, 15 cm of the prolapsed anal canal is in fact 30 cm. The sigmoid colon has prolapsed already. The size of thickness should be measured at the top of the prolapsed part. The thickness of the rectal wall is nearly the same, about 0.5—1 cm. On the prolapse of the rectum associated with a perineal median hernia, which causes the prolapsed anal canal to curve backward, the thickness of the wall differs greatly. The anterior wall becomes enlarged, a big prolapsed part is present. Then reposit the perineal median hernia and measure the size of the prolapsed rectum for comparison. When the small intestine and omentum are reposited, the total prolapsed part at once becomes smaller and the prolapsed axis straight. There is no obvious difference in the length and thickness of the wall. On repositing the perineal median hernia bowel sound is heard.

c. Measurement of the Median Space: Median space is one formed by the internal and external walls at the top of the rectal canal. Because the top of the inner and outer walls is at the same plane, it can be called the median space. Measure the inner and outer diameters of the median space to learn the size of the top of the prolapsed part. This is a measurement for the thickness. Generally, there is a slight difference in the thickness of walls. Measure how many fingers can be contained in the space. When there occurs a perineal median hernia, the median space is not in the middle, but in the posterior position. The anterior wall is very thick. Put a finger into the median space and feel the prolapsed rectal wall on both sides and the contents in it.

(2) Anal Digital Examination: Put the fingers into the rectal canal. First examine the power of the sphincters and produce the man—made prolapse of the rectum. Powerful contraction of the anus indicates the normal function of the sphincters, but easy inserting of the fingers into the anus and weekened contraction of

the anus show decreased function of the sphincters. When the rectal canal is squeezed and the anus opens big, it means declined function of the sphincters too. Now ask the patient to contract the anus to learn further the function of the sphincters. If you want to know the condition of prolapse, produce the man—made prolapse of rectum, i.e. ask the patient to increase the abdominal pressure, then the finger in the anus can touch the descending rectum. The anterior wall of the rectum goes down first in the sliding prolapse. For example, the anterior wall is pressed by fingers, then, when the abdominal pressure is increased, the prolapse of the rectum is not present. But when the other wall is pressed, prolapse is present on the increased abdominal pressure. All of the walls move down in the invagination prolapse. Any lateral rectal wall is pressed, prolapse of the rectum persists on the increased abdominal pressure. For those who have the inner prolapse of the rectum, sometimes the fold plica can be touched. If the fold plic is bigger, a sense of enlargement is felt on touching. Feel the inside of the rectum to see if there is any tumor or if there is hyperplasia of prostate in males. Do examinations as it is desired for any complication of the hemorrhoid and anal fistula.

4. Rectoscopy: Carefully examine the changes of the rectal walls. Strictly follow the rules of the examination when the anoscope is put into the anus. The cylinder should be withdrawn slowly and as the field of vision expands, carefully observe the change of the rectal wall, especially the plica and the protrusions. If the rectal wall totally moves downward, the annular fold may fill the whole field of vision. Rectoscopy is more significant for the internal prolapse of the rectum.

9.3.2 Differential Diagnosis

Chiefly make difference between the rectal mucosa prolapse and hemorrhoid prolapse.

1. Prolapse of Multiple or Big Internal Hemorrhoids and Prolapse of the Rectal Mucosa: On prolapse of the internal hemorrhoids, obvious boundaries between the hemorrhoids and congested hemorrhoidal mucosa, bright red and dark purple in color, are found. On the simple prolapse of the rectal mucosa radiative plicae are seen and the prolapsed mucosa is smooth and light red in color. If it is a annular prolapse, there is no obvious boundary of the swelling. But if it is confined to one aspect, difference shows because of the absence of the varicose vessel group. Sometimes mucosa prolapse is associated with the prolapse of the internal hemorrhoid, the prolapse of the internal hemorrhoid involves the moving downward of some mucosa. According to different case history, symptoms and signs, judge which one happens first. But sometimes it is difficult to tell.

2. Severe Subcutaneous Varicose of Vein of the Anus and Prolapse of the Rectal Wall: When the abdominal pressure is increased in condition of severe subcutaneous varicose of the vein of the anus, the rectal canal obviously moves downward due to large area pathological changes, but it shows the outer extension of the rectal canal, not real prolapse of it. The patient may wrongly think that something is falling. But clinically on the prolapse of the rectal canal there is no obvious varicose of the vein in the skin around the anus. On the increased abdominal pressure there is the prolapse of the rectal canal, and the dentate line is seen. However, on the prolapse of the rectal canal, there is no subcutaneous varicose of the vein of the anus, the dentate line

and prolapse of mucosa are seen.

9.4 Clinical Treatment

9.4.1 Internal Treatment

Medication can cure prolapse of the rectum in traditional Chinese medical therapy. The main purpose is to reinforce *Qi* and the lifting ability of the rectum. *Bozhong Yiqi Tang*(6)(modification) is usually administered with a large dose of Radix Astragali, Radix Codonopsia Pilousulae and Rhizoma Cimicifugae. The author uses *Zhiqiao Fugang Tang*(76)(modification) with some satisfactory result. But medication cannot exert quick effect and is not so effective to severe cases. Relapse occurs. It is important to regulate defecation, avoiding constipation and diarrhea.

9.4.2 External Treatment

1. Steaming and Washing Therapy

Prepare a decoction with such ingredients as Pericardium Oranati, Galla Chinensis, Calcined Alum, Fructus Aurantii, Radix Sophorae in single ingredient or compound ingredients. Steam and wash the affected part for 1-2 times daily.

2. External Application of Herbal Medicine: So many herbs can be given. But astringent herbs are mostly used. Commonly used herbs are Halloysitum Rubrum, Galla Chinensis, Fructus Mume, Semen Nelumbinis, Os Draconia Ustu, Herba Spirodelae and turtle head. Powder is prepared and applied to the affected part. Several ingredients are prepared together into powder, which covers the affected part, or the herbal powder mixed with water or vegetable oil or turtle blood is applied to the affected part.

3. Hot Compress: Heat a piece of brick and cover it with a towel, then apply it to the affected part for half an hour once, which is simple and convenient and is indicated for children.

4. Block Therapy: Block the peripheral anus or anterior sacrococcyx with Procaine to stop vicious circle and the prolapse of rectum. The dose is 60—100 ml 0.25—0.5% Procaine once a week until recovery for adults. The dose should be reduced appropriately for children.

5. Cauterization: An apparatus is used to cauterize the prolapsed mucosa. Cauterization is indicated for the prolapse of mucosa because when an eschar falls a scar is formed and the remaining mucosa is fixed. A high—frequency electric cautery or CO_2 laser is used for this purpose.

Technique: After routine sterilization and the local anesthesia, make the sphincter relax or dilation of the anus is applied to easily pull out the mucosa with a pair of tissue forceps. Fix both sides of it and clean the surface. Caterization is given to the space between the top of the prolapsed mucosa and dentate line from inside to outside and from outside to inside in 4—6 radiative cauterized lines to the deep layer of the mucosa until the tissue becomes burnt. Never hurt the deeper layer. After that remove the tissue forceps and push the burnt mucosa back. Put a piece of vaseline gauze or *Jiuhua Gao*(24) in the anus. Dressing changes daily until healing.

6. Ligation Therapy: It is indicated for the prolapse of the rectal mucosa. Ligation may be given to the mucosa on the right anterior, right posterior and left side. Technique is the same as that done to the internal hemorrhoids.

7. Injection Therapy: It is easy to be operated with fewer

sufferings, being safe and popularized. The efficacy is related to the drugs used, and the way they administered. The commonly used drugs are sclerosing agents, apocaustic astringents and smooth muscle stimulants, e.g. Alum, alcohol, Phenol Glycerite or vegetable oil, Sodium Morrhuate, Hydrpchoric acid, Urea Hydrochoiride, Ergot, Glucose, herbs in compound form. The drugs are given in the following ways.

(1) Submucose Injection: Point or cylindrical injection is conducted for the prolapse of the rectal mucosa or mild complete prolapse of the rectal wall.

Technique: First get the rectal canal to fall out of the anus, sterilize the mucosa and directly inject the drug in distal separate form. The dose depends on the drug administered. For instance, for each point 0.5 ml 5%Sodium Morrhuate is given. The injections are given in a circle around the anal canal. For each circle, 4—6 points are injected. Puncture is done from the distal to proximal part. Points injected between circles are not in parallel. After the injection push back the anal canal. Sometimes the anal canal is not made to fall out, an anoscope is used to dilate the anus and give the submucose injetion described as above. This is known as the submucose point injection. In recent years doctors in Chongqiang, Sichuan province, China, have developed an approach of direct injection. Several injections are given in parallel along the vertical axis of the rectal canal with a long needle and a large dose is injected The injected area looks vertically protruded. Better result is attained because the drug distribution is wider than that in the point injection. After the injection apply *Jiuhua Gao*(24) to the interior of the anus. Fix the dressing for several days without change.

(2) Peripheral Rectal Injection: The needle is directly inserted into the peripheral rectum instead of to the mucosa and the drug is injected into the submucosa and pheripheral rectal wall. On the injection, the anal canal is in the normal position. The following is a description of the Alum solution (77) injected into the peripheral rectum.

Indications: Complete prolapse of rectum.

Preparation of the Drug: 7%Potassium Aluminium Sulfate (pure Alum) solution is prepared with Sodium Citrate or some Procaine. The common Alum is not used because it is not pure in quality and tends to produce side—effect after the injection. The general concentration is 6—10%. The solution in ampule needs autoclaving with a pressure of 15 pounds for 15 minutes, because Alum cannot tolerate long high pressure. If precipitate is found, the solution must not be used.

Equipment and Materials: Only a few instruments are needed. Sterilization is desired as the surgery needs. Get ready a syringe, a 8 cm long needle for Alum injection. If a roll of gauze is used to fill, get ready a 8—10 cm rubber tube and a big piece of gauze, made into a roll of gauze for pressure.

Criteria of Efficacy: The Criteria of Efficacy of the Prolapse of the Rectum: Disappearance of symptoms and no presence of prolapse are considered as complete cure. This always has been the case. But the inner prolapse of the rectum is not be able to see, which causes difficulty in determining the efficacy. Through a long period practice, the author persists on the man—made prolapse of the rectum besides the above observation. This is a reliable judgment. The detailed criteria are as follows.

Complete Cure: No natural or man—made prolapse of the

rectum is found. On man—made prolapse of rectum, there is no remaining falling rectal wall of the middle and lower rectum. The rectal cavity is relatively empty and the sphincters are stronger.

Marked Cure: No natural prolapse of rectum is present, but on abdominal pressure, partial or complete prolapse of the rectal mucosa may occur. On the man—made prolapse of rectum, there is no presence of prolapse of the middle and lower part of the rectum. The rectal cavity seems enlarged. The strength of the sphincter is the same as before.

Improved: The patient has subjective relief of prolapse of rectum, but on the man—made prolapse of rectum, partial prolapse of ring plicae takes place. The strength of the sphincter is the same as before.

Injected Method: The patient is in a prone position with the buttocks elevated. After routine sterilization and the local infiltration anesthesia insert the needle at the left and right median positions, 1—2 cm away from the edge of the anus. At first the needle is in parallel to the anal canal. When it goes through the rectal ring, have it obliquely towards the lateral side. At the same time an index finger is put into the anus to guide the track of the needle. If the needle is too far away from the rectal mucosa possibly failed to reach, puncture the needle again. When the needle goes to the appropriate place, you can feel it obviously. Usually the needle goes 4—7 cm deep, and when no blood is found on drawing the plunger, inject two—fifth of the Alum solution, Then pull back the needle a little and continue the injection. Never inject the Alum solution into the sphincters to avoid causing pain and decreasing the efficacy. When the punctured point is far from the anal edge and the puncture is not close to the mucosa, poor fixation is found. But if the punctured point is too near the anal edge, the needle may penetrate the anal mucosa. The injection is also applied to the right anterior and posterior middle places when necessary, except the above places. For severe cases, the injection may be given to the right posterior, left anterior and left posterior places, but the anterior middle place. In general, separate injection is applied. For mild cases, it can be cured by injections on the left, right middle positions. But for severe cases, puncture one point and give the drug in several places, i.e. the fan-shaped injection is used. Twenty—sixty ml 7% Alum solution is for adults. Twenty—thirty ml is on the medium low dose, 60 ml is on the medium high dose. For some patients, 80 and 100 ml is given without any untoward effect. After the injection the injected mucosa becomes swollen. Knead the injected spots to flat and make the drug spread to a larger area. Finally, put a rubber tube covered with a piece of vaseline gauze into the anus and fix it with pressure. The size of the gauze roll should be in consistent with that of the rectal cavity and the degree of laxation of the anus. For adults, the diameter of the roll is 3—4 cm, for children, it is 1.5—2 cm thinner than that for adults. A piece of thread is tied to the rubber tube and the dressing to avoid its running into the upper part of the rectum. Otherwise it would be difficult to be taken out. The injection at a time is desired, but the second time of the injection may be suggested when necessary.

Points for Attention: Strictly follow the aseptic manipulation. Avoid penetrating puncture in the anterior prolapse of rectum. When the plunger is drawn back and no blood is present, inject the drug slowly. The dose must be enough.

Management before and after the Injection: Give the patient

soft diet one day before the treatment and on the day of treatment control the diet, and enema is given with 800 ml normal saline twice one day before the injection and stop bowel movements for two days. Another enema with 500 ml normal saline is given 3—5 hours before the injection. Have bed rest for 1—2 days after the injection. Treatment is given if there appear local or general disorders. The pressure of the gauze roll helps to fix its position and exert good effect on treatment. The author holds that the pressure of the gauze roll may serve as the routine management. The rubber tube covered with gauze may be put in the anus for 24—28 hours, the maximum is 60 hours. Short—duration pressure gives rise to bad effect. When the rubber tube is taken out, watch the contraction of the anus and judge the efficacy. Quick contraction of the anus and tight closure after the contraction refers to success and better fixation. On the contrary, it only shows poor fixation and it does not mean unsuccessful injection. But it does not say that the injection fails. Any anus looks as a cavity, because of complete relaxation of the anus. When the filling is taken out, the anus closes, which suggests the tension of the sphincter is strengthened. This is a sign of fixation. After the rubber tube being taken out, give 60—100 ml 50% Glycerin or castor oil for enema. On bowel movements the patient is not asked to squat down and increase the abdominal pressure, he should be in a bowing position. The Alum solution can fix the rectal canal, but it cannot strengthen the power of the sphincters. Then other measures are taken in the treatment, for example, according to the physique condition, administer drugs to stop constipation or diarrhea, and local hot compress, and the anal contraction exercises are also helpful. Acupuncture to aid the contracture of the anus and surgery for the astringent control of the sphincters are conducted when necessary. Ligate the rectal mucosa on prolapse of it.

Alum injection to treat prolapse of the rectum is one of the great achievements in traditional Chinese medicine, especially indicated for the adults' complete prolapse of rectum. It has far more advantages than abdominal surgery. But opinions vary about the Alum injection. Some people think that the injection therapy, including the Alum solution injection cannot cure the adults' complete prolapse of rectum. However, the author contends that efficacy of a large dose injection for once is far better than that of a small dose injection for several times. Practice proves it can completely cure prolapse of the rectum.

8. Surgery: Surgery has played an important role in the treatment of the prolapse of rectum, highly appraised at home and abroad. It is estimated that there are about 50—80 surgical operations for the prolapse of rectum, but they can be grouped under the following heads: (1)Tightening the anus to strengthen the sphincters; (2)Incising and repairing the prolapsed tissues; (3)Fixing the anal canal; (4)Strengthening the pelvic floor; (5)Closed rectum and bladder or sinking of rectum and uterus, and comprehensive application of several surgical operations. The operation may start from perineum, sacral part and abdominal perineum. Some are complicated and some are simple with differed efficacy. Among them tightening the anus to strengthen the sphincters may correct the relaxation of the anus, indicated for the prolapse of rectum associated with the extreme relaxation of the anus. In general it is only indicated for extreme relaxation of the anus to strengthen the tension of the sphincters. But it can-

not fix the prolapse of the rectal canal. It may prevent prolapse of mucosa due to the relaxation of the anus resulting in partial prolapse of mucosa through tightening the anus. This operation can be divided into two approaches: physiological tightening of the anus and the non-physiological tightening of the anus. The former refers to direct tightening of the anus or embedding the live skin-flap and fascia beneath the peripheral anus, which is consistent with the physiological need, thus it is named the physiological tightening of the anus. The latter refers to embedding unlive metal or non-metal wire or bend beneath the peripheral anus, which is inconsistent with the physiological need, thus it is termed nonphysiological tightening of the anus. According to the difference of operation, the surgery includes the following three kinds.

(1) Tightening the External Sphincters: It includes the simple tightening of the external sphincters or stitching of the anococcygeal groove.

Technique: After routine sterilization and the local or Yaoshu anesthesia, a radiative incision is made on one side or both sides of the anus, often about 1 cm away from the anal edge measured from the center of the anus. Cut the skin open and separate the subcutaneous tissues. Expose the external sphincters and insert vertically a pair of blood vessel forceps into the sphincter bundles and separate them. Then lift the separated muscular bundle and get a piece of fine silk thread going through the root of it and suture it, reducing $\frac{1}{3}$ of the pheripheral anus. The part above the tied thread is either cut off or embedded under the skin. The incision may be sutured or not. Dressing is applied to fix it. If it is an open wound, dressing is changed daily until healing. On doing stitching the anococcygeal groove make a "∧" incision 2 cm away from the posterior edge of the anus after routine sterilization and anesthesia. The incision should be bigger. Cut the skin and subcutaneous tissues open and separate the skin flap to the edge of the anus. Expose the anococcygeal ligaments and external sphincters. Separate the external sphincters and stitch and tighten them as described above. Or the skin flap is not separated, but at the edge of the wound a piece of silk thread is penetrating the sphincters, tighten it and suture two stitches. Then tighten the wound at the anal tail and suture it. The free skin flaps are cut off and the remaining part is in the shape of "△". Suture it together with the posterior skin at the lateral of the wound. After the operation, the anus can close naturally, and a tense sensation is felt on digital examination. Apply a piece of gauze to the incision and fix it.

(2) True Skin Embedding and Sphincteroplasty: Embed the skin flap beneath the anal peripheral skin to strengthen the power of the sphincters. The detailed technique is as follows.

The 1st Technique: After routine sterilization and the lumbar anesthesia a sword-shaped incision is made at the place left posterior or right posterior to the anus, about 10 cm away from the edge of the anus. The incision extends to the place about 1 cm away from the anus. Make the skin flap free, remove the epiderm and full layer of it and make it into a 8×1 cm skin flap, 0.2 cm thick. Then make a 1.5 cm vertical incision at the anterior middle part of the anus, insert a pair of curved vessel forceps into the cut, going through one side of the anus, and emerging from the site of the skin flap. Grip the skin flap and bring it to the anterior middle cut. Another vessel forceps goes through one side of the skin flap penducle and bring it to surround the other side of the anus and emerges from the root of the skin flap. Tighten it and suture the free skin flap and the root. Remove the remaining part of the skin flap and suture separately the cut of the skin flap. The anterior middle cut can be sutured or not. If the anus is desired to tighten far more, cut the skin flap and embed it beneath the skin of the peripheral anus.

The 2nd Technique: A sword—shaped incision is made at the place left posterior and right posterior to the anus, 5 cm away from the edge of the anus. The free skin flap is 4×1 cm, 0.2 cm thick. Then a vertical cut is made at the anterior middle part of the anus. The two free skin flaps are brought to the anterior middle cut with a pair of curved vessel forceps. Tighten them and suture them together with a piece of silk thread. Remove the remaining part and suture the joint of the two skin flaps with the tissues underneath. Suture separately the cut of the skin flap. Handle the anterior middle cut as above.

The 2nd technique is almost the same to the 1 st technique. In the 2nd technique, the skin flap is shorter and the cut at the lateral anus. The free flap does not go round the anus, but goes along its side to the anterior middle part and suture it. That is why the skin flap does not penetrate through the posterior middle subcutaneous edge of the anus. The skin flap is cut at the left and right posterior anus and suture it at the anterior middle anus so as to strengthen the contraction power of the anterior anus.

The 3rd Technique: A sword—shaped incision is made at the place left middle and right middle to the anus, 5 cm from the edge of the anus. The free skin flap is 4×1 cm, 0.2 cm thick.

Grip the skin flap with a pair of vessel forceps, making it go round half circle of the anus, pulling it out of the opposite incision and tightening it. Suture them respectively with the root of the opposite skin flap. Remove the remaining part and suture the joint point with the tissue underneath. Suture the incision with separated stitches.

The 3rd technique is similar to the previous two. But the skin flaps are at the left middle and right middle portions. They go round half circle of the anus and they go through the peripheral anus underneath. The above three should strictly follow aseptic operations to avoid infection.

(3) Anal Tightening: Tighten the peripheral anus with metal wire or non-metal thread or belt. Less reducing of anus is seen.

Anal Ligation with Metal Wire: Put a piece of stainless wire under the anus around the perianal skin, tighten it in the form of a ring. Now an index finger can pass the anus, for infants only the tip of the little finger can pass the anus. Because of the irritation caused by a foreign body the connective tissues begin to grow, which helps in tightening the anus. The stainless wire used may or may not be taken out several months later. Catgut and thick silk thread may replace the metal wire.

Tightening the Anus with a Rubber Belt: Put a soft, elastic rubber belt under the anus around the perianal skin. The operation is the same as that of the metal wire. The rubber belt is removed 2-3 months later. It serves either to tighten the anus or to produce a scarred tissue. It tends to cause pain and infection.

Tightening the Anus with a Fascia, etc.: Put a big thigh fascia, a silk or nylon belt under the anus around the perianal skin. Tighten the anus. The aseptic operation is similar to the previous ones. The anus can be better tightened with it than with other threads. Other operations are rarely applied at home because they tend to cause more injury.

9.4.3 Acupuncture Therapy

Points Selected: Baihui (DU20), Zusanli (ST36) Changqiang (DU1), Chengshan (BL 57), and Huaimen (on the border of the red and white flash on the middle of anus)

Manipulation: Moderate stimulation is given with retention of needles for 3—5 minutes. Treatment is given every other day and 10—15 treatments make a course.

Pricking Therapy: It is done as given to hemorrhoids. Moxibustion is applied to Baihui (DU20), Zusanli (ST36), Zhongwan (RN12) and Changqiang (DU1).

10 Rectal Polyp

Rectal polyp may be found in single or multiplicity. Children may have single rectal polyp and adults often have multiple polyps. Some have peduncle and some have not.

10.1 Etiology and Pathogenesis

It is produced by accumulation of blood stasis and noxious *Qi* due to blockage of the meridians resulting from unsmooth flow of *Qi* and pouring-down of pathogenic dampness and heat in the large intestine. Modern medicine contends the rectal polyp is a kind of benign tumor, the cause of which is yet unknown.

10.2 Clinical Manifestations

10.2.1 Classifications

According to the condition, there is rectal polyp with a peduncle, also known as rectal polyp or the peduncle type, and the rectal polyp without a peduncle, also called the sessile rectal, polyp. In terms of the number of polyp, the condition can be divided into solitary or multiple rectal polyp. The severest of the latter is called polyp disease. Infants often have solitary rectal polyp at the lower part of the rectum. A rectal polyp with a peduncle is known as the low solitary polyp with a peduncle. The above classification is of some clinical significance, because it indicates the common features of the rectal polyp. But a rectal polyp with of without a peduncle often coexists clinically. Careful examination must be given to the condition of a peduncle or a rectal polyp, to see whether it's a solitary or multiple occurrence. In terms of pathology, the rectal polyp can be classified into the following groups.

1. Adenomatoid rectal polyp also known as tubular adenomatoid rectal polyp, usually found in the rectal polyp. It is commonly seen at any age groups, therefore, clinically, the rectal polyp is sometimes called rectal adenoma, a result of excessive proliferation of the submucosal glands. Long clinical practice verifies that adenoma is a precancerous change. Its proliferation can be divided into four stages: The initial stage: Proliferation of the epithelial cells of the glands; 2nd stage: A swelling formed from the proliferated gland cells, or the formation of polyp; 3rd stage: Infiltration of the adenoma to other tissues, a phase of cancerous change; 4th stage: The adenoma severely affects and adheres to the surrounding tissues. In many years observation, there is only possible cancerous change for this kind of polyp.

At the initial stage, a protrusion as big as a granule or a piece of rice is present on the rectal mucosa. Then it grows bigger and bigger. Its size is as small as a pea, cherry, or as big as a red bayberry and walnut with a diameter of 0.5–1 cm in general. Some have or do not have peduncles, which vary in length and thickness. Different—sized peduncle does not have glandular tissue, it contains mucosa, submucosal tissue and blood vessels. Multiple polyps vary in size and distribution. The small ones distribute in a patch and the big ones grow as a cluster of grapes, mixed with big and small ones. Polyp is often delicate, red in color. and has a smooth surface. Ulcers of the surface of the polyp, dark red in color, may occur due to rubbing of feces or repeated prolapse. Sometimes a polyp may come off from its peduncle. Light red colored polyp is seen when there is fibrosis on the root of the peduncle, causing poor blood circulation.

2. Juvenile Polyp: It is frequently seen in children and young people and it is not easy to tell a juvenile polyp from an adenoma in shape, for fine grains are seen on the surface of it. It occurs solitarily or sporadically, usually with a peduncle. It grows at the lower part of the rectum with a peduncle. No carcinoma is developed from it.

3. Papilloma or Villous Tumor: This kind of polyp is seldem seen in infants but often in the elderly, developed from the rectal mucosal epithelial tissues of the rectal mucosa. It grows first on the surface of the mucosa, then the intestinal glands are involved. The polyp is dark red in color and has many papillomas or villous protrusions. The shape of the polyp varies greatly. Some are round, with rough surface and fine grains; some are lobulated, like sponge or jellyfish. Solitary big polyp is frequently found clinically. They are sessile. If the mucosa is pulled down, a big peduncle is found, and its end at the rectal wall is bigger than that at the polyp. When it prolapses by falling from the upper rectal canal to the rectal cavity, the polyp wanders greatly. There are many blood vessels on it, tending to bleed and develop to carcinoma with 30% of its potential. Recent research shows that the cells of papilloma secrete a substance, which causes the intestinal mucosa to congest and diarrhea due to more secretions of the intestine. In severe cases there may present dehydration acidosis or hypokalemia.

4. Proliferative Polyp: It is developed from the mucous

proliferation, frequently seen in the middle—aged. There is no obvious symptoms and potential of carcinoma. The polyp may degenerate or come off. Multiple polyps are all as big as soybeans.

5. Inflammatory Polyp: It is also called pseudo—polyp produced by inflammation, often accompanied by intestinal inflammation, e.g. chronic ulceric colitis, chronic dysentery and schitosomiasis.

6. Polyp in the Large Intestine: Polyp usually grows in the large intestine, especially in the rectum, sigmoid colon and ileocecum in young people. Family history should be considered.

10.2.2 Symptoms and Signs

Hematochezia: Prolapse of rectal polyp may be caused by hematochezia, with discharge of a small amount of blood, or stools with blood. In some cases, large amount of blood discharges. The blood is bright red or dark red in color, sometimes with mucus. Discharge of mucus or bloody mucus is seen in villous tumor or melena and diarrhea in severe cases.

Long rectal polyp may come out of the anus. Sometimes the polyp is only seen at the anus, and sometimes the peduncle falls out too. A big anal polyp should be reposited by fingers. Sometimes it incarcerates at the anus. Its size, solitary or group presence is described above. High rectal polyp may not come out of the anus and when there is no congestion and erosion no symptoms are present. Patients with protracted multiple rectal polyps may be debilitated due to anemia and wasting away.

10.3 Diagnosis and Differential Diagnosis

It is easy to determine a low solitary peduncled rectal polyp through learning of the history of hematochezia and the prolapsed polyp.

If the polyp does not move out, digital examination can be applied to all of the rectal walls. The polyp can be touched in children. The examination should be carefully done, feeling from the rectal wall to other places, and any part of the rectal canal if the finger can reach. Never feel it unsystematically and leave out a polyp. High polyp can be felt when the patient increases his abdominal pressure because it may move downward. If there are stools in the rectum, pass it first and then do the examination. Sometimes body posture should be changed for the examination. Anoscope examination is suggested for the appearance of the polyp and polyp at the upper part of the rectum can be seen. For multiple polyps sigmoidoscopy or fibro-colonoscopy can be employed to decide the location of a polyp.

Barium enema examination is not important in the examination of the rectal polyp. It is an approach for the colon polyp. Before the normal saline enema is given evacuate feces and gas first. Then the patient is asked to defecate for several times, discharging the stools or gas completely to avoid confusion of image. After that the patient is advised to have an hour's rest so as to get correct diagnosis because the irritation by the enema is relieved now. Thin Barium is used. In the process three observations are done. On Barium enema, do the first examination; after discharge of Barium, make a contrast examination, then the rectum is aerated and do a double contrast examination. A clear image can be got after the discharge of Barium and aeration. Three examinations are given before the Barium enema, after the discharge of Barium and aeration.

Differential Diagnosis: It is important to tell the difference between multiple rectal polyps of the initial stage and intestinal inflammation, such as the chronic proctilis and colitis. In both conditions there are granular prortusions, but the polyp can be found in the rectum in the former case, i.e. the growing rate of polyp in different areas varies.

10.4 Clinical Treatment

10.4.1 Internal Treatment

Oral taken medicinal herbs do not have much efficacy. Researches are being carried out in different parts of the country. The treating principle is eliminating heat and dampness with drugs sour in taste and astringency in property. But the inflammatory polyps may disappear after the medication. Swollen, congested mucosa of the multiple polyps can be alleviated or eliminated after medicines taken. The usually used prescriptions are *Chunpi Jiujing Jian*(78), compound *Wumei Wan* (79) and *Qinjiu Cangzhu Tang*(7).

10.4.2 External Treatment

1. Enema: Compound *Wumei Tang*(80) is given in enema for multiple rectal polyps, twice a day.

2. Ligation Therapy: Simple or penetrating ligation is applied when it prolapses naturally. After the ligation the polyp is not necessarily cut off, put it back to the anus to let it drop by itself. If it is tried to be removed, be sure to prevent the ligated thread from loosening. If the polyp does not move out naturally, ligate it after anesthesia. High rectal polyps are not visible. Pull the rectal wall of the polyp areas out and finally pull the polyps

out with a pair of tissue forceps. If it is a wide base polyp, grip the base of the polyp and some of the rectal mucosa, penetrate the normal mucosa at the base and ligate it with a piece of fine silk thread. Cut off the polyp, which is to be examined pathologically. Sometimes, apply simply ligation to make the polyp drop or wither.

Ligate the densely growing multiple polyps together with the healthy mucosa. The group of the polyps is lifted, a piece of thread goes through the normal mucosa under the polyps and ligate it. Several ligations may be done at a time. After healing, ligate other polyps until no presence of polyps. In addition, ligators can be used to place emulsive rings to the root of the polyps and make them wither.

3. Injection Therapy: When a sclerosing agent is used, the drug should be injected into the polyp to cause cirrhosis of it. If necrotizing agents are used, the drug should be injected at the root of the polyp to cause it to wither and drop.

4. Cauterization: The peduncle of a polyp is cauterized to cause dropping. Small sessile polyp can be cauterized directly, but cauterization must not reach the very depth in order not to damage the rectal wall. Other speific electric apparatus may be employed for this purpose.

5. Pinching—off Therapy: The polyp is pinched off by fingers. But if the peduncle of a polyp is big and in good blood circulation, give up this method, otherwise massive bleeding may produce.

6. Surgery: Surgery is indicated for high polyp, multiple polyps and sessile polyp. It is not so easy to remove via the anus the polyp at the upper part of the rectum, 8—12 cm away from it.

If the surgery is performed on the abdomen, the rectal canal must be cut open. Because it is at the lower position, it is difficult to be operated on and the patient may suffer from it. Dr. Zhao Shuoshi has developed a new way to remove this kind of polyp. The patient is in a lithotomy position. After routine sterilization and the peridural anesthesia and / or local anesthesia dilate the anal canal with fingers. The rectum is cleaned with cotton balls covered with Bromogeramine. Insert a bundle of 2−3 Foley urinary catheters of 30 ml to the place above the polyp. Flood water into the catheters, pull the catheters towards the edge of the anus, and the polyp moves downward. An anal retracter is used to enlarge the rectal canal and rectum, then grip the mucosa at the root of the polyp with a pair of blood vessel forceps. Suture the mucosa and cut off the polyp one by one. If bleeding is present, suture it again until cessation of hemorrhage.

This method may shorten the distance between the polyps and the edge of the anus, making it possible to perform the surgery from the anus. It is an easy and reliable approach.

If there is a big peduncle of the polyp, dilate the anus with an anal retractor after anesthesia, and full exposure of the polyp, then remove it and suture the wound. When it is a very high polyp and cannot be drawn out, incise the back rectal wall, ligate or remove it.

11 Prevention of Anorectal Diseases

11.1 Prevention of Hemorrhoids

It is very important to care and prevent anorectal diseases. It is pointed out in *Chuan Yan Jin Yan He Shu*(A Complete Manual of Experience in the Treatment of Sores) that " Care of hemorrhoids lies in less physical labor, no rage, control of sexual life and proper diet." These are instructions for prevention of hemorrhoids. Hemorrhoids are a specific problem of man. Since many causes produce hemorrhoids, comprehensive preventive measures should be taken.

11.1.1 Physical Exercises

Actively take part in physical exercises, like running, *Taijiquan*,etc. Those who stand or sit long at their work must regularly make exercise of the lower limbs and massage the hip muscles to promote smooth flow of Qi and blood and prevent local impeded circulation of blood.

11.1.2 Keeping off Anger and Worry

Strike a proper balance between work and rest and control sexual life. On an acute attack and treatment of hemorrhoid it is advised to have no sexual life at all.

11.1.3 Proper Diet

Take proper and regular diet, avoid food hot and pungent in

flavor. Eat more fruits and vegetables and drink much water to prevent its onset, or control its condition after an onset, or avoid recurrence. The following points should be observed. Varied grains, vegetables and animal meal are taken properly. Take vegetarian meals in the course of treatment.

11.1.4 Having Regular Bowel Movements Every Day

Make bowel movements once a day. The duration of it should be short. Treat constipation and diarrhea timely. Women should keep bowels open in pregnancy and after child delivery.

11.1.5 Keep Hygiene of the Anus

It is a way to avoid irritation. Frequently take bath and change underwears. The toilet paper should be clean and soft. Hip bath is an important way to keep off hemorrhoids. It not only makes the anus clean, but also promotes local circulation. Hip bath on attack of the disease or after the surgery may promote local blood circulation, subside inflammation and swelling, reducing sufferings and speeding up the healing.

11.1.6 Massage and Anus—Lifting Exercise

Massage is usually applied to the anus or sacrococcygeal region whereas the anus—lifting exercise is to contract the anus regularily, because it can activate the local blood circulation, increase the power of the sphincters and promote peristalis of the intestines to make bowel movements easy.

1. Massage: Before sleep at night, knead the anal region. There are two chief ways. Before sleep at night, knead the anal region with fingers in a squatting position. One of the hands is placed on one side of the hip. The index, middle and ring fingers are closed and slightly curved. Press the anus and massage it with the pad of the middle finger. The finger moves clockwise or

counterclockwise, forward or backward. Each cycle is called once. Knead the anus for about one hundred times. Do the massage every day before going to bed or every other day or with an interval of several days, or massage is applied to Changqiang (DU1) of the sacrococcygeal region to the posterior anus for 50—100 times until a hot sensation appears at the place.

2. Anus—Lifting Exercise: it is also called contraction of the anus. There are three patterns of exercise.

The first one is similar to the setting—up exercises to radio music, i.e. exercises of contraction of the anus in consistency with rhythm, also known as the anal healthy exercises. The second is an anus—lifting exercise in consistence with breathing. The third is contraction of the anus, muscles of the hip and perineum, a comprehensive anus—lifting exercise.

(1) Anal Setting—up Exercise: Get ready a basin of warm or cold water. After bowel movements put the anus into the water. Push the anus upward with the index finger or insert the finger halfway into the anus. Then lift the anus at a frequency of 1 second for 64 times. The exercise is done once a day, or do it wthout a finger in the anus.

(2) *Qigong* Anus—Lifting Exercise: It is in fact a *Qigong* exercise, which, quite effective to hemorrhoids, should be popularized. The exercise should strictly follow its practising rules. Please see the detailed description as follows.

a. The patient may be in a sitting, standing or lying position. On breathing in, swell the abdomen with relaxing the anus and on breathing out contract the adbomen and the anus. Each exercise lasts 15—20 minutes, once or twice a day. A warm sensation appearing in the abdomen or anus indicates a better result. Another approach is that the patient first is to relax himself. On breathing in, contract the anus with the tongue tip on the palate and keeping the breath for a while. On breathing out, relax the anus. Fifteen minutes make an exercise, twice a day in the morning and evening.

b. Anus—Lifting and Massage Designed by Lin Xiande from Nanjing: The exercise is done in the morning and in the evening. The patient is in a supine position with his mind concentrating on his anus. While breathing in he lifts his anus, leading *Qi* to his *Dantian,* then breathe out and relax the anus. After a ten-minute practice, the patient squats and massages his anal region for another 5 minutes. Any time in the day constantly lift your anus to prevent constipation and hemorrhoids.

c. Yan Zijie Exercise: It is an exercise designed by Yang Ze from Shandong province, who has learned it from his teacher Yan Zijie, pupil of Han Qichang and the 15 generation successor of the five plum-blossom patterns associated with his own experience in prevention and treatment of hemorrhoids.

Technique: The patient is in a supine position on a high pillow, half closing of his eyes and mind concentrating on the *Dantian*. The tongue tip is put on the palate and breathe naturally.

Anus—Lifting: On breathing in, strongly lift the anus while *Qi* is led upward. On breathing out relax the anus and *Dantian*. Twenty-seven times make an exercise.

Kneading *Dantian:* Mind concentration is on Point Laogong (PC8) and rub both hands until presence of a hot sensation. Cover *Dantian* with the right hand and the left hand is put on the right one. Knead counterclockwise the abdomen for 81 times.

Regulating *Yin—Yang:* Direct the middle fingers to both Baihui (DU20) for 1 minute, then to Huiyin (RN1) for 1 minute. Mind concentration is on *Dantian*. On breathing in, lift the anus and on breathing out, relax the anus.

Regulating the *Dai* Meridian: Hold hands in front of the chest in a sitting position with two legs crossed. Turn the body from ldft to right and from right to left for 9 times respectively with natural breathing.

Requirement: Completely relax yourself and calm down. Do the exercise slowly with even long breathing. Exert even force to knead the point and saliva is swallowed gradually. The swallowed saliva is sent to *Dantian* by mind. Do the exercise twice a day. This exercise is good for smooth blood circulation around the perianal region, tightening of the sphincters and promoting peristalsis of the stomach and intestines. When there is abundant *Qi* in the *Dantian*, the spleen and stomach can be strengthened. *Yang* can go up to relieve sinking of organs. Working on Baihui (DU 20) and Huiyin (RN1) may lead *Yang Qi* to descend and *Yin Qi* to ascend. A harmonious *Dai* Meridiaan controls the other meridians and tendons function well and *Qi* does not descend. The above technique can strengthen *Qi* and send *Yang* upward, replenishing *Qi* and *Yang*, regulating *Qi* and blood, removing stasis and killing pain.

(3) Anus—Lifting and Other Exercises:

a. Sitting Position: Cross the feet with arms akimbo. Stand up, put arms down, close the legs and lift the anus for 5 seconds. Then sit down again and relax yourself.

b. Standing Position: Cross the legs with arms akimbo. Stand up on toes, close the legs and lift the anus for 5 seconds and then relax yourself.

c. Supine Position: Cross the legs with the heels and shoulders on the bed. Close the legs and lift the anus for 5 seconds and then relax yourself.

Do any of the exercises twice a day, in the morning and evening, and repeat the movement 10—20 times for each exercise.

d. Supine—Genuflexion Position: Flex the legs and have the heels close to the hip. Put the hands under the head. Keep the metalarsus and shoulder to touch the bed. On breathing in, lift the perineal muscles and the pelvis, making the trunk in the form of a bridge for 3 seconds. On breathing out, relax the whole body. Repeat the movement 10—20 times.

e. Squatting Position: Stand naturally, lift the anus while squatting for 5 seconds. Stand up and relax the body. Repeat the movement for 1 minute, once or twice a day.

11.1.7 *Daoyin*

As described in *Zhu Bing Yuan Hou Lun,* (General Treatise on the Cause and Symptoms of Diseases), the following exercise is to keep fit and disperse *Qi*, a way to treat hemorrhoids.

Stand on the left leg and the right one is flexed. hold the flexed leg with arms and get it close to the chest. Several minutes later, stand straight. Then stand on the right leg and flex the left one and do the movements again. The exercise should be done 28 times continuously to prevent hemorrhoids.

11.2 Prevention of Anal Fistula

Anal fistula is a result of the rectal inflammation because bacteria tend to attack the lower part of the rectum, leading to its infection with purulence. There is no ideal prevention. Comprehensive measures to prevent hemorrhoids can improve the local blood circulation and local resistance to disease. It may lessen the incidence of the anal fistula. In case of an attack, it is essential to have hip bath. In the initial stage or for inflammatory anal fistula the patient should take bed rest ,and proper diet and keep bowels open.

11.3 Prevention of Anal Fissure

A rational treatment may cure the condition. But radical cure is difficult to attain. Thus it is important to prevent anal fissure and its relapse. The local inflammation and mechanical injury are chief cause of the anal fissure and they are cause and effect. It is significant to remove or alleviate the anal inflammation and avoid mechanical injury and diarrhea. Keep bowels open is the best prevention. Others are proper diet and local massage. Do the same anus-lifting *Qigong* exercise for hemorrhoids. In the presence of the anal fissure, stools are desired to pass. Never have constipation. Try to have a regular defecation habit, once a day. If bowel movements take place every two, three or more days constipation tends to occur because long staying of stools in the colon and rectum causes absorption of water. Constipation must be timely handled, resuming normal bowel movements as quick as possible when there is the anal fissure, avoid passing of hard stools to reduce the local irritation and sufferings. When one passes hard stools, never give extra abdominal pressure to avoid injury of the sphincters. Fingers are used to slightly knead the anus to dilate the sphincters. When part of the hard stools is passed, withdraw the remaining part into the anus. Repetition of the process may dilate the anus. Too hard stools are difficult to pass, break the part passed with the help of hands covered with toilet paper. Gradually removing the dry stools may avoid anal fissure. Keep bowels open constantly. Pregnant women and women after child birth should pay special attention to free bowel movements. Keep hygiene of the anus and timely treat intestinal infections. Diarrhea which may increase sufferings should be timely treated. In the presence of the anal fissure loose stools are desired to pass.

11.4 Prevention of Prolapse of Rectum

Most cases of prolapse of rectum are of deficiency type. Spontaneous cure is only seen in infants alongside its development and growth. Such cure is seldom found in adults and the elderly. Comprehensive measures should be taken to prevent and treat the condition. Diarrhea is the chief cause of prolapse of rectum in children, brought about by disturbance of nervous nourishment. It is significant to lessen the incidence by the prevention and proper treatment of diarrhea. In the presence of prolapse of rectum, diarrhea must be kept away for fear of deterioration of the condition. Keep bowels open because constipation can deteriorate the condition too. Shorten the duration of defecation. Keep a standing or bowing position on defecation. The prolapsed rectum should be pushed back timely. Keep the anus clean constantly. Anus—lifting and *Qigong*exercise are helpful to it.

11.5 Prevention of Rectal Polyp

The rectal polyp is a kind of benign tumor and there is no better prevention so far. The best way is to do physical exercise to improve health and strengthen resistance to the disease according to the integrated concept in traditional Chinese medicine. The *Qigong* exercises can keep fit and ward off diseases. Try to do the exercise to see if the condition can be avoided.

Formula Index

1–5% Alumen Injection　　**1-5%明矾注射液(54)**54,314

1%*Alumen* Injection(based on experience)
Ingredients:
Alumen(used in medicine)　1 g　　医用明矾(*Yiyongmingfan*)
Dilute Hydrochloric Acid　8 ml　　稀盐酸(*Xiyansuan*)
1% Novocaine　　　　　　92 ml　　普鲁卡因(*Pulukayin*)

Administration: Solution is made and sterilized with high pressure. It is used as an injection to wither the internal hemorrhoid.

制用法：上药制成溶液，高压灭菌，用于内痔注射。使内痔萎缩。

4%*Mingfan Yinghua Ji*(An injection is made by the Hospital for Hemorrhoid and Fistula, Jishan, Shanxi Province)**4%明矾硬化剂**(山西稷山痔瘘医院)

Ingredients:
Alumen	4 g	明矾(*Mingfan*)
Glycerin	26 or 34 ml	甘油(*Ganyou*)
Berberine	0.05 g	黄连素(*Huangliansu*)
Novocaine	0.25 g	普鲁卡因(*Pulukayin*)
Benzyl alcohol	2 g	苯甲醇(*Benjiachuen*)
Distilled water	(to reach 100ml)	蒸馏水(*Zhengliushui*

Administration: Dissolve the above powder in the distilled water, put the liquid into Glycerin and boil it for ten minutes. Clarified liquid by filter paper is got and PH adjusted to neutral. Filter it again through a No. 3 glass-filter. Put the liquid in a 10 ml ampoule, boil it for 45 minutes for sterilization. The drug becomes a clear yellow liquid, used for an injection, indicated for internal hemorrhoid and withering of the hemorrhoids.

制用法：将几种粉剂置入蒸馏水中溶解，再加入甘油中煮沸10分钟，放置后取澄液用滤纸滤过，调整PH使呈中性，再经3号玻璃滤球滤过，封装于10 ml安瓿，后煮沸消毒45分钟，药液黄色澄清。适用于内痔注射，使痔核萎缩。

7%Alum Injection　　7% 明矾注射液(77)　　　167,372

Ingredients:
Potassiun-Aluminiun Sulfate　　7　g　硫酸钾铝
　　　　　　　　　　　　　　　　　　　(*Liusuanjialu*)
Sodium Citrate　　　　　　　1.5 g　枸橼酸钠
　　　　　　　　　　　　　　　　　　(*Juyuansuanna*)
Normal Saline or distilled water 100 ml　生理盐水
　　　　　　　　　　　　　　　　　　(*Shengliyanshui*)

Administration: The above agents are made into a solution. After autoclaving the solution is available for injection.

Indication: Prolapse of rectum.

制用法：上药制成溶液，高压灭菌。注射用。

主治：直肠脱垂。

10%Calcium Chloride Injection　　10%氯化钙注射液(58)

78,316

Ingredients:

10%Calcium Chloride	40 ml	氯化钙 (*Luhuagai*)
Novocaine	0.8 g	普鲁卡因 (*Pulukayin*)
Carbolic Acid(pure)	0.4 ml	纯石碳酸 (*Chuenshitansuan*)
Adrenaline	20 drops	肾上腺素 (*Shenshangxiansu*)

Administration: A solution is made from the above materials and sterilized by high pressure. It is indicated for the injection to internal hemorrhoid to wither it.

制用法：上药制成溶液，高压灭菌。适用于内痔注射，可使痔核枯死。

"603" *Xiaozhi Ye* 603 消痔液(56) 75,314

Ingredients:

Citric Acid(powder)	50 g	枸橼酸粉 (*Juyuansuanfen*)
Procaine Hydrochloride (powder)	20 g	普鲁卡因 (*Pulukayin*)

Administration: Add 800 ml distilled water to dissolve the above powder, then another 200 ml distilled water is added. When the powders are dissolved, stir it and filter it for several times. Put it in ampoules and flowsteam sterilization is adopted for 30 minutes. It is indicated for internal hemorrhoid.

制用法：取枸橼酸粉 50 克，盐酸普鲁卡因粉 20 克，加注射用水 800 ml，溶解后再加注射用水至 1000 ml，搅匀，先用布氏漏斗初滤，再用 3 号或 4 号垂溶漏斗精滤，分装安瓿，以流通蒸汽灭菌 30 分钟备用。适用于内痔注射，使痔核萎缩。

Bazheng San 八正散(34) 50,298

Ingredients:
Semen Plantaginis	9 g	车前子(*Cheqianzi*)
Herba Dianthi	9 g	瞿麦(*Qumai*)
Herba Polygoni Avicularis	9 g	萹蓄(*Bianxu*)
Fructus Gardeniae	9 g	栀子(*Zhizi*)
Caulis Akebiae	9 g	木通(*Mutong*)
Talcum	15 g	滑石(*Huashi*)
Radix et Rhizoma Rhei	6 g	大黄(*Daihuang*)
Tip of Radix Glycyrrhizae	3 g	甘草梢(*Gancaoshao*)
Medulla Junci	1.5 g	灯芯(*Dengxin*)

Administration: A decoction is made and taken.
Indication: Dysuria.
用法：水煎服。
主治：小便不利。

Buzhong Yiqi Tang 补中益气汤(6) 13,45,59,68,164
274,295,304,310,371

Ingredients:
Radix Astragali seu Hedysari	15–30 g	黄芪(*Huangqi*)
Radix Codonopsis Pilosulae	15–30 g	党参(*Dangshen*)
Rhizoma Atractylodis Macrocephalae (roasted)	10–20 g	炒白术(*Chaobaizhu*)
Radix Angelicae Sinensis	10–20 g	当归(*Danggui*)

Rhizoma Cimicifugae	10–20 g	升麻 (*Shengma*)
Radix Bupleuri	6 g	柴胡(*Chaihu*)
Pericarpium Citri Reticulatae	6 g	陈皮(*Chenpi*)
Radix Glycyrrhizae	6 g	甘草(*Gancao*)

Administration: A decoction is made and taken.

Indication: Nourishing *Qi* and lifting the middle–*burner* for prolapse of rectum caused by deficiency of *Qi*.

用法：水煎服。

主治：能补气升提，适用于气虚脱肛者。

Chixiaodou Danggui San 赤小豆当归散(2)   9,273

Ingredients:

Semen Phaseoli	30 g	赤小豆(*Chixiaodou*)
Radix Angelicae Sinensis	9 g	当归(*Danggui*)

Administration: A decoction is made and taken.

Indication: Clearing away damp–heat and regulating blood for hematochezia due to accumulation of damp–heat.

用法：水煎服。

主治：清湿热和营血，用于湿热蕴结的便血症。

Chunpi Jiucu Jian 椿皮酒醋煎(78)   182,382

Ingredients:

Cortex Ailanthi	250 g	椿根白皮(*Chuengenbaipi*)
Yellow wine	250 ml	黄酒(*Huangjiu*)
Vinegar	250 ml	醋(*Cu*)
Water	250 ml	水(*Shui*)

Administration: A decoction is made and taken.

Indication: Chronic enteritis and multiple polyps.

用法：水煎服。

主治：慢性肠炎、多发性息肉等。

Danggui Yuliren Tang 当归郁李仁汤(18)　　　14,275

Ingredients:
Radix Angelicae Sinensis	当归(Danggui)
Semen Pruni	郁李仁(Yuliren)
Fructus Gleditsiae	皂角仁(Zaojiaoren)
Fructus Aurantii Immaturus	枳实(Zhishi)
Radix Gentianae Macrophyllae	秦艽(Qinjiu)
Fructus Cannabis	麻仁(Maren)
Radix Rehmanniae(raw)	生地(Shengdi)
Rhizoma Atractylodis	苍术(Cangzhu)
Radix et Rhizoma Rhei	大黄(Daihuang)
Rhizoma Alismatis	泽泻(Zexie)

Administration:　A decoction is made and taken.

用法：水煎服。

Fufang Jingjie Xiyao 复方荆芥洗药(38)　　59,69,102
　　　　　　　　　　　　　　　　　　　　　　143,394,311
　　　　　　　　　　　　　　　　　　　　　　332,358

Ingredients:
Herba Schizonepetae	10–15 g	荆芥(Jinjie)
Radix Ledebouriellae	10–15 g	防风(Fangfeng)
Speranskia Tuberculate	15–30 g	透骨草(Tougucao)
Lignum Sappan	15–30 g	苏木(Sumu)
Herba Potentillae Chinensis	15–30 g	蛤蟆草(Hamacao)
Radix Aconiti(raw)	9 g	生川乌(Shengchuanwu)
Radix Aconiti Kusnezoffii(raw)	9 g	生草乌

		(Shengcaowu)
Flos Lonicerae:	12 g	双花(Shuanghua)
Radix Sophorae Flavescentis	12 g	苦参(Kushen)
Pericarpium Zanthoxyli (for sharp pain)	9 g	川椒(Chuanjiao)

Administration: A decoction of 1000 ml is made for bath of the affected part, 2–3 times a day, lasting for half an hour for each time.

Indication: Diminishing inflammation and stopping pain, promoting blood circulation and subsiding swelling, indicated for an acute attack of swollen and painful fistula.

制用法：上药水煎至 1000 ml，入盆内乘热熏洗患处，每日 2～3 次，每次半小时左右。

主治：消炎止痛，活血消肿。适用于痔瘘肿痛急性发作等。

Fufang Wumei Tang 复方乌梅汤(80) 182,382

Ingredients:

Fructus Mume	12 g	乌梅(Wumei)
Pumex	12 g	海浮石(Haifushi)
Galla Chinensis	6 g	五倍子(Wubeizi)
Fructus Schisandrae	6 g	五味子(Wuweizi)
Concha Ostreae	30 g	牡蛎(Muli)
Spica Prunellae	30 g	夏枯草(Xiakucao)
Radix Arnebiae seu Lithospermi	15 g	紫草(Zicao)
Rhizoma Dryopteris	15 g	贯众(Guanzhong)

Administration: A decoction is made and concentrated to 150–200 ml, 50 ml is used for enema each time, once or twice a day.

Indication: Intestinal mutiple polyps, etc.

用法：将上药浓煎为 150~200 ml，每用 50 ml，保留灌肠，每日 1~2 次。

主治：适用于肠道多发性息肉等。

Fufang Wumei Wan   复方乌梅丸(79)   182,382

Ingredients:

Carbonized Fructus Mume	250 g	乌梅炭(Wumeitan)
Bombyx Batryticatus slightly roasted	250 g	僵蚕(Jiangcan)
Honey	0.5 kg	蜂蜜(Fengmi)

Administration: The above ingredients are made into honey bolus. Take 9 g each time, three times a day.

Indication: Hematochezia, intestinal multiple polyps.

制用法：蜜丸，每次服 9 克，每日服 3 次。

主治：用于便血、肠道多发性息肉。

Guipi Tang   归脾汤(43)   68,310

Ingredients:

Radix Astragali seu Hedysari	15 g	黄芪(Huangqi)
Radix Codonopsis Pilosulae	15 g	党参(Dangshen)
Semen Ziziphi Spinosa(roasted)	10 g	炒枣仁(Chaozaoren)
Rhizoma Atractylodis Macrocephalae(roasted)	10 g	炒白术(Chaobaizhu)
Radix Angelicae Sinensis	10 g	当归(Danggui)
Poria cum Ligno Hospite	10 g	茯神(Fushen)
Arillus Longan	10 g	龙眼肉(Longyanrou)
Radix Polygalae	6 g	远志(Yuanzhi)
Radix Glycyrrhizae	6 g	炙甘草(Zhigancao)

(roasted with honey)
Radix Aucklandiae 3 g 木香(*Muxiang*)
Rhizoma Zingiberis 生姜(*Shengjiang*)
  Recens(three pieces)
Fructus Ziziphi Jujubae(a few) 大枣(*Dazao*)

Administration: A decoction is made and taken.

Indication: Nourishing the heart and spleen, supplementing *Qi* and enriching blood. The indication is the same as that of *Shiquan Dabu Tang*.

用法：水煎服。

主治：能养心健脾、益气补血。适应症同十全大补汤。

Heye Wan(a patent medicine) 荷叶丸(44) 68,310

Administration: Take 1–2 boluses each time and 2–3 times a day.

Indication: Severe hematochezia.

每次服1~2丸，每日服2~3次。适用于大便下血重者。

Hongfen Yougao 红粉油膏(26) 45,59,294,304

Ingredients:
Hydrargyri Oxydum Rubrum 30 g 红粉(*Hongfen*)
Cinnabaris 90 g 朱砂(*Zhusha*)
Sesame oil 250 g 香油(*Xiangyou*)
Vaseline 250 g 凡士林(*Fanshilin*)

Administration: Heat and melt vaseline in sesame oil. Put the powder of the first two drugs into it to prepare ointmental gauze.

Indication: Removing the necrotic tissues and promoting granulation, indicated for hemorrhoid and fistula on dressing change.

制用法：将凡士林、香油共加热至全溶化时，再将前两药混合研细之药粉放入搅匀，并制成油膏纱布备用。

主治：祛腐生肌，适用于痔瘘换药。

Honghua Taoren Tang 红花桃仁汤(19) 14,275

Ingredients:
Cortex Phellodendri	黄柏(*Huangbai*)
Radix Rehmanniae(raw)	生地(*Shengdi*)
Rhizoma Alismatis	泽泻(*Zexie*)
Rhizoma Atractylodis	苍术(*Cangzhu*)
Radix Angelicae Sinensis	当归(*Danggui*)
Radix Stephaniae Tetrandrae	汉防己(*Hanfangji*)
Radix Ledebouriellae	防风(*Fangfeng*)
Polyporus Umbellatus	猪苓(*Zhuling*)
Herba Ephedrae	麻黄(*Mahuang*)
Flos Cathami	红花(*Honghua*)
Semen Persicae	桃仁(*Taoren*)

Administration: A decoction is made and taken.

用法：水煎服。

Hongsheng Dan (a patent medicine) 红升丹(成药)(68)

121,143,344,358

Administration and Indication: The drug is pounded into powder to apply to the affected part, or the drug is inserted into the anal fistula to remove the necrotic tissue and promote granulation.

用时研细粉涂患处。亦可制成红升丹条，用于痔瘘插药。具有祛腐生肌作用。

Huaijiao Wan (from *Chuangyang Lingyan Quanshu*- A Complete Manual of Experience in the Treatment of Sores)　槐角丸《疮疡经验全书》(11)　　13,274

Ingredient: Fructus Sophorae(stalk discarded). Pound it into powder, put it into an ox-gall, and dry it at a ventilating place, then pound it into powder. Pills are made with honey and 40 pills are taken before meals each time with *Pingwei San*(Decoction for Stomach Relief).

Indication: Hemorrhoidal bleeding

槐角去梗为末入乌牛胆内，挂透风处干后为末，炼蜜为丸。每次服40丸，平胃散作汤送下。

Huaijiao Wan (from *Zhizhi Fang*, Essential Recipe)　槐角丸(直指方)(12)　　14,275

Ingredients:

Fructus Sophorae	30 g	槐角(*Huaijiao*)
Radix Ledebouriellae	15 g	防风(*Fangfeng*)
Radix Sanguisorbae	15 g	地榆(*Diyu*)
Radix Angelicae Sinensis	15 g	当归(*Danggui*)
Fructus Aurantii	15 g	枳壳(*Zhiqiao*)
Herba Euqiseti Hiemalis	15 g	木贼(*Muzei*)
Poria cum Ligno Hospite	15 g	茯神(*Fushen*)

Administration: The above are pounded into powder, which are made pills as big as the fruit of Chinese parasol free with alcohol. Take 30 pills each time with rice water.

上药为末，酒面糊丸梧子大，每次服30丸，米饮下。

Huaijiao Wan(from the imperial hospital)　槐角丸(御药院)(12)

Ingredients:

Fructus Sophorae(roasted)	1000 g	炒槐角 (*Chaohuaijiao*)
Radix Astragali seu Hedysari	120 g	黄芪(*Huangqi*)
Fructus Aurantii(fried)	120 g	炒枳壳 (*Chaozhiqiao*)
Radix Rehmanniae Praeparata	120 g	熟地(*Shudi*)
Radix Angelicae Sinensis	120 g	当归(*Danggui*)
Radix Ledebouriellae	120 g	防风(*Fangfeng*)
Radix Aucklandiae	30 g	木香(*Muxiang*)

Administration:　The above are pounded into powder, and pills as big as the fruit of Chinese parasol tree made with wheat flour. Take 60 pills each time with warm boiled water before or after meals.

上药为末，面糊丸桐子大，每次服60丸，不拘时，温水饮下。

Huaijiao Wan(from *Waike Qixuan*,—The Revelations of the Mystery of External Diseases)　槐角丸《外科启玄》(12)

Ingredients:

Fructus Sophorae	60 g	槐肉(*Huairou*)
Radix Angelicae Sinensis	30 g	当归(*Danggui*)
Radix Ledebouriellae	30 g	防风(*Fangfeng*)
Fructus Aurantii(fried)	30 g	炒枳壳(*Chaozhiqiao*)
Radix Scutellariae	30 g	黄芩(*Huangqin*)
Radix Sanguisorbae	15 g	地榆(*Di yu*)

Administration:　The above are pounded into powder and

pills as big as the fruit of Chinese parasol tree is made with alcohol. Take 50 pills each time before breakfast or with warm boiled water.

Indication: Hematochezia caused by fistula and hemorrhoids.

上药为末酒糊丸桐子大，每次服50丸，空腹或白汤送下。主治痔瘘下血。

Huaijiao Wan(from Yangke Xuancui— The Selected Works on Sores) 槐角丸《疡科选粹》(12)

Ingredients:

Fructus Sophorae	60 g	槐角(Huaijiao)
Radix Rehmanniae(raw)	60 g	生地(Shengdi)
Radix Angelicae Sinensis	30 g	当归(Danggui)
Radix Astragali sea Hedysari	30 g	黄芪(Huangqi)
Colla Corii Asiai	150 g	阿胶(Erjiao)
Rhizoma Coptidis	30 g	黄连(Huanglian)
Rhizoma Ligustici Chuanxiong	150 g	川芎(Chuanxiong)
Radix Scutellariae	30 g	黄芩(Huang)
Fructus Aurantii	30 g	枳壳(Zhiqiao)
Radix Gentianae Macrophyllae	30 g	秦艽(Qinjiu)
Radix Ledebouriellae	30 g	防风(Fangfeng)
Fructus Forsythiae	30 g	连翘(Lianqiao)
Radix Sanguisorbae	30 g	地榆(Diyu)
Rhizoma Cimicifugae	30 g	升麻(Shengma)
Radix Angelicae Dahuricae	15 g	白芷(Baizhi)

Administration: The above are pounded into powder and pills made with honey or alcohol. Take 50 pills each time at first and then take 50-80 pills each time with warm alcohol.

上药为细末，蜜丸或酒糊丸，每次服 50 丸，渐至 80 丸。温酒下。

Huaijiao Wan(from the proved prescription)　槐角丸(经验方)(12)

Ingredients:

Fructus Sophorae	90 g	槐角(Huaijiao)
Flos Sophorae(fried)	90 g	炒槐花(Chaohuaihua)
Radix Rehmanniae(raw)	90 g	生地(Shengdi)
Radix Scutellariae	90 g	黄芩(Huangqin)
Cortex Phellodendri	90 g	黄柏(Huangbai)
Radix Angelicae Sinensis	90 g	当归(Danggui)
Cacumen Biotae(burnt)	90 g	侧柏炭(Cebaitan)
Radix Schizonepetae	60 g	荆芥(Jingjie)
Herba Ledebouriellae	60 g	防风(Fengfeng)
Fructus Aurantii(fried)	60 g	枳壳(Zhiqiao)
Radix Sanguisorbae(burnt)	60 g	地榆炭(Diyutan)
Rhizoma Coptidis	30 g	黄连(Huanglian)
Radix et Rhizoma Rhei(raw)	30 g	生大黄(Shengdaihuang)
Rhizoma Ligustici Chuanxiong	30 g	川芎(Chuanxiong)

Administration: The above are pounded into powder and bolus is made with honey, each weighs 9 grams. One or two is taken each time and two to three times a day.

Indication: Removing heat from blood to stop bleeding and keeping bowels open to relieve constipation and pain, indicated for hematochezia, constipation due to heat in the intestines and anal swelling and pain.

制法：共为细粉，炼蜜为丸，每丸9克。
用法：每次服1～2丸，每日服2～3次。
主治：凉血止血、润便止痛。适用于大便下血，肠热便秘，肛门肿痛等。

Huaijiao Wan(from Yangke Xuancui— The Selected Works on Sores) 槐角丸《疡科选粹》(13)   14,275

Ingredients:
Fructus Sophorae(roasted with honey)   槐角(*Huaijiao*)
Radix Angelicae Sinensis(roasted with honey) 当归(*Danggai*)
Cortex Lycii Radicis(roasted with honey)   地骨皮(*Digubi*)

Administration: Equal portion of the above is pounded into powder and pills are made. Take 20 pills each time with warm boiled water before meals, three times a day.

槐角、当归、地骨皮炙各等分。上药为末，制水丸，每次服20丸，食前温水下，每日服3次。

Huaijiao Yuan(traditional prescription) 槐角圆(正统方) (10)   13,68,274,310

Ingredients:

Fructus Sophorae(roasted)	1000 g	炒槐角(*Chaohuaijiao*)
Radix Sanguisorbae	500 g	地榆(*Diyu*)
Radix Angelicae Sinensis (soak it in alcohol for one night and toast it)	500 g	当归(*Danggui*)
Radix Ledebouriellae	500 g	防风(*Fangfeng*)
Radix Scutellariae	500 g	黄芩(*Huangqin*)
Fructus Aurantii	500 g	枳壳(*Zhiqiao*)

Administration: The above are pounded into powder, and made into pills as big as the fruit of Chinese parasol tree with alcohol. Take 30 pills each time with rice water.

Indication: Pain, itching, discharge of pus and blood, swelling and damp-heat.

制用法：上药为末、酒糊圆为梧桐子大，每次服 30 丸，米饮下。

主治：治肠风疮内小虫，里急下脓血，止痒痛，消肿聚，驱湿毒。此方即当今应用之槐角丸主方。

Huaizi Wan 槐子丸(8) 13,274

Ingredients:

Semen Sophorea	120 g	槐子(Huaizi)
Lacquer(dried)	120 g	干漆(Ganqi)
Radix Evodiae	120 g	吴荑根(Wuyugen)
Radix Evodiae(peel)	120 g	吴荑皮(Wuyupi)
Radix Gentianae Macrophyllae	60 g	秦艽(Qinjiu)
Radix Angelicae Dahuricae	60 g	白芷(Baizhi)
Cortex Cinnamomi	60 g	桂心(Guixin)
Radix Scutellariae	60 g	黄芩(huangqin)
Radix Astragali seu Hedysari	60 g	黄芪(Huangqi)
Radix Cynanchi Atrati	60 g	白薇(Bailian)
Concha Ostreae	60 g	牡蛎(Muli)
Os Draconis	60 g	龙骨(Longgu)
Omphalia	60 g	雷丸(Leiwan)
Flos Caryophyili	60 g	丁香(Ding xiang)
Fructus Tribuli	60 g	蒺藜(Jili)
Radix Aconiti Praeparata	60 g	附子(Fuzi)

Administration: The above are pounded into powder, and pills as big as the fruit of Chinese parasol tree made. Take 20 pills each time and three times a day.

Indication: Hemorrhoids

制用法：上药共研为细末，蜜丸，如梧子，每次 20 丸，每日服 3 次。

主治：适用于痔。

Huangcu Huji 黄醋糊剂(66) 102,332

Ingredients:

Radix et Rhizoma Rhei (powder)(proper amount)　大黄粉(*Daihuangfen*)

Vinegar(proper amount)　醋(*Cu*)

Administration: The above are mixed into a paste. Before application of the paste to the affected part, apply *Suanxiao Huji* to the affected part first. In general, cover the affected part with the drug and dress it for 24 hours. After that repeat the medication. If there appear blisters or erosion cease using *Suanxiao Huji,* and use *Huangcu Huji* only. The therapeutic effect is not good if *Suanxiao Huji* is not applied first.

Indication: Same as (65).

制用法：上药调成稠糊称黄醋糊剂，涂于患处。用前先涂蒜硝糊剂，后再更换黄醋糊剂，一般涂 1 厚层，外盖 1 薄膜，再敷纱布包扎，24 小时后，重复上述处理，即与蒜硝糊剂交替敷用。如皮肤出现水疱、糜烂，停用蒜硝糊剂，单独涂布黄醋糊剂。开始应用时如不先涂蒜硝糊剂，直接应用此糊，则效果较差。

主治：同(65)

Huanglian Biguan Wan   黄连闭管丸(4)   12,120,274,344

Ingredients:
Rhizoma Picrorhizae (ground into powder)	30 g	胡黄连(*Huhuanglian*)
Squama Manitis (fried in sesame oil to yellow color)	15 g	穿山甲(*Chuanshanjia*)
Concha Haliotidis (forged)	15 g	煅石决明(*Duanshijueming*)
Flos Sophorae (slightly fried)	15 g	炒槐花(*Chaohuaihua*)

Administration: The above are pounded into powder and bolus is made with honey, 3 grams are taken for each time with rice water before breakfast and supper. In cases with hard projections around the fistula, add 20 silkworm cocoons(in powder form and be fried)to the above ingredients and make bolus for administration.

Indication: Anal fistula not fit for surgery.

制用法：上药为末，炼蜜为丸，如麻子大，每服3克，空腹清米汤送下，早晚日服2次。如瘘之四边有硬肉突起者，加蚕茧20个炒末和入药中服用。

主治：肛瘘不宜手术者。

Huanglian Chushi Tang   黄连除湿汤(62)   102,332

Ingredients:
Rhizoma Coptidis	3 g	黄连(*Huanglian*)
Radix Scutellariae	3 g	黄芩(*Huangqin*)
Rhizoma Ligustici Chuanxiong	3 g	川芎(*Chuanxiong*)

Radix Angelicae Sinensis	3 g	当归(*Danggui*)
Radix Ledebouriellae	3 g	防风(*Fangfeng*)
Rhizoma Atractylodis	3 g	苍术(*Cangzhu*)
Cortex Magnoliae Officinalis	3 g	厚朴(*Houpu*)
Fructus Aurantii	3 g	枳壳(*Zhiqiao*)
Fructus Forsythiae	3 g	连翘(*Lianqiao*)
Radix et Rhizoma Rhei	6 g	大黄(*Daihuang*)
Mirabilite	6 g	朴硝(*Puxiao*)
Radix Glycyrrhizae	1.5 g	甘草(*Gancao*)

Administration: A decoction is made and taken.

Indication: Perianal abscess(at the initial stage), downward pouring of damp-heat to the anus, swelling, pain of anus and constipation.

用法：水煎服。

主治：脏毒初起，湿热流注肛门，结肿疼痛，大便秘结者。

Huanglian Jiedu Tang 黄连解毒汤(41) 68,310

Ingredients:

Equal portion of the following:

Rhizoma Coptidis	黄连(*Huanglian*)
Radix Scutellariae	黄芩(*Huangqin*)
Cortex Phellodendri	黄柏(*Huangbai*)
Fructus Gardeniae	山栀(*Shanzhi*)

Administration: A decoction is made and taken.

Indication: Clearing away heat and detoxicating, indicated for hematochezia due to blood-heat, abscess of anus, an acute attack of fistula.

用法：水煎服。

主治：能清热解毒，用于血热妄行之便血，肛周脓肿和肛瘘急性发作等。

Huangtu Tang 黄土汤(1)   9,272

Ingredients:

Radix Glycyrrhizae	9 g	甘草(*Gancao*)
Radix Rehmanniae(dried)	9 g	干地黄(*Gandihuang*)
Rhizoma Atractylodis Macrocephalae	9 g	白术(*Baizhu*)
Radix Aconiti Praeparata	9 g	炮附子(*Paofuzi*)
Colla Corii Asini	9 g	阿胶(*Ejiao*)
Radix Scutellariae	9 g	黄芩(*Huangqin*)
Oven yellow earth	24 g	灶中黄土(*Zaozhonghuangtu*)

Administration: A decoction is made and taken.

Indication: Warming *Yang* and invigorating the spleen, nourishing blood and checking bleeding to treat hematochezia due to deficiency of spleen *Qi*.

用法：水煎服。

主治：有温阳健脾，养血止血之功，用于脾气虚寒所致便血。

Huanzhi San 唤痔散(23)   18,72,277,312

Ingredients:

Radix Aconiti Kusnezoffii(raw)	3 g	生草乌(*Shengcaowu*)
Corium Erinacei (burnt with the original property retained)	3 g	刺猬皮(*Ciweipi*)
Alumen Exsiccatum	15 g	枯矾(*Kufan*)
Salt(roasted)	9 g	炒食盐(*Chaoshiyan*)
Moschus	1.5 g	麝香(*Shexiang*)

Borneolum Syntheticum　　0.6 g　冰片(*Bingpian*)

Administration: The above are pounded into powder and made into paste with water. A cotton ball covered with it is put into the anus.

Indication: Internal Hemorrhoids are treated with *Kuzhi San* and the above drug is used to cause quick prolapse of the internal hemorrhoid by irritating it.

制用法：上药为细末，装瓶备用。用水调成糊状，以棉球蘸药纳肛内。

主治：内痔以枯痔散治疗，如痔核不脱出时，以此药刺激痔体使迅速增大脱出。

Huazhi Wan(a patent medicine)　　化痔丸(45)　　68,310

Administration: Take 25 pills each time and twice or three times a day.

每次服 25 粒，每日服 2～3 次。

Hulian Zhuidu Wan　　胡连追毒丸(67)　　120,344

Ingredients:
Rhizoma Picrorhizae(sliced)　30 g　胡黄连(*Huhuanglian*)
　(roasted with Rhizoma Zingiberis Recens juice)
Corium Erinacei　　　　　　30 g　刺猬皮(*Ciweipi*)
　(roasted to yellow colour)
Moschus　　　　　　　　　0.6 g　麝香(*Shexiang*)

Administration: The above are pounded into powder and bolus is made. Take 3 g each time with alcohol before meals.

Indication: Anal fistula. First take the drug to remove pus, then take it after taking *Huanglian Biguan Wan* to have better effect.

制用法：上药为末，软饭为丸，麻子大，每服3克食前酒下。

主治：治痔瘘。先用此丸追尽脓毒，后服黄连闭管丸，自然取效。

Huzhi Gao　护痔膏(52)　　　　　　　　　　72,312

Ingredients:

Rhizoma Bletillae	9 g	白芨(*Baiji*)
Gypsum Fibrosum	9 g	石膏(*Shigao*)
Rhizoma Coptidis	9 g	黄连(*Huanglian*)
Moschus	0.6 g	麝香(*Shexiang*)
Borneolum Syntheticum	0.6 g	冰片(*Bingpian*)

Administration: The above are pounded into powder, which is mixed with egg white and applied to the affected part.

Indication: When an internal hemorrhoid is treated by *Kuzhi San*, this drug is applied to the healthy tissues around the hemorrhoid to avoid injury of the surrounding tissues.

制用法：上药为细末，装瓶备用。用鸡蛋清调膏，涂局部。

主治：内痔以枯痔散治疗时，以此膏敷贴所枯痔核周围正常组织，免受腐蚀。

Jichang San(proved recipe)　鸡肠散(经验方)(49)

68,310

Ingredients:

Fructus Amomi	9 g	砂仁(*Sharen*)
Panax Ginseng	9 g	紫叩(*Zikou*)
Pericarpium Citri Reticulatae	9 g	陈皮(*Chenpi*)

Cotex Cinnamomi	9 g	边桂(*Biangui*)
Semen Cardamomi Rotundi	9 g	肉豆蔻(*Roudoukou*)
Semen Myristicae	9 g	力参(*Lishen*)
Radix Ginseng	9 g	瓦松(*Wasong*)
Chicken intestine	one or two	鸡肠(*Jichang*)

Administration: The above seven ingredients are pounded into powder. Semen Myristicae is roasted to remove fat. Wash the chicken intestine, clean and dry it, which is later burnt and pounded into powder. Take a spoonful of the chicken intestine and 6—9 g powder of herbal drugs with 150 ml boiled warm yellow wine. Take it every other day. For mild cases, 1—2 doses are enough, but for severe cases, take several doses.

Indication: Stopping bleeding and diminishing inflammation, indicated for hematochezia due to hemorrhoid and an attack of fistula with dischange of pus.

制用法：上7味药肉豆蔻须炙去油，共为细末装瓶备用。鸡肠末制法，先将鸡肠内粪便缕出，用一细圆棍长约1尺许，将鸡肠内面翻至外面，重新洗净，然后凉干或晒干，再在瓦上焙焦，后研细末。取鸡肠末1汤匙，再加上方中药面6～9克，用黄酒150ml冲服。服时先将黄酒烧开，将药粉放入搅匀，待温后一次服完。一般隔日服1次，轻者1～2次即愈，重者可服几次。

主治：能止血、消炎，适用于痔疮便血，肛瘘发作出脓水。

Jichang San (from *Jinzhou Yanfang Xuan*—The Selected Proved Prescriptions in Jinzhou) 鸡肠散《锦州验方选》(49)　　68,310

Ingredients, administration and indication:

Take 1/3 meter intestine of a chicken and put a scolopendra into it. Have 50 intestines of chickens with scolopendra well done by steaming. Dry and pound them into powder. Take 0.3 g each time, three times a day, indicated for hematochezia due to hemorrhoid and chronic enteritis.

鸡肠1尺许，内装蜈蚣1条，取装有蜈蚣的鸡肠50根，蒸熟，干后研细粉，每次服0.3克，每日服3次。治痔便血、慢性肠炎等。

Jiedu Xiyao　解毒洗药(64)　　102,332

Ingredients:

Herba Taraxaii	30 g	公英(*Gongying*)
Radix Sophorae Flavescentis	12 g	苦参(*Kushen*)
Cortex Phellodendri	12 g	黄柏(*Huangbai*)
Momordica Cochinchinensis	12 g	木鳖子(*Mubiezi*)
Flos Lonicerae	12 g	双花(*Shuanghua*)
Fructus Forsythiae	12 g	连翘(*Lianqiao*)
Radix Angelicae Dahuricae	12 g	白芷(*Baizhi*)
Radix Paeoniae Rubra	9 g	赤芍(*Chishao*)
Cortex Moutan Radicis	9 g	丹皮(*Danpi*)
Radix Glycyrrhizae(raw)	9 g	生甘草(*Shenggancao*)

Administration:　A decoction is made for bath.

Indication:　Clearing away toxic heat, promoting blood circulation and subducing swelling, removing the necrotic tissue and draining the pus away. It has the same action as *Fufang Jingjie Xiyao*.

用法：水煎外熏洗。

主治：具有清热解毒、活血消肿、去腐排脓作用。临床应用同复方荆芥洗药。

Jiuhua San　九华散(24)

44,55,69,73,77,88,90,143,
165,166,294,301,311,313,
316,323,324,358,372

Ingredients:
Pulvis Talci	620 g	滑石粉(*Huashifen*)
Os Draconis	120 g	龙骨(*Longgu*)
Borax	90 g	月石(*Yueshi*)
Bulbus Fritillariae Cirrhosae	18 g	川贝(*Chuanbei*)
Vermilion	18 g	银珠(*Yinzhu*)
Borneolum Syntheticum	18 g	冰片(*Bingpian*)

In an alternate prescription, Borneolum Syntheticum and Vermilion are replaced by Cinnabaris.

Administration: The above are pounded into powder for use.

一方银珠为朱砂，无冰片。

制法：上药共研细粉，装瓶备用。

Jiuhua San　九华散(24)

Ingredients:
Pulvis Talci	15 g	滑石粉(*Huashifen*)
Os Draconis	15 g	龙骨(*Longgu*)
Borax	9 g	月石(*Yueshi*)
Bulbus Fritillariae Thunbergii	9 g	浙贝(*Zhebei*)

Borneolum Syntheticum 3 g 冰片(Bingpian)
Cinnataris 3 g 朱砂(Zhusha)
Moschus 麝香(Shexiang)

Administration: Same as the above.
制用法同上。

Jiuhua Gao 九华膏(24)

Ingredients: Compound *Jiuhua San* and vaseline to form a 30% ointment.

Indication: Hemorrhoids.

用九华散以凡士林配成 30%油膏。适用于痔疮换药。

Kuzhi Ding 枯痔丁(21) 15,72,275,313

Ingredients:
Compound of Arsenium 8 g 砒矾化合物(Pifanhuahewu)
Trioxidum and Alumen (the proportion is 1∶2)
Glutious rice flour 16 g 糯米粉(Nuomifen)
Cinnabaris 2 g 朱砂(Zhusha)
Realgar 4 g 雄黄(Xionghuang)
Commiphora Myrrha 1 g 没药(Moyao)

Administration: Mix Arsenicum Trioxidum with Alumen and pound them into powder. Calcine the compound for 2 or 3 hours. Don't stop calcining until the white smoke replaces the black smoke. When it is cooled, the compound is mixed with Cinnabaris, Realgar and Commiphora Myrrha, and all of them are pounded into powder. Glutinous rice flour is added and boil them to paste. Medicated nails as long as 2 to 3 cm are made. Dry them at a cool place for use.

Indication: Internal hemorrhoids.

制用法：先将白砒、明矾2药研碎混合，盛于瓦罐内，放火上烧炼，经2～3小时，至黑烟消失出现白烟时，即停止烧炼，凉后取出白色砒矾化合物。将此药8克，加朱砂2克，雄黄4克，没药1克，共研细粉，后加糯米粉16克，用水煮成稠糊，搓制药丁，长约2～3 cm，阴干备用。

主治：用于内痔插药。

Kuzhi San　枯痔散(20)　　　　　　　　　　　15,275

Ingredients:

Alumen	90 g	明矾(Mingfan)
Chalcanthitum	15 g	胆矾(Danfan)
Melanterite	9 g	皂矾(Zaofan)

Administration: The above are pounded into powder, and paste is made for external application to the hemorrhoid surface. The healthy tissues around the hemorrhoids should be covered with a piece of vaseline gauze.

Indication: Withering the hemorrhoids, indicated for prolapsed and incarcerated internal hemorrhoids.

制用法：上药分别研细粉调匀即可。外敷痔面，周围健康组织以凡士林纱布保护。

作用：枯脱痔组织。适用于内痔脱垂嵌顿。

Liangxue Dihuang Tang (from Piwei Lun—The Treatise on Stomach and Spleen)　凉血地黄汤(40)　67,310

Ingredients:

Cortex Phellodendri	6 g	黄柏(Huangbai)
Rhizoma Anemarrhenae	6 g	知母(Zhimu)
Pericarpium Citri Reticulatae Viride	3 g	青皮(Qingpi)
Fructus Sophorae	3 g	槐子(Huaizi)

Radix Rehmanniae Praeparata 15 g 熟地黄(Shudihuang)
Radix Angelicae Sinensis 15 g 当归(Danggui)
Administration: A decoction is made and taken.
Indication: Severe hematochezia, hemorrhoid and fistula.
用法: 水煎服。
主治: 肠澼痔瘘病甚者。

Liangxue Dihuang Tang (from *Wai Ke Zheng Zong*—The Orthodox Manual of External Diseases) 凉血地黄汤《外科正宗》(40)

Ingredients:
Rhizoma Ligustici Chuanxiong 3 g 川芎(Chuanxiong)
Radix Angelicae Sinensis 3 g 当归(Danggui)
Radix Paeoniae Alba 3 g 白芍(Baishao)
Radix Rehmanniae 3 g 生地(Shengdi)
Rhizoma Atractylodis Macrocephalae 3 g 白术(Baizhu)
Poria 3 g 茯苓(Fuling)
Rhizoma Coptidis 1.5 g 黄连(Huanglian)
Radix Sanguisorbae 1.5 g 地榆(Diyu)
Radix Ginseng 1.5 g 人参(Renshen)
Fructus Gardeniae 1.5 g 山栀(Shanzhi)
Radix Trichosanthis 1.5 g 花粉(Huafen)
Radix Glycyrrhizae 1.5 g 甘草(Gancao)
Administration: A decoction is made and taken.
Indication: Perianal abscess, anal pain, hematochezia, dizziness, and weakness of the low back and legs.
用法: 水煎服。

主治：脏毒，肛门疼痛，大便坠重便血，头晕、眼花、腰膝无力者。

Liangxue Dihuang Tang(from *Wai Ke Da Cheng*— A Complete Book of External Diseases) 凉血地黄汤《外科大成》(40)

Ingredients:

Radix Rehmanniae	15 g	生地(*Shengdi*)
Fructus Sophorae	10 g	槐角(*Huaijiao*)
Radix Sanguisorbae	10 g	地榆(*Diyu*)
Radix Angelicae Sinensis	10 g	当归(*Danggui*)
Radix Paeoniae Rubra	10 g	赤芍(*Chishao*)
Fructus Aurantii	10 g	枳壳(*Zhiqiao*)
Radix Trichosanthis	10 g	花粉(*Huafen*)
Radix Scutellariae	10 g	黄芩(*Huangqin*)
Herba Schizonepetae	6 g	荆芥(*Jinjie*)
Rhizoma Coptidis	6 g	黄连(*Huanglian*)
Radix Glycyrrhizae	6 g	甘草(*Gancao*)
Rhizoma Cimicifugae	3 g	升麻(*Shengma*)

Administration: A decoction is made and taken.

Indication: Clearing away heat and cooling blood, indicated for internal hemorrhoids with massive bleeding.

用法：水煎服。

主治：能清热凉血，治血箭痔。

Maoyan Caogao 猫眼草膏(27)   45,59,294,304

Ingredients and administration: Liquid extract is made from Herba Euphorbiae Lunulatae and then concentrated into jelly. A piece of gauze covered with the jelly is used to be filled in the wound and sinus, or apply it directly to the wound.

Indication: Removing the necrotic tissues and promoting granulation, indicated for tuberculous anal fistula on dressing change. General inflammatory anal fistula can be covered with the drug, when much exudate comes out of the infected wound. When new tissues grow, it may cause pain owing to its irritative action.

组成制用法：取洁净猫眼草熬汁，滤过浓缩至成流膏时为止。以流膏纱布条敷盖创面或填塞创口及窦道。亦可直接涂布。

主治：祛腐生肌。适于结核性肛瘘换药。一般炎性肛瘘如创面组织腐败重分泌物多时，亦可应用。此药刺激性大，用后尤其创面转新时，可引起疼痛。

Maren Wan 麻仁丸(70)   142,357

Ingredients:
Fructus Cannabis	60 g	麻子仁(*Maziren*)
Radix et Rhizoma Rhei	60 g	大黄(*Daihuang*)
Semen Pruni Armeniacae	30 g	杏仁(*Xingren*)
Cortex Magnoliae Officinalis	30 g	枳实(*Zhishi*)
Fructus Aurantii Immaturus	30 g	厚朴(*Houpu*)
Radix Paeoniae Alba	30 g	芍药(*Shaoyao*)

Administration: The above are pounded into powder and pills as big as the fruit of Chinese parasol tree made with honey. Take 10 pills (equal to 3 g) each time and 3 times a day.

Indication: Constipation due to intense heat in the intestines. It should be careful to give for constipation in the deficiency syndrome.

制用法：上药为细末，炼蜜为丸，如梧子大。每服10丸(3克)，日服3次。

主治：肠热便秘。虚证便秘慎用。

Maren Zipi Wan 麻仁滋脾丸(71)   142,357

Ingredients:

Fructus Cannabis	240 g	媡仁(*Huomaren*)
Radix Angelicae Sinensis	240 g	当归(*Danggui*)
Radix et Rhizoma Rhei (praeparata)	500 g	熟军(*Shujun*)
Fructus Aurantii	120 g	枳实(*Zhishi*)
Cortex Magnolicae Officinalis	120 g	厚朴(*Houpu*)
Semen Pruni Armeniacae	120 g	郁李仁(*Yuliren*)
Semen Pruni	120 g	杏仁(*Xingren*)
Radix Paeoniae Alba	90 g	白芍(*Baishao*)

Administration: The above are pounded into powder and boluses are made with honey. Every bolus weighs 9 g. Take one bolus a day.

Indication: Constipation due to intense heat in the intestines. It should be careful to give for constipation in the deficiency syndrome. It is contraindicated for pregnant women.

制用法：上药为细末，炼蜜为丸，每丸9克。每次服1丸，日服1次。

主治：肠热便秘。虚证便秘慎用，孕妇忌服。

Meilan Changxiao Zhitong Ji 美兰长效止痛剂(30)

46,296

Ingredients:

Methylene Blue	0.2 g	亚甲兰(*Yajialan*)
Novocaine	2 g	普鲁卡因(*Pulukayin*)

Distilled water for injection   100 ml   注射用水 (Zhushe Yongshui)

Administration: The above are made into sterilized injection, or mix Methylene Blue, Novocaine(2%), Lidocaine(2%) and Bupivacaine(0.25%) to make an analgesic agent.

Indication: Healing wound, discarding pain after surgery or used in the block therapy for anal fissure.

制用法：上药溶解过滤，分装安瓿，高压灭菌备用。也可用市售美兰液与2%普鲁卡因、2%利多卡因、0.25%布比卡因配成适当浓度的美兰止痛剂。

主治：适用于创口封闭，术后止痛和肛裂封闭治疗等。

Mingfan Ye 明矾液(37)   55,301

Ingredients and administration: 0.5%—3% suspension is made from Alumen for enema. The dosage is applied according to the condition.

Indication: Stopping bleeding, especially for hematochezia due to internal hemorrhoids and post-operative hemorrhage.

制用法：取一般明矾适量，用普通水配成0.5~3%混悬液，灌肠用。用量多少视病情而定。

主治：止血。用于内痔便血及痔瘘术后续发性出血。

Neizhi Kutuo You 内痔枯脱油(57)   78,316

Ingredients:

Table salt   8 g   食盐(Shiyan)
Glycerin   100 ml   甘油(Ganyou)
Carbolic Acid   2 ml   石碳酸(Shitansuan)

Administration: Put table salt in Glycerin and dissolve it by heating. Mix the solution with Carbolic Acid, and sterilize it by high pressure. It is used for the internal hemorrhoid injection to wither it.

制用法：食盐入甘油内加热溶解，与石炭酸混合，高压灭菌备用。适用于内痔注射，使痔核估死。

Niuhuang San 牛黄散(73)

Ingredients:

Calculus Bovis	0.3 g	牛黄(*Niuhuang*)
Margarita	0.3 g	珍珠(*Zhenzhu*)
Morneolum Syntheticum	0.3 g	冰片(*Bingpian*)
Moschus	0.3 g	麝香(*Shexiang*)
Concha Haliotidis	3 g	石决明(*Shijueming*)
Resina Boswelliae Carterii	3 g	乳香(*Ruxiang*)
Myrrha	3 g	没药(*Moyao*)
Os Draconis	3 g	龙骨(*Longgu*)
Concha Ostreae	3 g	牡蛎(*Muli*)
Fel Ursi	1.5 g	熊胆(*Xiongdan*)
Calomelas	1.5 g	轻粉(*Qingfen*)
Rhizoma Coptidis	9 g	黄连(*Huanglian*)

Administration: First, roast Resina Boswelliae Carterii and Myrrha to remove their oil, then pound the fifth, the eighth, the ninth and the twelfth ingredients into powder. Finally, put the first, second, third, fourth, tenth and eleventh ingredients to the mixture. Pound them into powder, which is placed in a bottle. Spray it to the wound or fill the wound or sinus with it.

Indication: Diminishing inflammation and promoting granulation, indicated for dressing change after anal surgical operation.

制用法：先将乳香、没药炒去油，同石决明、龙骨、牡蛎、黄连共研细末，再将熊胆、轻粉、牛黄、珍珠、冰片、麝香加入，研为极细末，装瓶密闭备用。以喷药器向创口喷撒药粉适量，或蘸药粉填塞创口和窦道。

主治：能消炎、生肌，肛门术后换药用。

Qingge San 青蛤散(39)   59,304

Ingredients:

Cyclina Sinensis(forged)	15 g	煅青蛤(*Duanqingge*)
Gypsum Fibrosum(forged)	15 g	煅石膏(*Duanshigao*)
Calomelas	9 g	轻粉(*Qingfen*)
Cortex Phellodendri	9 g	黄柏(*Huangbai*)
Indigo Naturalis	4.5 g	青黛(*Qingdai*)

Administration: The above are pounded into powder and put into a bottle for use. A wet lesion is covered with the powder, but a dry lesion is covered with the drug mixed in sesame oil.

Indication: Clearing away damp-heat and alleviating itching, indicated for eczema of anus.

制用法：上药共为细粉，装瓶备用。患处湿者则干擦，干者可用香油调涂。

主治：祛湿止痒，肛门湿疹可用。

Qinjiu Baizhu Wan 秦艽白术丸(14)   14,68,275,310

Ingredients:

Radix Gentianae Macrophyllae	30 g	秦艽(*Qinjiu*)
Semen Persicae	30 g	桃仁(*Taoren*)
Fructus Gleditsiae(burnt with the original property retained)	30 g	皂角仁(*Zaojiaoren*)
Tip of Angelicae Sinensis	15 g	当归梢(*Dangguishao*)

Rhizoma Alismatis	15 g	泽泻(Zexie)
Fructus Aurantii Immaturus	15 g	枳实(Zhishi)
Rhizoma Atractylodis Macrocephalae	15 g	白术(Baizhu)
Radix Sanguisorbae	9 g	地榆(Diyu)

Administration: Pills are made and take 50-70 pills each time with water before meals.

制用法：上药制丸如鸡头仁大，每服50～70丸，白汤下，空腹服。

Qinjiu Cangzhu Tang 秦艽苍术汤(7) 13,67,182
274,310,382

Ingredients:

Radix Gentianae Macrophyllae	3 g	秦艽(Qinjiu)
Semen Persicae	3 g	桃仁(Taoren)
Fructus Gleditsiae(burn it with the original property retained and pound it into powder)	3 g	皂角仁(Zaojiaoren)
Rhizoma Atractylodis	2 g	苍术(Cangzhu)
Radix Ledebouriellae	2 g	防风(Fangfeng)
Cortex Phellodendri	1.5 g	黄柏(Huangbai)
Tip of Angelicae Sinensis	1 g	当归梢(Dangguishao)
Rhizoma Alismatis	1 g	泽泻(Zexie)
Semen Arecae	0.5 g	槟榔(Binglang)
Radix et Rhizoma Rhei(small amount)		大黄(Daihuang)

If there is pus on the lesion, five Flos Althaeae Roseaes (without calyx), Pericarpium Citri Reticulatae Viride(1.5 g) and Radix Aucklandiae(1 g) should be added.

Administration: A decoction is made and taken.

Indication: Clearing away damp-heat and eliminating the swelling, indicated for swollen fistula, bearing-down pain and chronic enteritis.

用法：水煎服。

主治：能祛湿热，消肿坠。适用于痔瘘肿痛、下坠不适，慢性肠炎等。

Qinjiu Danggui Tang 秦艽当归汤(17)   14,275

Ingredients:

Radix Gentianae Macrophyllae	秦艽(*Qinjiu*)
Radix et Rhizoma Rhei	大黄(*Dahuang*)
Fructus Aurantii Immaturus	枳实(*Zhishi*)
Rhizoma Alismatis	泽泻(*Zexie*)
Radix Angelicae Sinensis	当归(*Danggui*)
Fructus Gleditsiae	皂角仁(*Zaojiaoren*)
Rhizoma Atractylodis Macrocephalae	白术(*Baizhu*)
Flos Carthami	红花(*Honghua*)
Semen Persicae	桃仁(*Taoren*)

Administration A decoction is made and taken.

水煎服。

Qinjiu Fangfeng Tang 秦艽防风汤(15)   14,275

Ingredients:

Radix Gentianae Macrophyllae	4.5 g	秦艽(*Qinjiu*)
Radix Ledebouriellae	4.5 g	防风(*Fangfeng*)
Radix Angelicae Sinensis	4.5 g	当归(*Danggui*)
Rhizoma Atractylodis Macrocephalae	4.5 g	白术(*Baizhu*)

Radix Glycyrrhizae(roasted with honey)	1.8 g	炙甘草(Zhigancao)
Rhizoma Alismatis	1.8 g	泽泻(Zexie)
Cortex Phellodendri	1.5 g	黄柏(Huangbai)
Radix et Rhizoma Rhei	0.9 g	大黄(Daihuang)
Coxtex Cinnamomi	0.9 g	桂皮(Guipi)
Radix Bupleuri	0.6 g	柴胡(Chaihu)
Rhizoma Cimicifugae	0.6 g	升麻(Shengma)
Semen Persicae	30 g	桃仁(Taoren)
Flos Carthami(small amount)		红花(Honghua)

Administration: A decoction is made and taken. 水煎服。

Qinjiu Qianghuo Tang 秦艽羌活汤(16)　　14,275

Ingredients:

Radix Gentianae Macrophyllae	3.6 g	秦艽(Qinjiu)
Rhizoma seu Radix Notopterygii	3.6 g	羌活(Qianghuo)
Radix Astragali seu Hedysari	3 g	黄芪(Huangqi)
Radix Ledebouriellae	2.1 g	防风(Fangfeng)
Rhizoma Cimicifugae	1.5 g	升麻(Shengma)
Radix Glycyrrhizae (fried with honey)	1.5 g	炙甘草(Zhigancao)
Herba Ephedrae	1.5 g	麻黄(Mahuang)
Radix Bupleuri	1.5 g	柴胡(Chaihu)
Rhizoma Ligustici	0.9 g	藁本(Gaoben)
Herba Asari(small amount)		细辛(Xixin)
Flos Carthami(small amount)		红花(Honghua)

Administration: A decoction is made and taken.

水煎服。

Qinjiu Wan 秦艽丸(32)   48,68,297,310

Ingredients:
Flos Lonicerae	150 g	金银花(Jinyinhua)
Radix Gentianae Macrophyllae	90 g	秦艽(Qinjiu)
Radix Ledebouriellae	90 g	防风(Fangfeng)
Rhizoma Cimicifugae	60 g	升麻(Shengma)
Rhizoma Atractylodis	90 g	苍术(Cangzhu)
Rhizoma Alismatis	90 g	泽泻(Zexie)
Radix Angelicae Sinensis	90 g	当归(Danggui)
Cortex Phellodendri	30 g	黄柏(Huangbai)
Radix Glycyrrihizae	30 g	甘草(Gancao)

Administration: The above are pounded into powder, and pills made with water. Take 10 pills each time and 2 to 3 times a day.

Indication: Clearing away damp-heat and subduing the swelling, indicated for swollen anus and a bearing-down sensation.

制用法：共为细末，水丸，如梧桐子大。每次服10克，每日服2～3次。

主治：祛湿热、消肿坠。适用于肛门肿痛、下坠不适等。

Quedu Tang 却毒汤(51)   69,311

Ingredients:
Mirabilitum	30 g	焰硝(Yanxiao)
Herba Orostachyos	15 g	瓦松(Wasong)
Herba Portulacae	15 g	马齿苋(Machixian)

Radix Glycyrrhizae(raw)	15 g	生甘草(Shenggancao)
Galla Chinensis	9 g	五倍子(Wubeizi)
Pericarpium Zanthoxyli	9 g	川椒(Chuanjiao)
Radix Ledebouriellae	9 g	防风(Fangfeng)
Cacumen Biotae	9 g	侧柏叶(Cebaiye)
Fructus Aurantii	9 g	枳壳(Zhiqiao)
Caulis Allii Fistulosi	9 g	葱白(Congbai)
Rhizoma Atractylodis	9 g	苍术(Cangzhu)

Mirabilitum may be replaced by mirabilite.

Administration: A decoction is made and while hot it is used for steam-bath and medicated bath, once or twice a day.

Indication: Swelling and pain of hemorrhoid and fistula due to an acute attack and inflammation.

焰硝可以朴硝代土。

用法：煎汤乘热熏洗坐浴，每日 1～2 次

主治：适用于痔瘘肿痛急性炎症发作。

Runchang Pian 润肠片(72)   142,357

Ingredients:

Pig's gallbladder(fresh)	30	鲜猪胆(Xianzhudan)
Radix et Rhizoma Rhei (powder)	1000 g	生大黄粉(Shengdaihuangfen)

Administration: The above are pounded into powder and tablets made. Every tablet weighs 0.3—0.5 g. Take 2 tablets each time, twice or three times a day before meals.

Indication: Diarrhea and constipation.

制用法：共研匀制成片剂，每片 0.3—0.5 克。每次 2 片，每日服 2—3 次，饭前服。

主治：缓泻，适用于一般性便秘。

Runchang Wan 润肠丸(69) 142,357

Ingredients:

Radix et Rhizoma Rhei	15 g	大黄(*Daihuang*)
Radix Angelicae Sinensis(end)	15 g	归尾(*Guiwei*)
Rhizoma seu Radix Notopterygii	15 g	羌活(*Qianghuo*)
Semen Persicae	30 g	桃仁(*Taoren*)
Fructus Cannabis	30 g	麻仁(*Maren*)

Administration: All the ingredients except the last one as big as the fruit of Chinese paraol free which is pounded into paste, are pounded into powder and pills made with honey. Take 50 pills each time with water before meals.

Indication: Constipation.

制用法：上药除麻仁另研如泥外，捣细炼蜜为丸，如梧桐子大。每服50丸，空腹服，白汤送下。

主治：大便秘涩。

Sanhuang Tang 三黄汤(60) 102,332

Ingredients:

Radix et Rhizoma Rhei	9 g	大黄(*Daihuang*)
Radix Scutellariae	6 g	黄芩(*Huangqin*)
Rhizoma Coptidis	6 g	黄连(*Huanglian*)

Administration: A decoction is made and taken at a draft.

Indication: Clearing away heat, toxic substances and dampness, indicated for perianal abscess or an acute attack of anal fistula.

用法：水煎顿服。

主治：能清热解毒利湿，适用于肛周脓肿或肛瘘急性发作。

Sanmiao San (Wan)　三妙散(丸)(61)　　　102,322

Ingredients:

Rhizoma Atractylodis		苍术(*Cangzhu*)
(Steeped in the rice-washed water) 180 g		
Cortex Phellodendri		
(roasted with alcohol)	120 g	黄柏(*Huangbai*)
Radix Achyranthis Bidentatae	60 g	牛膝(*Niuxi*)

Administration: The above are pounded into powder and pills as big as the fruit of Chinese parasol tree made. Take 9 g each time with light salty water, twice or three times a day.

Indication: Clearing away heat and dampness, indicated for anal pain or an attack of fistula due to downward pouring of damp-heat.

制用法：共为细末，水丸如梧桐子大，每次服9克，淡盐汤送下，每日服2—3次。

主治：能清热利湿，治湿热下注，肛痛或肛瘘发作。

Sanpin Yitiaoqiang　三品一条枪(22)　　　15,275

Ingredients:

Alumen	60 g	明矾(*Mingfan*)
Arsenicum Trioxidum	45 g	白砒(*Baipi*)
Realger	7.2 g	雄黄(*Xionghuang*)
Resina Boswelliae Carterit	5.6 g	乳香(*Ruxiang*)

Administration: Alumen and Arsenicum Trioxidum are pounded into powder, put them in a pot and calcine them until white smoke appears. When it is cooled, 30 grams of the compound are got. Add Realger and Resina Boswelliao Carterit to the compound, and pound them into powder, and paste is made, and it is prepared into thin sticks. Put them at a cool place for use.

Indication: Internal hemorrhoid and anal fistula.

制用法：将砒矾2味共为细末，入小罐内，加炭火煅红，青烟已尽，即起白烟，片刻小罐上下红彻，住火取罐放置一夜，将药取出，约得净药30克，再加雄黄、乳香研细粉，调稠糊，搓细条，阴干备用。用时插入患处。

主治：用于内痔、肛瘘插药。

Shengfu Tang 生肤汤(29) 45,59,295,304

Ingredients:

Caulis Lonicerae	30 g	忍冬藤(*Rendongteng*)
Radix Astragali seu Hedysari(raw)	15 g	生黄芪(*Shenghuangqi*)
Rhizoma Dioscoreae	15 g	山药(*Shanyao*)
Radix Ophiopogonis	15 g	麦冬(*Maidong*)
Radix Codonopsis Pilosulae	12 g	党参(*Dangshen*)
Rhizoma Atractylodis Macrocephalae	12 g	白术(*Baizhu*)
Poria	12 g	云苓(*Yunling*)
Radix Rehmanniae	12 g	生地(*Shengdi*)
Radix Rehmanniae Praeparata	12 g	熟地(*Shudi*)
Radix Paeoniae Alba	12 g	杭芍(*Hangshao*)
Radix Angelicae Sinensis	12 g	当归(*Danggui*)

Administration: A dedcoction is made and taken.

Indication: Invigorating *Qi*, nourishing blood and *Yin* to promote production of body fluid, indicated for delayed healing of wound.

用法：水煎服。

主治：能补气养血、滋阴生津。适于创口愈合迟缓者。

Shengji Yuhong Gao　生肌玉红膏(25)　　44,55,143
　　　　　　　　　　　　　　　　　　　　　294,301,358

Ingredients:

Radix Angelicae Sinensis	60 g	当归(Danggui)
Cera Chinensis	60 g	白蜡(Baila)
Radix Glycyrrhizae	36 g	甘草(Gancao)
Radix Angelicae Dahuricae	15 g	白芷(Baizhi)
Calomelas	12 g	轻粉(Qingfen)
Resina Draconis	120 g	血竭(Xuejie)
Radix Arnebiae seu Lithospermi	6 g	紫草(Zicao)
Sesame oil	500 ml	香油(Xiangyiu)

Administration: Put Radix Angelicae Sinensis, Radix Angelicae Dahuricae, Radix Arnebiae seu Lithopermi and Radix Glyeyrrhizae in sesame oil. Fry them and discard the dross. Calomelas and Resina Draconis are ground into powder which, with Cera Chinensis, is put into the oil and mix them up. Ointmental gauze is made to be applied to the wound or to be filled in sinus of the cut.

Indication: Promoting granulation, indicated for anal fistula on dressing change.

制用法：先将当归、白芷、紫草、甘草4味入油内炸枯去渣，再将血竭、轻粉研细，同白蜡共入油内搅均即可。并制成油膏纱布备用。以油膏纱布敷盖创面或填塞刀口窦道。

主治：生肌。适于肛瘘换药。

Shiquandabu Tang　十全大补汤(28)　　45,59,68,295
　　　　　　　　　　　　　　　　　　　　　304,310

Ingredients:

Radix Astragali seu Hedysari	15 g	黄芪(*Huangqi*)
Radix Codonopsis Pilosulae	12 g	党参(*Dangshen*)
Rhizoma Atractylodis Macrocephalae(fried)	9 g	炒白术(*Chaobaizhu*)
Poria	9 g	茯苓(*Fuling*)
Radix Rehmanniae Praeparata	9 g	熟地(*Shudi*)
Radix Paeoniae Albae	9 g	白芍(*Baishao*)
Radix Angelicae Sinensis	9 g	当归(*Danggui*)
Rhizoma Ligustici Chuanxiong	6 g	川芎(*Chuanxiong*)
Radix Glycyrrhizae	6 g	甘草(*Gancao*)
Cortex Cinnamomi	3 g	肉桂(*Rougui*)

Administration: Decoction is made and taken.

Indication: For patients with hemorrhoids or fistula of the deficiency symdrome, or delayed healing of wounds after surgery.

用法：水煎服。

主治：痔瘘虚证患者或术后创口愈合迟缓者。

Shoukou San 收口散(75) 143,358

Ingredients:

Gypsum Fibrosum(forged)	30 g	煅石膏(*Duanshigao*)
Rubber(forged)	15 g	煅橡皮(*Duanxiangpi*)
Os Draconis(forged)	3 g	煅龙骨(*Duanlonggu*)
Calomelas	1.5 g	轻粉(*Qingfen*)
Borneolum Syntheticum	0.9 g	冰片(*Bingpian*)
Margarita(forged)	0.6 g	煅珍珠(*Duanzhenzhu*)

Administration: The above are pounded into powder and stored in a bottle. Its administration is the same as *Niuhuang San*(73).

Indication: Promoting granulation and healing the wound.

制用法：上药共为极细末，装瓶备用。用法同牛黄散(73)。
主治：能生肌收口。

Siwu Tang 四物汤(3) 12,274

Ingredients:

Radix Rehmanniae Praeparata	9 g	熟地(*Shudi*)
Radix Angelicae Sinensis	9 g	当归(*Danggui*)
Radix Paeoniae Alba	9 g	白芍(*Baishao*)
Rhizoma Ligustici Chuanxiong	4.5 g	川芎(*Chuanxiong*)

Administration: Nourishing blood and increasing volume of blood for hematochezia caused by insufficiency of blood.

用法：水煎服。
主治：有养血补血之功，用于血虚便血。

Suanxiao Huji 蒜硝糊剂(65) 102,332

Ingredients:

Bulbus Allii(fresh better)	3 portions	大蒜(*Dasuan*)
Mirabilite	1 portion	芒硝(*Mangxiao*)

Administration: The above are pounded into thick paste. Thickness is believed to be suitable when there appears something like thread during raising the paste. Too much Bulbus Allii makes thin paste while too much Mirabilite makes thick paste. Apply the paste to the affected part of an adult, lasting for 1–2 hours. In children, half an hour's application is enough. Then remove the paste and red color is seen on the place where the paste was applied, which makes it easy for yellow vinegar paste to penetrate to the deep layers.

Indication: Abscess and inflammation, or deeper abscess.

制用法：将蒜硝共捣如泥，即成稠糊，用物将稠糊挑起，出现拔丝现象则稠稀适宜。蒜多则成稀糊，芒硝多则呈膏状。如大蒜存放时间较久水份较少时，在捣蒜硝时可加水适量，使成稠糊。用时如患处皮肤较脏，可先用盐水擦拭，然后将此糊涂于患处，一般成人涂药可持续1～2小时，小儿因皮肤细嫩可涂半小时。后将药糊去掉，因药物作用可使皮肤潮红，便于黄醋糊剂向组织深部渗透。

主治：脓肿炎块等，深部脓肿亦可用。

Tongpao Tang　通脬汤(35)　　　　　　　　　　50,298

Ingredients:

Cortex Cinnamomi	4.5 g	官桂(*Guangui*)
Radix Astragali seu Hedysari	15 g	黄芪(*Huangqi*)
Radix et Rhizoma Rhei	15 g	生军(*Shengjun*)
Poria	10 g	茯苓(*Fuling*)
Resina Boswelliae Carterii	10 g	乳香(*Ruxiang*)
Commiphore Myrrha	10 g	没药(*Moyao*)
Caulis Akebiae	10 g	木通(*Mutong*)
Radix Angelicae Dahuricae	10 g	白芷(*Baizhi*)
Rhizoma Alismatis	10 g	泽泻(*Zexie*)
Semen Plantaginis	10 g	车前子(*Cheqianzi*)
Cortex Phellodendri	10 g	黄柏(*Huangbai*)
Radix Achyranthis Bidentatae	5 g	牛膝(*Niuxi*)

Administration: (1) For oral medication: A decoction is made and taken, twice a day, in the morning and evening; (2) Hot compress: Roast the drugs of the decoction with some ginger, scallion and vinegar, or a little bran. Put them into a cloth pocket and apply it to the lower abdomen; (3)Enema: The above ingredients are decocted and concentrated to 50 ml. Put 50 ml. liquid paraffin in it for enema.

Indication: Dysuria.

用法: (1)内服法: 水煎服, 每日 1 剂, 早晚各服 1 次。(2)熨炙法: 将第 2 煎的药渣加生姜、葱、醋适量, 也可加入少量麦麸, 同入锅中炒热, 用布袋装好, 熨小服。(3)灌肠法: 本方加水浓煎 50 毫升再加入液状石蜡 50 毫升灌肠。

主治: 小便不利。

Wuling San 五苓散(33)　　　　　　　　　　50,298

Ingredients:

Poria	9 g	茯苓(*Fuling*)
Polyporus Umbellatus	9 g	猪苓(*Zhuling*)
Rhizoma Atractylodis Macrocephalae	9 g	白术(*Baizhu*)
Rhizoma Alismatis	12 g	泽泻(*Zexie*)
Ramulus Cinnamomi	3 g	桂枝(*Guizhi*)

Administration: A decoction is made and taken.

Indication: Dysuria.

用法: 水煎服。

主治: 小便不利。

Xiangya Huaguan Wan 象牙化管丸(5)　　　12,120, 274,344

Ingredients:

Ivory	60 g	真象牙(*Zhenxiangya*)
Rhizoma Picrorhizae	60 g	胡黄连(*Huhuanglian*)
Fructus Sophorae	60 g	槐实(*Huaishi*)
Rhizoma Coptidis	30 g	川黄连(*Chuanhuanglian*)
Radix Angelicae Sinensis	30 g	当归(*Danggui*)

Poria	30 g	白茯苓(*Baifuling*)
Radix Sanguisorbae(burned)	30 g	蕉地榆(*Jiaodiyu*)
Corium Erinacei	30 g	刺猬皮(*Ciweipi*)
Radix Scutellariae	15 g	黄芩(*Huangqin*)
Resina Boswelliae Carterii	12 g	乳香珠(*Ruxiangzhu*)

Administration: The above are pounded into powder and pills as big as the fruit of Chinese parasol tree are made, 30 to 40 pills are taken each time with warm boiled water before meals and take it once or twice a day.

Indication: Treating all kinds of anal fistula, such as gangrenous fistula, honey comb fistula, multiple anal fistula and carbuncle of the buttocks. Patients who are not fit for surgery are advised to take 1-2 packages of pills to cure the fistula or alliviate the suffering. When taking the pills, one should abstain from chilli, alcohol, beef and mutton.

制用法： 上药共为细末，蜜为丸，如梧桐子大。每服30～40丸，饭前开水送下。每日服1～2次。

主治： 肛门部一切瘘疮如通脊瘘、坏疽瘘、蜂窝瘘、穿臀瘘、臀痈等，凡不适宜割治者，宜服此药1～2料，多能治愈或减轻疮势与痛苦。服药期间忌食辣椒、酒、牛羊肉等。

Xiaohuashi Wan 小槐实丸(9) 13,274

Ingredients:

Fructus Sophprae	1500 g	槐子(*Huaizi*)
White sugar	1000 g	白糖(*Baitang*)
Alumen	500 g	矾石(*Fanshi*)
Sulphur	500 g	硫黄(*Liuhuang*)
Radix et Rhizoma Rhei	300 g	大黄(*Daihuang*)
Lacquer(dried)	300 g	干漆(*Ganqi*)

Os Draconis 300 g 龙骨(Longgu)

Administration: The above are pounded into powder and pills as big as the fruit of Chinese parasol free made. Take 20 pills each time with alcohol, three times a day. Then the dosage increases to 30 pills each time.

Indication: Hemorrhoids.

制用法：上 7 味如法制丸如梧子，酒服 20 丸，每日服 3 次，稍增至 30 丸。

主治：适用于痔。

Xiaoyan zhitong San 消炎止痛散(53) 73,313

Ingredients:
Calamina(forged)	15 g	煅甘石(Duanganshi)
Pulvis Talci	15 g	滑石粉(Huashifen)
Pb_3O_4	6 g	章丹(Zhangdan)
Resina Draconis	3 g	血竭(Xuejie)
Acacia Catechu	3 g	儿茶(Ercha)
Cinnabaris	3 g	朱砂(Zhusha)
Resina Boswelliae Carterii	1.5 g	乳香(Ruxiang)
Borneolum Syntheticum	0.9 g	冰片(Bingpian)

Administration: The above are pounded into powder and put into a bottle for use.

Indication: Diminishing inflammation and pain, promoting granulation.

制用法：上药共研细粉装瓶备用。

作用：消炎止痛生肌。

Xiaozhiling Injection 消痔灵注射液(55)   75,314

Ingredients:

Tannic Acid	0.15 g	柔酸(*Rousuan*)
Potassium Aluminum Sulfate	4 g	硫酸钾铝(*Liusuanjialu*)
Sodium Citrate	1.5 g	枸橼酸钠(*Juyuansuanna*)
Low Molecular Dextran	10 ml	右旋糖酐(*Yiuxuantanggan*)
Glycerin	10 ml	甘油(*Ganyiu*)
Chlorbutanol	0.5 g	三氯叔丁醇(*Sanlushudingchun*)
Distilled water(to reach 100 ml)		蒸馏水(*Zhengliushui*)

Administration: (1)Dissolve Sodium Citrate in 50 ml warm distilled water; (2) Add Potassium Aluminum Sulfate to it, and dissolve it in the above solution by stirring. Tannic Acid and Chlorbutanol are put in the Glycerin and melted by heating them on water bath. Mix the first and second solutions, with low Molecular Dextran and add distilled water up to 100 ml. A No. 4 sintered glass funnel is used to filter the final solution and put it in 10 ml ampoules, boil it for 30 minutes for sterilization. It is used for injection to internal hemorrhoid to make it wither.

制用法：将枸橼酸钠溶于50 ml温蒸馏水中，加入硫酸钾铝搅拌溶解。另加柔酸、三氯叔丁醇溶解于甘油中，溶时可水浴上加热。将两者混合加低分子右旋糖酐，再加蒸馏水至足量。用4号垂溶漏斗过滤后封装10 ml安瓿，煮沸灭菌30分钟。适用于内痔注射，使痔核萎缩消失。

Xiaozhi Pian 消痔片(47)   68,310

Ingredients:

Radix Rehmannia	150 g	生地(*Shengdi*)

Fructus Sophorae	120 g	槐角(Huaijiao)
Flos Sophorae Immaturus	120 g	槐米(Huaimi)
Fructus Meliae Toosendan	90 g	川连(Chuanlian)
Radix Angelicae Sinensis	90 g	当归(Danggui)
Radix Paeoniae Rubra	90 g	赤芍(Chishao)
Squama Manitis	90 g	山甲珠(Shanjiazhu)
Spina Gleditsiae	90 g	牙皂(Yazao)
Rhizoma Ligustici Chuanxiong	60 g	川芎(Chuanxiong)
Radix Paeoniae Alba	60 g	杭芍(Hangshao)
Alumen Exsiccatum	60 g	枯矾(Kufan)
Radix Sanguisorbae	30 g	地榆(Diyu)
Radix et Rhizoma Rhei(raw)	15 g	生大黄(Shengdaihuang)

Administration: The above are pounded into powder and 0.5 g tablets are made. Take 5-10 tablets each time, twice or three times a day.

Indication: Cooling blood and stopping bleeding, relaxing the bowels and alleviating pain, indicated for hematochezia, constipation due to internal heat (mostly in the bowel) and swelling and pain of anus.

制用法：共为细粉制成片剂，每片0.5克。每次5～10片，每日服2～3次。

主治：凉血止血、润便止痛。适用于大便下血，肠热便秘，肛门肿痛等。

Xijiao Dihuang Tang 犀角地黄汤(42) 68,310

Ingredients:

Cornu Rhinoceri	1.5 g	犀角(Xijiao)
Radix Rehmannia	30 g	生地(Shengdi)
Cortex Moutan Radicis	9 g	丹皮(Danpi)

Radix Paeoniae Alba　　　9 g　芍药(*Shaoyao*)

Administration: A decoction is made and taken.

Indication: Clearing away heat and detoxicating, indicated for hematochezia due to blood-heat, abscess of anus, an acute attack of fistula.

用法：水煎服。

主治：能清热解毒，用于血热妄行之便血，肛周脓肿和肛瘘急性发作等。

Xinliuhao Kuzhi Ye 新6号枯痔液(59)　　　78,316

Ingredients:

Calcium Chloride (for injection)	12 g	氯化钙(*Luhuagai*)
Ammonium Chloride (for medicine)	3 g	氯化铵(*Luhuaan*)
Distilled water	100 ml	注射用水(*Zhusheyongshui*)

Administration: The above are dissolved and filtered. Put them into ampoules, have flowsteam sterilization for an hour or boiling sterilization for half an hour.

Indication: Internal hemorrhoid, in order to make it wither.

制用法：上药溶解过滤，分装安瓿，流通蒸汽消毒1小时或煮沸消毒半小时备用。适用于内痔注射，可使痔核枯死。

Zanglian Wan(from *Zhengzhi Zhunsheng*— The Standards of Diagnosis and Treatment) 脏连丸(46)　　68,310

Ingredients and administration: 240 g powder of Rhizoma Coptidis is put into a section of the clean large intestine of a hog, 1.2 *Chi* in length. Tie the two ends up. Cook the section of the large intestine in a pot with 1.25 kg alcohol. When the alcohol is nearly dried, take the intestine out and smash it. Then small pills are made. 70 pills are taken each time with warm alcohol before breakfast. Or mix Rhizoma Coptidis powder with some yellow wine and put the mixture into a section of the large intestine of a hog. Tie up the two ends of it and steam it. Cut it open and dry it in the sun, then smash it into powder to make bolus with honey. Teng of the bolus is taken each time, twice or three times a day.

Indication: Hemorrhoid, hematochezia, pain and a bearing-down sensation of anus.

黄连净末240克，用公猪大肠尽头一段长1尺2寸，温汤洗净，将黄连末灌入肠内两头以线扎紧，用时将酒2斤半放砂锅内煮，酒将干为度，取起脏药共捣如泥，如药湿再晒1时许复捣丸如桐子大，每服70丸空腹温酒送下。亦可用黄酒将黄连末拌匀装入大肠内，两端扎紧，上锅蒸熟，再剖开晒干，同大肠共研细末炼蜜为丸，每服10克，日服2～3次。主治痔无论新久，便血作痛肛门坠重者。

Zanglian Wan(from *Wai Ke Qi Xuan*—The Revelations of the Mystery of External Diseases) 脏连丸《外科启玄》(46)

Ingredients and administration:

Rhizoma Coptidis	30 g	胡黄连(*Huhuanglian*)
Spica Schizonepetae	30 g	荆芥穗(*Jinjiesui*)
Radix Sanguisorbae	30 g	地榆(*Diyu*)
Flos Sophorae	45 g	槐花(*Huaihua*)
Auricularia Auricula of Pagodatree	45 g	槐树木耳(*Huaishumuer*)

The above are pounded into powder. Take a live crucian carp (weighing about 300 grams). Only the carp meat is mixed with the herb powder. Then put the mixture into a section of a pig large intestine. 1.5 *Chi* in length and steam it well. Take it in two times before breakfast. For persistent cases the mixture is dried under the sun and pills are made with honey. Take 3 grams each time with alcohol or water before breakfast.

Indication: Persistent hemorrhoid and fistula.

上药为细末用活鲫鱼1尾，重300克，去肠刺，取肉捣如泥和作团，用健猪大肠头1尺5寸，翻过去油洗净装前药扎定煮熟，空心食之，至重不过2次。如患病年久日远，以药末晒干为末，蜜丸桐子大，每服3克，空心酒下或白汤下。主治多年痔瘘。

Zangsuan Fang 脏蒜方(50) 68,310

Ingredients:

1/3 meter large intestine of a pig		猪大肠(*Zhudachang*)
Garlic clove(dozens)		蒜(*Suan*)
Refined sugar	125 g	白糖(*Baitang*)
Brown sugar	125 g	红糖(*Hongtang*)

Administration: Clean the intestine and put the garlic and sugar in it. Tie the two ends of the intestine up and cook it well. One intestine is a dose. Generally, a dose is taken a day, three doses can be taken successively or finish the doses in 2-3 days.

Indication: Hematochezia due to hemorrhoid.

制用法：将肠洗净，蒜糖装肠内，肠两端以线扎紧，煮熟，肠烂即可。一个为1剂，一般1天吃1剂，可连吃3剂，如1天未能吃1剂，可随便吃，2~3天吃完亦可。

主治：痔疮便血。

Zhining (a patent medicine)　痔宁(48)　　　68,310

Administration: Take 5 tablets each time and twice or three times a day.

每次服 5 片：每日服 2～3 次。

Zhiqiao Fugang Tang　枳壳复肛汤(76)　　164,371

Ingredients:
Fructus Aurantii(raw)　　　30 g　生枳壳(*Shengzhiqiao*)
Radix Astragali Seu Hedysari　15 g　黄芪(*Huangqi*)
Radix Codonopsis Pilosulae　15 g　党参(*Dangshen*)
Rhizoma Cimicifugae　　　10 g　升麻(*Shengma*)
Radix Glycyrrhizae(raw)　　10 g　生甘草(*Shenggancao*)

Administration: A decoction is made and taken.

Indication: Invigorating *Qi* and lifting prolapsed organs, indicated for prolapse of rectum.

用法：水煎服。

主治：能补益升提，适用于直肠脱垂。

Zhitong Rushen Tang　止痛如神汤(31)　　47,48,68,
296,297,310

Ingredients: It is pointed out in *Wai Ke Qi Xuan* (The Revelation of the Mystery of External Diseases) that *Zhitong Rushen Tang* is *Qinjiu Cangzhu Tang* with modification. Both are formed by the same ingredients, except differed dosage of Radix et Rhizoma Rhei. Li Dongyuan advocated a little dose of it but Shen Douyuan administered 3 grams of it. In the *Yizong Jinjian* (The Golden Mirror of Medicine), 3.6 grams of Radix et Rhizoma Rhei are given.

组成:《外科启玄》说:"止痛如神汤即秦艽苍术汤加减"。实际药味全同,只有大黄量有别,李东垣为大黄少许,申斗垣将大黄定为3克,《医宗金鉴·外科心法要诀》大黄为3.6克。

Zhixue San 止血散(36)   51,97,123,124,146,300,328,345, 346,360

Ingredients:

Resina Draconis	9 g	血竭(Xuejie)
Acacia Catechu	9 g	儿茶(Ercha)
Resina Boswelliae Carterii	9 g	乳香(Ruxiang)
Myrrha	9 g	没药(Moyao)
Rubber	3 g	橡皮(Xiangpi)
Margarita	0.3 g	珍珠(Zhenzhu)
Borneolum Syntheticum	0.3 g	冰片(Bingpian)

Administration: Cut the rubber into thin pieces, roast them until they are brown in color. Roast Resina Boswelliae, Carterii and Myrrha to remove their fat, pound them and Acacia Catechu into powder. Then other ingredients are added. All of them are made into powder for use. Fill the cut with a piece of vaseline gauze covered with the drug.

Indication: Alleviating pain and stopping bleeding, diminishing inflammation and promoting granulation, indicated for bleeding after surgery.

制用法:先将橡皮切片炒黄,乳香、没药炒去油,同儿茶共研细末,再将血竭、珍珠、冰片加入,研为细粉装瓶密闭备用。以凡士林纱条,蘸药粉填塞创口即可。

主治:止血止痛、消炎生肌。适用于手术止血或疮疡出血外敷。

Zhushe San 珠麝散(74) 143,358

Ingredients:

Margarita	0.3 g	珍珠(*Zhenzhu*)
Borneolum Syntheticum	0.3 g	冰片(*Bingpian*)
Moschus	0.3 g	麝香(*Shexiang*)
Concha Haliotidis	3 g	石决明(*Shijueming*)
Resina Boswelliae Carterii	3 g	乳香(*Ruxiang*)
Myrrha	3 g	没药(*Moyao*)
Os Draconnis	3 g	龙骨(*Longgu*)
Concha Ostreae	3 g	牡蛎(*Muli*)
Rubber	3 g	橡皮(*Xiangpi*)
Calomelas	1.5 g	轻粉(*Qingfen*)
Rhizoma Coptidis	9 g	黄连(*Huanglian*)

Administration: Cut the rubber into pieces and roast them. roast Resina Boswelliae Carterii and Commiphore Myrrha to remove their fat and the three ingredients with Concha Haliotidis. Os Draconis, and Concha Ostreae are pounded into powder. Add the remainings to the mixture, pound them into fine powder, which is placed in a bottle for use.

Indication: Same as *Niuhuang San*(73)

制用法：先将橡皮切片炒黄，乳香、没药炒去油，同石决明、龙骨、牡蛎、黄连共研细末，然后再将轻粉、珍珠、冰片、麝香加入，研为极细末，装瓶密闭备用。用法、主治同牛黄散(73)。

Ziyin Chushi Tang   滋阴除湿汤(63) 102,332

Ingredients:

Rhizoma Ligustici Chuanxiong	3 g	川芎(*Chuanxiong*)
Radix Angelicae Sinensis	3 g	当归(*Danggui*)
Radix Paeoniae Alba	3 g	白芍(*Baishao*)
Radix Rehmanniae Praeparata	3 g	熟地(*Shudi*)
Radix Bupleuri	2.4 g	柴胡(*Chaihu*)
Radix Scutellariae	2.4 g	黄芩(*Huangqin*)
Rhizoma Anemarrhenae	2.4 g	知母(*Zhimu*)
Pericarpium Citri Reticulatae	2.4 g	陈皮(*Chenpi*)
Bulbus Fritillariae Thunbergii	2.4 g	贝母(*Beimu*)
Rhizoma Alismatis	1.5 g	泽泻(*Zexie*)
Cortex Lycii Radicis	1.5 g	地骨皮(*Digupi*)
Radix Glycyrrhizae	1.5 g	甘草(*Gancao*)
Rhizoma Zingiberis Recens	3 slices	生姜(*Shengjiang*)

At present, the amount of ingredients administered according to the condition (6–10 g in general) except the last one.

Administration: A decoction is made and taken.

Indication: Nourishing *Yin* and clearing away dampness, indicated for perianal abscess of the deficiency syndrome.

现临床应用，除生姜用量仍为3片外，其他各药味可据不同症证灵活应用，一般为6~10克。

用法：水煎服。

主治：能滋阴除湿，适用于肛痈虚证者。

15

肛门直肠病学

序

《英汉实用中医药大全》即将问世，吾为之高兴。

歧黄之道，历经沧桑，永盛不衰。吾中华民族之强盛，由之。世界医学之丰富和发展，亦由之。然而，世界民族之差异，国别之不同，语言之障碍，使中医中药的传播和交流受到了严重束缚。当前，世界各国人民学习、研究、运用中医药的热潮方兴未艾。为使吾中华民族优秀文化遗产之一的歧黄之道走向世界，光大其业，为世界人民造福，徐象才君集省内外精英于一堂，主持编译了《英汉实用中医药大全》。是书之问世将使海内外同道欢呼雀跃。

世界医学发展之日，当是歧黄之道光大之时。

吾欣然序之。

     中华人民共和国卫生部副部长
       兼国家中医药管理局局长
     世界针灸学会联合会主席
     中国科学技术协会委员
     中华全国中医学会副会长
     中国针灸学会会长

            胡熙明
           1989年12月

序

中华民族有同疾病长期作斗争的光辉历程，故而有自己的传统医学——中国医药学。中国医药学有一套完整的从理论到实践的独特科学体系。几千年来，它不但被完好地保存下来，而且得到了发扬光大。它具有疗效显著、副作用小等优点，是人们防病治病，强身健体的有效工具。

任何一个国家在医学进步中所取得的成就，都是人类共同的财富，是没有国界的。医学成果的交流比任何其他科学成果的交流都应进行得更及时，更准确。我从事中医工作30多年来，一直盼望着有朝一日中国医药学能全面走向世界，为全人类解除病痛疾苦做出其应有的贡献。但由于用外语表达中医难度较大，中国医药学对外传播的速度一直不能令人满意。

山东中医学院的徐象才老师发起并主持了大型系列丛书《英汉实用中医药大全》的编译工作。这个工作是一项巨大工程，是一种大型科研活动，是一个大胆的尝试，是一件新事物。对徐象才老师及与其合作的全体编译者夜以继日地长期工作所付出的艰苦劳动，克服重重困难所表现出的坚韧不拔的毅力，以及因此而取得的重大成绩，我甚为敬佩。作为一个中医界的领导者，对他们的工作给予全力支持是我应尽的责任。

我相信《英汉实用中医药大全》无疑会在中国医学史和世界科学技术史上找到它应有的位置。

中华全国中医学会常务理事
山东省卫生厅副厅长

张奇文
1990年3月

出版前言

中国医药学是我中华民族优秀文化遗产之一，建国以来由于党和国家对待中医药采取了正确的政策，使中医药理论宝库不断得到了发掘整理，取得了巨大的成绩。当前，世界各国人民对中国医药学的学习和研究热潮日益高涨，为促进这一热潮更加蓬勃的发展，为使中国医药学能更好地为全人类解除病痛服务，就必须促进中医中药在世界范围内的传播和交流，而要使这一传播和交流进行得更及时、更准确，就必须首先排除语言障碍。因此，编译一套英汉对照的中医药基本知识的书籍，供国内外学习、研究中医药时使用，已成为国内外医药学界和医药学教育界许多人士的迫切需要。

多年来，在卫生部门的号召下，在"中医英语表达研究"方面，已经作出了一些可喜的成绩。本书《英汉实用中医药大全》的编辑出版就是在调查上述研究工作的历史和现状的基础上，继续对中医药英语表达作较系统、较全面的研究，以适应中国医药学对外传播交流的需要。

这部"大全"的版本为英汉对照，共有21个分册，一个分册介绍论述中国医药学的一个分科。在编著上注意了中医药汉文稿的编写特色，在内容上注意了科学性、实用性、全面性和简明易读。汉文稿的执笔撰写者主要是有20年以上实践经验的教授、副教授、主任医师和副主任医师。各分册汉文稿撰写成后，均经各学科专家逐一审订。各分册英文主译、主审主要是国内既懂中医又懂英语的权威人士，还有许多中医院校的英语教师及医药卫生部门的专业翻译人员。英译稿脱稿后，经过了复审、终审，有些译稿还召开全国22所院校和单位人员参加的英译稿统稿定稿研讨会，对英译稿进行细致的研讨和推敲，对如何较全面、较系统、较准确地用英语表达中国医药学进行了探讨，从而推动整个译文达到较高水平，因此，这部"大全"可供中医院校高年级学生作为泛读教材使用。

这部"大全"的编纂得到了国家教育委员会、国家中医药管理局、山东省教育委员会、山东省卫生厅等各部门有关领导的支持。在国家教委高等教育司的指导下，成立了《英汉实用中医药大全》编译领导委员会。还得到了全国许多中医院校和中药生产厂家领导的支持。

希望这部"大全"的出版，对中医院校加强中医英语教学，对国内卫生界培养外向型中医药人才，以及在推动世界各国人民对中医药的学习和研究方面，都将产生良好的影响。

高等教育出版社

1990年3月

前　言

　　《英汉实用中医药大全》是一部以中医基本理论为基础，以中医临床为重点，较为全面系统、简明扼要、易读实用的中级英汉学术性著作。它的主要读者是：中医药院校高年级学生和中青年教师，中医院的中青年医生和中医药科研单位的科研人员，从事中医对外函授工作的人员和出国讲学或行医的中医人员，西学中人员，来华学习中医的外国留学生和各类进修人员。

　　由于中国医药学为我中华民族之独有，因此，英译便成了本《大全》编译工作的重点。为确保译文能准确表达中医的确切含义，我们邀集熟悉中医的英语人员、医学专业翻译人员、懂英语的中医药人员乃至医古文人员于一堂，共同翻译、共同对译文进行研讨推敲的集体翻译法，这样，就把众人之长融进了译文质量之中。然而，即使这样，也难确保译文都能尽如人意。汉文稿虽反映了中国医药学的精髓和概貌，但也难能十全十美。我衷心地盼望读者能提出批评和建议，以便《大全》再版时修改。

　　参加本《大全》编、译、审工作的人员达200余名，他们来自全国28个单位，其中有山东、北京、上海、天津、南京、浙江、安徽、河南、湖北、广西、贵阳、甘肃、成都、山西、长春等15所中医学院，还有中国中医研究院，山东省中医药研究所等中医药科研单位。

　　山东省教育委员会把本《大全》的编译列入了科研计划并拨发了科研经费，山东省卫生厅和一些中药生产厂家也给了很大支持，济南中药厂的资助为编译工作的开端提供了条件。

　　本《大全》的编译成功是全体编译审者集体劳动的结晶，是各有关单位主管领导支持的结果。在《大全》各分册即将陆续出版之际，我诚挚地感谢全体编译审者的真诚合作，感谢许多专家、教授、各级领导和生产厂家的热情支持。

愿本《大全》的出版能在培养通晓英语的中医人才和使中医早日全面走向世界方面起到我所期望的作用。

主编　徐象才

于山东中医学院

1990年3月

目 录

说明 ... 267
1 中医学对肛肠病学的贡献 ... 269
　1.1 病名及其源流 ... 269
　1.2 对肛肠解剖学的研究 ... 269
　1.3 对肛肠生理病理学的研究 ... 270
　1.4 对病因学的认识 ... 270
　1.5 辨证 ... 271
　　1.5.1 分类 ... 271
　　1.5.2 证候、体征、脉象、归经等 ... 272
　1.6 治疗 ... 272
　　1.6.1 内治法 ... 272
　　1.6.2 外治法 ... 275
　　1.6.3 针灸与导引法 ... 277
　1.7 调护及预防 ... 278
2 肛门直肠病检查法 ... 279
　2.1 病人体位 ... 279
　　2.1.1 侧卧位 ... 279
　　2.1.2 伏卧位 ... 279
　　2.1.3 截石位 ... 279
　　2.1.4 膝胸位或膝肘位 ... 279
　　2.1.5 屈膝仰卧位 ... 279
　　2.1.6 蹲位 ... 279
　　2.1.7 站立躬身位 ... 280
　　2.1.8 倒置位 ... 280

- 2.1.9 骑伏位 ········· 280
- 2.2 检查步骤 ········· 280
  - 2.2.1 问诊 ········· 280
  - 2.2.2 视诊 ········· 280
  - 2.2.3 指诊 ········· 280
  - 2.2.4 肛镜检查 ········· 281
  - 2.2.5 探针检查 ········· 281
  - 2.2.6 隐窝钩内口定位 ········· 281
- 2.3 病历书写和检查记录 ········· 282
  - 2.3.1 病历书写格式 ········· 282
  - 2.3.2 病程记录书写要求 ········· 282
  - 2.3.3 局部检查常用图示、符号及表示法 ········· 284

3 肛门直肠麻醉方法 ········· 286

- 3.1 针刺麻醉 ········· 286
  - 3.1.1 取穴 ········· 286
  - 3.1.2 针麻前准备 ········· 286
  - 3.1.3 操作方法 ········· 286
  - 3.1.4 优缺点 ········· 286
- 3.2 局部麻醉 ········· 286
  - 3.2.1 适用 ········· 286
  - 3.2.2 麻醉方法 ········· 287
  - 3.2.3 操作要求 ········· 287
  - 3.2.4 优缺点 ········· 287
- 3.3 腰俞穴麻醉 ········· 287
  - 3.3.1 适应证 ········· 287
  - 3.3.2 常用药物 ········· 287
  - 3.3.3 麻醉方法 ········· 288
  - 3.3.4 麻醉效果 ········· 288
  - 3.3.5 腰俞穴麻醉临床应用的一些具体问题 ········· 288

3.4 其他麻醉 ... 292
3.4.1 腰麻 ... 292
3.4.2 腰骶段硬脊膜外麻醉 ... 292
3.4.3 冷冻麻醉 ... 292
3.4.4 静脉麻醉、全身麻醉等 ... 292

4 肛门直肠手术前后处理与术后反应并发症的处理 ... 293
4.1 肛门直肠手术前后处理 ... 293
4.1.1 术前准备 ... 293
4.1.2 术后处理 ... 293
4.2 术后反应与并发症的处理 ... 295
4.2.1 疼痛 ... 295
4.2.2 坠胀 ... 296
4.2.3 排尿障碍 ... 297
4.2.4 出血 ... 298
4.2.5 发热 ... 303
4.2.6 局部肿胀 ... 304
4.2.7 湿疹及皮炎 ... 304
4.2.8 创口愈合迟缓 ... 304
4.2.9 肛门狭窄及大便失禁 ... 305

5 痔 ... 306
5.1 病因病机 ... 306
5.1.1 整体与内因 ... 306
5.1.2 局部与外因 ... 306
5.2 临床表现 ... 307
5.2.1 分类 ... 307
5.2.2 症状与体征 ... 309
5.2.3 归经及其关联 ... 309
5.3 诊断和鉴别诊断 ... 309
5.4 临床治疗 ... 310

	5.4.1	内治法	310
	5.4.2	外治法	310
	5.4.3	针灸与磁疗	329

6 肛门直肠周围脓肿 ... 331
6.1 病因病机 ... 331
6.2 临床表现 ... 331
6.3 临床治疗 ... 332
6.3.1 内治法 ... 332
6.3.2 外治法 ... 332

7 肛瘘 ... 333
7.1 病因病机 ... 333
7.2 临床表现 ... 333
7.2.1 分类 ... 333
7.2.2 症状与体征 ... 335
7.3 诊断和鉴别诊断 ... 336
7.3.1 问诊 ... 336
7.3.2 视诊 ... 336
7.3.3 触诊 ... 337
7.3.4 探针检查 ... 338
7.3.5 肛镜及隐窝钩检查 ... 339
7.3.6 管道液体注入法 ... 340
7.3.7 X线摄片 ... 341
7.3.8 了解内外口关系和管道曲直的有关规则 ... 341
7.3.9 病理切片检查 ... 343
7.4 临床治疗 ... 344
7.4.1 内治法 ... 344
7.4.2 外治法 ... 344

8 肛裂 ... 353
8.1 病因病机 ... 353

- 8.1.1 解剖学因素 ········· 353
- 8.1.2 炎性因素 ········· 353
- 8.1.3 机械性损伤 ········· 354
- 8.1.4 其他因素 ········· 354
- 8.2 临床表现 ········· 354
  - 8.2.1 临床分期 ········· 354
  - 8.2.2 症状与体征 ········· 355
- 8.3 诊断和鉴别诊断 ········· 356
- 8.4 临床治疗 ········· 356
  - 8.4.1 内治法 ········· 356
  - 8.4.2 外治法 ········· 358
  - 8.4.3 针刺与磁疗 ········· 362

9 直肠脱垂 ········· 363
- 9.1 病因病机 ········· 363
  - 9.1.1 滑动疝学说 ········· 363
  - 9.1.2 肠套叠学说 ········· 363
- 9.2 临床表现 ········· 364
  - 9.2.1 分类 ········· 364
  - 9.2.2 症状与体征 ········· 366
- 9.3 诊断和鉴别诊断 ········· 368
  - 9.3.1 诊断 ········· 368
  - 9.3.2 鉴别诊断 ········· 370
- 9.4 临床治疗 ········· 371
  - 9.4.1 内治法 ········· 371
  - 9.4.2 外治法 ········· 371
  - 9.4.3 针灸疗法 ········· 378

10 直肠息肉 ········· 379
- 10.1 病因病机 ········· 379
- 10.2 临床表现 ········· 379

    10.2.1 分类 ··· 379
    10.2.2 症状和体征 ··· 381
  10.3 诊断和鉴别诊断 ··· 381
  10.4 临床治疗 ··· 382
    10.4.1 内治法 ··· 382
    10.4.2 外治法 ··· 382

11 肛肠疾病的预防保健 ·· 384
  11.1 痔病的预防保健 ··· 384
    11.1.1 加强锻炼,增进健康 ··························· 384
    11.1.2 精神调养与起居 ································· 384
    11.1.3 注意饮食调节 ····································· 384
    11.1.4 保持大便通畅,养成定时大便的习惯 ··· 384
    11.1.5 保持肛门局部清洁,减少刺激 ············· 384
    11.1.6 按摩与提肛 ··· 385
    11.1.7 导引法 ··· 387
  11.2 肛瘘的预防保健 ··· 388
  11.3 肛裂的预防保健 ··· 388
  11.4 直肠脱垂的预防保健 ································· 389
  11.5 直肠息肉的预防保健 ································· 389

附方索引（英汉对照） ······································ (194—251)
英汉实用中医药大全(书目) ·································· 390

说　　明

　　肛门直肠病学是《英汉实用中医药大全》的第 15 分册。

　　中医对痔瘘等肛肠疾病的诊治有悠久历史，独特的理论体系和丰富的临床实践。

　　本分册主要内容为：中国医药学对肛肠病学的贡献，痔、肛周脓肿、肛瘘、肛裂、直肠脱垂、直肠息肉等常见肛肠病的病因、病机、辨证和治疗，以及检查、麻醉方法、手术前后处理和常见方药等。

　　本分册汉文稿经中国中医药学会肛肠分会主任委员丁泽民主任医师审阅。在山东泰安英文稿统稿会上，上海中医学院孙祥燮教授和河南中医学院的李震声教授帮助审查了英文稿。

1 中医学对肛肠病学的贡献

祖国医学历史悠久,是我国劳动人民长期与疾病作斗争的经验总结。在几千年的发展中,肛肠病学逐渐成为一门专门学科,具有独特的理论体系和丰富的临床经验,在祖国医学宝库中占有重要地位。根据历史文献作一初步介绍。

1.1 病名及其源流

痔、瘘病名早在西周时期(公元前 11 世纪～公元前 770 年)即已提出。战国时期对痔的记述已比较明确,《庄子·列御寇》(公元前 770 年～公元前 403 年)载:"庄子曰:秦王有病召医,破痈溃痤者得车一乘,舐痔者得车五乘,所治愈下,得车愈多……"此故事所言之痔,原为贬意语。相传战国的宋国使臣曹商在秦国向秦惠王献媚取宠,得车 100 乘,而向庄子显示其功。庄子对其为人非常厌恶,用此奇辨以挫曹商。此虽为庄子讽刺曹商,但说明在 2000 年前已知痈(大疮)、痤(小疮)、痔等病,并有疗痔之法。关于病名,有痔病、五痔、痔疮、痔疾、痔核、痔瘘、肛漏(瘘)等。痔核一词,首见于明朝《医学正传》(公元 1515 年)一书,距今约 400 余年。一些病名已交流海外,至今仍被采用。

1.2 对肛肠解剖学的研究

我国古代医学家对解剖学亦有突出贡献,早在商周时期,对人体即做过实地解剖。如《灵枢·经水篇》曰:"者夫八尺之士,皮肉在此,外可度量切循而得之,其死可解剖而视之……"。《难经·四十四难》说:"大肠小肠会为阑门,下极为魄门。"早在汉代

(公元前206年~公元前220年)已知阑门(回盲瓣)为大小肠之分界处,其形似闸门能阻拦肠内容物之运行,故曰阑门,同时观察到消化道的最下端为魄门(肛门),前人认为肺与大肠为表里,肺藏魄,故大肠之末端称魄门,又名肛门。明代《医宗必读》一书附有大肠之图谱,此图与现代结肠图形极为相似。从大量文献可知,前人对肠管的形态学如大小、长短、容积、血液供给及与周围组织的关系等都有较详细的描述。历代著述以《灵枢》和《难经》为主,《灵枢》所称之回肠又名大肠,即今回肠和结肠大部分,所称之广肠即今乙状结肠、直肠和肛门。肛门一词首见于《难经》。肛肠一词首见于《太平圣惠方》(公元982年~公元992年),距今约1000年,可为世界肛肠一词最早应用者。直肠一词,可能为《难经》注解者杨玄操提出,如是则出自唐代,明、清时期已广泛应用。

1.3 对肛肠生理病理学的研究

祖国医学对肛肠生理病理学的研究,论述颇多。综括历代所述:大肠为阳腑,属金,主津主收,本性燥,为传道之官,变化出焉。其特点泻而不藏,实而不满。肛门为肺大肠之候,主行道,无化物之功,《内经》曰:"魄门亦为五脏使,水谷不得久藏。"前人认为大肠司传送糟粕之功能,主管疏泄而不藏精,并能吸收水分,其喜燥恶湿。如功能失调,可引起便秘、腹泻等症。

1.4 对病因学的认识

先贤对痔瘘的病因记述颇为详尽,早在2000多年前即认为痔是血管病变,如《素问·生气通天论》(公元前240年)说:"因而饱食,筋脉横解,肠澼为痔。"《素问》认为痔乃筋脉横解,为痔的血管曲弦学说世界最早提出者。《太平圣惠方》提出血热妄行理论。金元时期(公元1127年~1168年)刘完素、李东垣认为痔因大肠、肺、肝、脾等脏腑功能失调,李东垣又倡导湿、热、风、燥四气相合而为病。《丹溪心法》认为"痔者皆因脏腑本虚"。《疮疡经验全书》说："人生素不能饮酒亦患痔者，脏腑虚故也；亦有父子相传者……"提出脏腑虚损与遗传因素对痔的影响。《外科启玄》倡导"痔者沸也"的瘀滞学说。《外科正宗》提出"夫痔者乃素积湿热"等。这对后世均有一定影响。前人对痔瘘的病因论述甚详，可综括为：整体与内因，局部与外因两方面，且互为影响而发病。这些病因学论点为前人长期临床经验的总结，应用已数世纪直至今日仍指导临床辨证论治，为后人所推崇和依循。

1.5 辨证

1.5.1 分类

痔的分类在秦汉时期有 4 痔分类，如《五十二病方》有牡痔、牝痔、脉痔、血痔。隋朝《诸病源候论》（公元 610 年）提出牡痔、牝痔、脉痔、肠痔、血痔、酒痔、气痔，且每种都有具体的描述，后人常将前 5 种痔称 5 痔。5 痔论点在我国肛肠病学史上，对学术的发展曾起过积极的作用。后人应用达几个世纪之久，历代不少医家以 5 痔为基础，加以发挥，而有 7 痔、8 痔、10 痔、11 痔等。值得注意的是，今人应用的内痔、外痔病名，早在唐代我国医学家即已提出。如《外台秘要》（公元 752 年）引用许仁则对痔的观察说："此病有内痔，有外痔，内但便即有血，外有异。外痔下部有孔，每出血从孔中出。"此后，病名逐渐繁多，金元时期提出 25 痔，明朝提出 24 痔，其中有里外痔（混合痔）病名，均绘有痔形图谱。至清朝除 5 痔外，25 痔、24 痔同时并用，清朝同治 12 年（公元 1873 年）我国第 1 本痔瘘专著《马氏痔瘘科七十二种》提出 72 种痔，其中有"裂肛痔"（肛裂）一病。由此可见前人在痔病分类方面，积累了丰富的经验。但因受当时条件所限，痔中还包括其他肛门直肠病。瘘的分类，《五十二病方》虽有肛瘘之病，但未细分，自秦汉至晋、隋、唐、肛瘘多以痔病名而总括之。宋朝《太平圣惠方》将痔和肛瘘明确区分。《疮疡经验全书》（公元 1569 年）对肛瘘有进一步认识，如曰："又有肛门左右，别有一窍出脓血，名曰单漏。"从字义讲，单漏即单纯之瘘管，非多管也，或为今称之单纯性肛瘘。此后亦有不同之分类法。

1.5.2 证候、体征、脉象、归经等

前人对痔瘘的症征如肿痛下坠、便血、脱垂、作痒、出脓水、病变形状、部位等均有详尽的描述。对大肠病诊脉的位置《内经》取尺部候大肠；唐《千金要方》提出了于右手寸口诊大肠之脉；亦有从趺阳脉诊大肠者。关于脉之状况，有细弱沉迟芤等虚证之脉象和洪大、弦数等实证之脉象。关于归经及其关联，大肠病与大肠经、肺经、肝、脾、肾经、膀胱经、任、督二脉、胆经等经脉有关。对于类证鉴别，也辨之甚详，如金元时期《兰室秘藏》一书说：大肠末端肿胀为湿因引起，疼痛重为风因引起，大便燥结难解是火邪所致。通过实践，明朝《外科大成》又进一步发挥，使李东垣倡导的湿因局部见肿，风因致痛，火邪使大便热结不通的湿热风燥临床见证更为完善，而提出："如其肿者湿也，痛者火也，痒者风也，闭结者火燥也"的论点。对证轻重顺逆之描述亦较全面，因而对疾病预后的判断，较为可靠。

1.6 治疗

痔、瘘等肛肠病治法甚多，有内治法、外治法、针灸法、导引法等，外治法中包括枯痔、结扎、挂线、手术、烟熏、熏洗、导便等。如《五十二病方》除内治法外，还载有手术、敷药、药浴、烟熏、熨灸、角法（似拔火罐）等多种疗法。然而历代强调内治，外治法到明清时期才有更大发展。现以治法归纳如下。

1.6.1 内治法

《五十二病方》即载有内治方药。东汉张仲景著《金匮要略》（公元 205 年）中说："下血,先便后血,此远血也,黄土汤(1)主

之。""下血，先血后便，此近血也，赤小豆当归散（2）主之。"对便血之先后进行了区别，并拟定了代表方药。关于治则，金元四大家（刘完素、张从正、李东垣、朱震亨）均主张清热泻火、凉血。李东垣又提出和血润燥，疏风止痛之法，如《兰室秘藏》说："其疾甚者，当以苦寒泻火，以辛温和血润燥疏风止痛，是其治也。"《丹溪心法》说："痔疮专以凉血为主。"《疮疡经验全书》说："大法以凉血为主，徐徐取效。"而《医学真传》说："其治法总则宜温补不宜凉泻，温补则血循经脉，补益则气能统血。"认为治痔之法应以补益为主。关于肛瘘的治疗，其治则及用药与痔病相近，唯更强调补益。如《儒门事亲》说："夫痔漏肿痛……同治湿法而治之。"《丹溪心法》说："漏疮，先须服补药生气血，用参、术、芪、芎、归为主，大剂服之。"《疮疡经验全书》说："治之须以温补之剂补其内，生肌之药敷其外。"《医学入门》说："漏流脓血初是湿热，久是湿寒，初起宜凉血清热燥湿，病久则宜涩窍杀虫温补。"《外证医案汇编》说："所以治漏之法，如堤之溃，如屋之漏，不补其漏，安能免乎，治漏者，先固气血为先，气旺内充，而能收蓄，使其不漏，可无害矣，津液日增，虚损可复。……今后六方，奇脉久漏空虚者，以有情之品填之，久漏胃弱，以甘温之品固之，阴虚阳亢，滋阴药中佐苦以坚之，土不生金者，甘温培中，兼酸以收之，各方中莲子、芡实、诃子、中白固摄真元者，皆补漏之法也。"关于脱肛之治疗，其治则均以《内经》"虚则补之""酸主收"等为准绳，《景岳全书》说："内经曰，下者举之。徐之才曰，涩可去脱。皆治脱肛之法也。"

关于用药前人积累了极其丰富的经验。除《五十二病方》、《金匮要略》外，《神农本草经》365味药中有30余味能治痔瘘。《备急千金要方》治五痔方26首。《太平圣惠方》治五痔方213首，加治便血方共220首。《普及方》所载痔瘘方药甚多，其中肠风下血方136，脏毒下血方225，诸痔方800余，加肛门赤痛等共1200余张。《古今图书集成·医部全录》治痔瘘及脱肛方 240 方，单方验方 300 余，方共 500 余张。前人积累方药之多，如汗牛充栋，这些方药包括秘方、验方等，是我国古代医学家长期实践的结果。

痔疮所用药物，《医学正传》说："治法以苦寒泻火，芩、连、栀子、槐花之类。以辛温和血，当归、川芎、桃仁之类。风邪在下，以秦艽、防风、升麻之类提之。燥热弗郁以大黄、枳壳、麻仁之类润之。"《本草纲目》载："李东垣随证用药凡例：下部见血，须用地榆为之使。下部痔瘘，苍术、防风为君，甘草、芍药佐之，详证加减。"《证治汇补》治便血，"主以四物汤 (3)。风加荆芥、防风；湿加苍术、秦艽；热加槐角、芩、连；寒加木香、干姜；气（滞）加香附、枳壳；瘀加桃仁、韭汁；久虚者加参、芪、术、草；下陷加升麻、柴胡；虚热加阿胶、生地；虚寒加附子、炮姜。"

肛瘘用药，多服参芪等补剂，也可服黄连闭管丸 (4)、象牙化管丸 (5) 等。脱肛用药，《疮疡经验全书》说："血虚脱肛以四物汤为主，气虚脱肛以参芪归术为之，血热以凉血为主，四物汤加黄柏"该书对虚人脱肛以补中益气汤 (6) 加减用药亦较全面。《景岳全书》说："故古人之治此者，多用参、芪、归、术、川芎、甘草、升麻之类，以升之补之。或兼用五味、乌梅之类，以固之涩之。"在肛肠病所用方药中，槐角丸、秦艽苍术汤 (7) 均为名方，应用已久。槐角丸为滋阴凉血、清利湿热的代表方剂，不仅医家常用，而为世人所知，当今大有槐角丸遍及天下之势。《备急千金要方》有槐子丸 (8) 和小槐实丸 (9)，《千金翼方》称槐子圆和小槐实圆，但药味与今不同。《太平惠民和剂局方》（公元 1107 年）所载槐角圆 (10) 即今槐角丸之主方，作者称其为正统方。《疮疡经验全书》有槐角丸 (11) 方，但药味反槐角、乌牛胆二味，实为胆槐丸，《医学入门》称槐胆丹。后人应用药味与此方全同，药量遵其比例者，均为槐角圆或正统槐角丸，如药味全同，药量不一，或药量有增减者，可属正统槐角丸

类方 (12)。如药味不同为非正统槐角丸 (13)。秦艽苍术汤为李东垣所订,自金元至明、清直至今日,颇受医家称道,《兰室秘藏》载有 7 张痔瘘方药,即秦艽白术丸 (14)、秦艽苍术汤、秦艽防风汤 (15)、秦艽羌活汤 (16)、秦艽当归汤 (17)。当归郁李仁汤 (18)、红花桃仁汤 (19) 等。作者根据临床体会结合后世对秦艽苍术汤的认识,认为此方更能体现东垣"辛温和血润燥疏风止痛"的立法。并将其定为痔瘘内治法的首要治则,以此方为代表方剂。将秦艽白术丸等定为秦艽苍术汤的类方。此二方药及其部分类方为前人所创,经多世纪应用,效果较好,在原方基础上加减变通,不仅扩大了其类方范围,也扩大了适应证。目前除治疗痔瘘外还用治全身其它系统疾病,实为肛肠病学药物学中之明珠。

1.6.2 外治法

1. **枯痔法** 为祖国医学主要的传统疗法,在历史的发展中,对痔瘘病的治疗曾起过重要作用。早在宋朝即已应用,明、清时期倍受推崇。所用药物有枯痔散 (20),枯痔丁 (21) 等。枯痔方药以《外科正宗》(公元 1617 年) 所载的"三品一条枪"(22) 为主方,枯药大部含砒,须经特殊炼制,方能应用。不论涂药或插药,从组织枯脱到创口愈合以及反应与并发症的处理等方面,前人均积累了丰富的经验。枯痔散疗法因疗程长,痛苦较大,目前已较少采用。枯痔丁疗法,从药丁制作,临床应用到实验研究等,均有较大发展,仍为当今主要外治法之一。

2. **结扎,挂线法** 亦为主要传统疗法。结扎法始于宋朝,距今约 1000 年。是治疗痔核的重要方法。挂线法是治疗肛瘘的有效方法。从结扎和挂线器材到临床应用,论述颇详,直至目前仍有较大的实用价值,且早已交流至海外。通过不断的研究,以切开配合挂线法治疗高位复杂性肛瘘,取得满意效果,是我国肛肠学科近代取得的突出成就。

3. **手术法** 祖国医学以手术治疗痔瘘,始于秦汉时期,如

《五十二病方》载:"牡痔居窍旁……以小角角之,如熟二斗米顷,而张角,絜以小绳,剖以刀。其中有如兔髋,若有坚血如抇末而出者,即已。令。"此文较详细的描述了牡痔的手术疗法,即先在痔上施以类似后人拔火罐疗法的角法,拔火罐毕,系以小绳,再以刀剖之,痔中可见兔丝子样物或坚硬血块破碎而出,即愈。此疑为血栓外痔之手术。另例为肛瘘手术:"巢塞直(朘)(肛瘘)者,杀狗,取其脬,以穿龠入直(朘)中,炊(吹)之引出,徐以刀去其巢,冶黄黔(芩)而娄(屡)傅之。"此文言痔瘘患者手术时先杀狗将狗之膀胱套在竹管上,插入直肠吹胀,将直肠下端患处引出,然后以刀慢慢切割去除病患。术后以黄芩末屡敷之。早在 2000 年前,先贤即创用此别具一格的手术方式,术后结合应用中药治疗,可谓先进之至。《外科图说》又曰:"至于治痔一法,全要审其形势如何,若小而收根分株者易治,上以麻药,施以利刃,用絮止血,应手取效,何难之有。……若久年漏证,初诊探以银丝方能知其横飘直柱,以及浅深曲直之由通肛过桥之重症。然后每日用柳叶刀开其二三分,开后用絮止血,约半日去絮,乃上药版。通肛则用湾刀。若素有血证不可开,劳病脉数不可开,肛门前后不可开,髫龄以及耄年均不可开……。"此文较详细记载了肛瘘的切割法,并提出了手术的禁忌症,如血液病、肺结核活动期、病变在肛门前后位、年龄较小或老年均不适于手术。由此可见其经验甚为丰富。清朝除痔瘘手术外,对先天性肛门闭锁和肛门直肠异物也进行手术处理。前人对肛肠病的诊疗亦采用了适宜的体位。

为了使手术顺利进行,使用了麻醉药物,研制了专科器械,如《外科图说》载有外科刀剪钳各式物件图,器械共 30 余件,其中痔瘘专科器械有探肛筒(肛镜)、银丝(从图形看为两端球头银丝)、治管银针、过肛针、穿肛针套(挂子)、弯刀(似今探针镰形刀)、拖刀(弯刀之一种)、勾刀、柳叶刀等,其他除各种剪钳外,还有换药、制药、检查、灸炙等器械。《医门补要》的作者赵濂创制了拔脓管,对疮疡排脓颇为方便。书中介绍说:"其管以薄铜,卷如象筋粗,式长二寸余,要中空似细竹,急焊其缝,一头锉平,一头锉斜尖式,用时要尖头插患孔内,少顷则脓自管中射出如箭。"为了无菌操作,宋朝即应用了煮沸消毒手术器械和器械存放之法。如《卫济宝书》说:"……打炼刀一枚,小钩一个,右用桑白皮、紫藤香煮一周时,以紫藤香末藏之。"

4. 导便　汉朝即应用肛门栓剂和灌肠术,如张仲景用蜜煎导法,取蜜微火煎如饴,捻作锭如枣核样,纳谷道中,又用猪胆一个取汁和醋少许灌入谷道中,片刻大便自通。药物多用竹管灌入直肠。明朝创用喷药导便法。取竹管一头插入谷道中,一头套入猪膀胱,药先放竹管内,用手着力一捻猪脬,药即喷入直肠。导便药物较多,有胆汁、蜂蜜、香油、醋、葱汁、复方中药液以及温水等。《回春方》采用头低脚高位灌肠法,用药比例香油温水各半,以竹筒为灌肠器,早在明代导便之法已如此先进。

另外在枯痔和手术前,为使肠道清洁便于操作,在明代即用中药缓泻或峻泻,以准备肠道。如《外科正宗》说:"……凡疗内痔者,先用通利药荡涤脏腑,然后再用唤痔散(23)涂入肛门……。"《医学纲目》说:"凡医痔之法,且如明日要下手,今日先与此药(通便方),所以宽大肠,使大便软滑,不与痔相碍,且不泻泄。"此即术前应用峻泻和缓泻法之例。

1.6.3 针灸与导引法

针灸是治疗痔瘘等肛肠病的重要方法,受到历代重视。晋朝《针灸甲乙经》(公元282年)载:"痔痛,攒竹主之。痔,会阴主之,……脱肛下(利),刺气街主之。"《针灸资生经》(公元1220年)载:"何教授汤薄有此疾(痔病)积年,皆一灸除根。汤薄因传此法,后观灸经,此穴疗小儿脱肛泻血(便血),盖歧伯灸小儿法也。后人因之以灸大人肠风泻血尔,若灸肠风,长强为要穴。"前人常用穴位有:长强、承山、八髎、足三里、气海、百会等。近年通过研究除体针外又有耳针等,并发现了新的有效穴位如气衡等，而针刺麻醉可用于痔瘘手术。导引是养生防病的医疗方法，《诸病源候论》、《保生秘要》等均有记述。如按其法练习，可治五痔等病。

1.7 调护及预防

历代一向重视痔瘘患者的调护，注意饮食起居等方面的宜忌。如元朝《外科精义》提出：要注意饮食调节，切忌酒辛热肥腻之物，饮食应清淡，忌房事，少思虑。《疮疡经验全书》说："少劳，戒怒，远色，忌口，斯能愈矣。"《医学正传》说："自宜慎口节欲，依法调治，无有不安者也。"对适宜之饮食包括药膳和禁忌之食物，不再举例。为了减轻患病后的痛苦，前人亦积累了不少经验，如《直指方》说，患痔下坠，即不能坐，又不容行，站立其坠愈甚，惟高枕，仰卧，心平气定，其肿自收。《疡医大全》介绍：治痔瘘等症，患者欲坐不能，须铺极厚芦花坐垫，中开一洞，将患处坐向洞中，自无压挤伤疮之患。此康复保健之法，至今仍可采用。

痔瘘的予防甚为重要，祖国医学强调整体调治，《内经》中即提出预防为主的原则。《诸病源候论》养生方说，导引法有补养宣导之功。故推之如常人经常练习，则可防痔。《马氏痔瘘科七十二种》说："…，且求其永远除根，不能再犯者更属寥寥，若男在十六岁、女在十四岁以前先用无形化痔丹一料，化尽先天之毒涣清后天之气，则一生不染痔疮之患。此丹防患未然诸疮不生。"可见当时对预防痔瘘也进行了研究。

2 肛门直肠病检查法

2.1 病人体位

2.1.1 侧卧位

患者侧卧,上腿屈曲靠近腹部,下腿稍伸直,或两腿全曲使臀部和肛门暴露。有左侧卧位和右侧卧位两种,可按习惯不同而采用。此体位舒适,体弱或手术时间较长时宜用,适于检查或手术。

2.1.2 伏卧位

患者伏卧,腿略低,两下肢分开,如将臀部垫高,则称臀高伏卧位。此体位亦舒适,体弱或手术时间较长时宜用,适于检查或手术。手术时为充分暴露肛门,可用宽胶布牵开两臀。

2.1.3 截石位

患者仰卧,下肢屈曲抬高并向两侧分开。此体位能充分暴露肛门,但上下台费时,适于检查或手术。如做示教手术,观察空间较小。又因患者两腿抬高,助手活动不便。

2.1.4 膝胸位或膝肘位

患者跪伏,头低臀高。如胸部着床称膝胸位;肘部着床称膝肘位。此体位虽不太舒适,但能充分暴露局部,适于一般检查和结肠镜检查。

2.1.5 屈膝仰卧位

患者仰卧,用自己的两手将两腿抱起屈膝,使臀部暴露。此适于检查。

2.1.6 蹲位

患者蹲踞并用力努挣。此体位可检查内痔脱垂、直肠脱垂等。

2.1.7 站立躬身位

患者站立，弯腰向前，两手可扶床边或椅橙，胸下可垫被褥。适于检查。此体位不需特殊设备，简便易行，但暴露不够充分。

2.1.8 倒置位

又称颠倒位，或折刀式。患者伏卧于床，通过床的调整使头低臀高，两膝跪于床端，适于检查和手术。但上下台不便，如头过低时则感不适。

2.1.9 骑伏位

患者骑于特制木马式床上，背向检查者，露出臀部后将上身伏于台面，头略转向一侧，两臂自然下垂，握住台身两边的下撑。适于检查、手术和换药。此体位能充分暴露肛门，上下台方便。经多年实践认为对检查、换药和一般手术尤为适宜。但手术时间较长时，手术结束后少数患者因起立下床可发生姿式性虚脱。

特制木马式床，为山东中医学院附院设计，原为木制，现已改制为万能手术床。

2.2 检查步骤

2.2.1 问诊

耐心听取患者对病情的叙述，根据不同的病情，询问时应有重点。除注意局部病情外，并对全身健康状况作重点了解。注意有无高血压病、冠心病、糖尿病以及肝、肾疾病和肺结核病等。

2.2.2 视诊

患者取一定体位后暴露肛门，对好灯光，亦可利用自然光线，进行检查。检查时，分开患者两臀，查看病变区和肛门自然外貌。

2.2.3 指诊

指诊是检查痔、瘘等病的重要方法。检查时先触摸肛外，有无压痛、波动或条索状物，如有条索状物应触摸其行径。然后将戴有指套并沾润滑剂的食指慢慢伸入肛内，触摸肛管壁有无柔软隆起或坚硬肿物等。如有瘘管，可在齿线区触摸内口，并注意括约肌力和直肠环情况。

2.2.4 肛镜检查

将肛镜涂滑润剂，慢慢插入肛内，抽出镜心，对好灯光，并徐徐外退，注意观察直肠和肛管内变化，如粘膜色泽，有无溃疡，痔核位置、大小、数目等。

2.2.5 探针检查

为检查肛瘘的主要措施。取粗细适宜的球头探针，由肛瘘外口缓慢轻柔地插入瘘管，探查管道行径、长度和深度，另手食指戴指套沾滑润剂后，伸入肛道，与探针对应检查。如瘘管平行或近平行肛管时，肛内手指可于管道顶端对应外之肠壁，感触探针冲撞。

2.2.6 隐窝钩内口定位

是确定肛瘘内口的重要方法。以二叶镜扩开肛门，取钩长不同的隐窝钩，先后予以钩探。先取钩小者（0.5 cm），首先钩探所窥见的或指诊时所触及的明显病变区，再沿齿或慢慢检查，如遇内口，则容易钩入。如肛隐窝发炎变深时，可取钩长者（1 cm）予以鉴别。如为肛隐窝仅可钩入一定深度，如为瘘管内口常可顺利吞没全钩，且钩的方向与肛外触得的瘘管方向一致，这是因为隐窝钩经内口钩入瘘管之故。

其他检查措施如肛瘘内口美兰染色，局部 X 线造影拍片，乙状结肠镜和纤维结肠镜检查等，可视不同病情而采用。局部检查后，应对全身重点检查，一般可作血常规和出凝血时间，或仅查白细胞和出凝血时间，必要时查大小便常规、血沉、血型、肝功、胆固醇等。特殊检查如心电图、脑血流图等，应酌情而定。

2.3 病历书写和检查记录

检查后应详细记写病历或填写专科记录表，并以图表示。

2.3.1 病历书写格式

门诊病人可用表式病历记录；住院病人应写完整病历。

2.3.2 病程记录书写要求

1. 时间

(1) 入院后当日要记录。

(2) 术前要记录，如全身情况一向较好，局部病情稳定，且距术日较近时，入院后当日记录可作术前记录。

(3) 手术日要记录，一般为术后记写，书写次数不限。

(4) 术后记录，一般病人术后每日记1次，连记3日后，每周记两次直至痊愈。如全身或局部病情较重或有明显不适，应随时记录，至病情稳定或症状好转后再按一般病人记录。

2. 记写内容

病程记录记写病人住院期间的诊疗过程，也就是患者住院后通过各种治疗，病情由重转轻直至痊愈或由轻转重直至死亡的真实记写。痔瘘等肛肠病目前主要采用中西医结合的治疗手段，为了突出中医特点，除注意手术和与其有关的现代医学的记录外，应以四诊和辨证施治为主来记写。具体的要求：

(1) 入院后当日记录，实际是简要的入院记录。一般习惯先于左上角记写书写日期，紧接记录所写内容。其内容主要包括患者因何病入院，住院后经全身和局部检查，提出了怎样的诊断依据和治疗方案，并准予以实施。如病情较重，对治疗和护理中的注意事项和实施措施可一一开列清楚。

(2) 术前记录。对合并有全身其他系统疾病的患者，应有术前记录。入院后因全身或局部情况尚不具备手术条件需进行一阶段调治，当通过调治已具备手术条件时，即应写明近日全身和局部情况，进行手术有何依据，便于与入院时比较对照。如全身情况较好，局部病情稳定且距手术日较近，入院后当日记录可作为术前记录。

(3) 手术日记录。记写术中和术后当日情况，如术中患者全身有何不适，局部有无疼痛，如发生明显反应应记写术中处理情况。所取体位、消毒、麻醉、切割等详细情况在手术记录中记写，术后病程记录中不再重复。回病房后主要记写全身和局部情况。全身情况仍然是手术刺激的结果或麻醉后体位变化引起的，如头痛、头晕、心悸、出大汗、恶心呕吐等。如需继续测量血压或术中输液输血等情况亦应记录。局部情况主要记写常见反应与并发症，如疼痛、坠胀、出血、排尿障碍（小便难、尿潴留）、腹胀气等，并记写处理措施和缓解过程。

(4) 术后记录。自术后次日起记写全身、局部病况和处理。全身方面手术刺激引起的证候将逐渐减轻，但因受凉、组织刺激（吸收热）和感染等又会出现新的症状和体证。全身记录内容除上述情况外，应记写有无发热恶寒，口苦否。欲饮否，是否出虚汗，食睡情况，小便通利否，是否尿痛尿频，小便颜色，大便何时解下，干或稀，有无带血和滴血或出黑血块。局部内容除上述者外，应记录创口情况，有无炎肿等。

根据全身和局部情况制定治疗措施时应辨证施治，对症状体证进行综合分析，提出治则和方药。如需兄弟科室协助解决要提出会诊意见和请求。上级医师和兄弟科室的意见应认真记写。治疗期间如需进行特殊检查，应写明理由，检查后要记录结果。医生交接班期间，应写交接班记录，交班记录近似阶段小结，对重病人应提出注意事项，接班记录则较简单，可按一般病程记录记写。此外，因病情变化需要转科时，应写转出记录或转入记录。

转出记录，主要记写患者转出理由和应注意的事项及会诊医生的转科意见。转入记录，记录内容较多，格式同入院记录，即转科后的新写入院记录，叙述时应注明因何故由哪科转来。转院记录，格式与入院记录同，但主要记录入院期间的诊疗情况，目前全身和局部情况，转出理由等。

(5) 出院记录。即治疗结束时的系统记录，包括一般项目，入院日期，住院日数，入院后诊疗情况，出院时全身、局部情况，主要治疗手段，治疗结果，手术次数，疗程，今后注意事项等。

2.3.3 局部检查常用图示、符号及表示法

1. 肛管横面示意图，如图 (1)

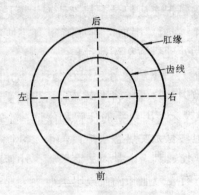

图 1　肛管横面示意图

2. 肛门会阴示意图，如图 (2)

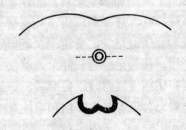

图 2　肛管会阴平面示意图

3. 常用符号及表示法，如图 (3)

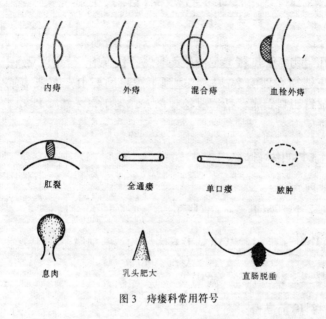

图3 痔瘘科常用符号

3 肛门直肠麻醉方法

肛门和肛管皮肤感觉锐敏而直肠下段又有括约肌,故该区手术时应选择合理麻醉法,并达到下述目的要求,即术中镇痛完善,做到切割无痛;括约肌松弛良好,便于充分暴露术区;无内脏牵拉反应。

3.1 针刺麻醉

3.1.1 取穴

1. 耳针:神门、肺、直肠下段、直肠上段、肌松等。
2. 体针:承山、气衡(手太阴肺经穴,前臂掌侧中上$\frac{1}{4}$与上$\frac{1}{4}$交界处是穴)、长强、骶侧等。

3.1.2 针麻前准备

向患者介绍针麻特点,解除思想顾虑,树立信心。术前可视情况给用小量杜冷丁、非那根等。

3.1.3 操作方法

取穴后进针捻转,出现酸麻胀感时再接针麻仪,刺激强度以患者能耐受为限,一般诱导30分钟左右。

3.1.4 优缺点

安全,无副作用,但镇痛不全,括约肌松弛欠佳。

3.2 局部麻醉

3.2.1 适用

适于一般痔瘘手术。用药:0.5%~2%普鲁卡因;1~2%利多卡因；0.15~0.5%布比卡因。
3.2.2 麻醉方法
1. 肛周浸润：多用于混合痔或内痔结扎。浸润方法见图4和图5。

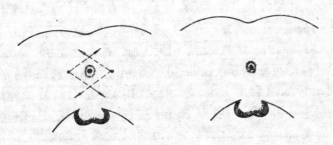

图4 肛周浸润麻醉分层浸润法　　图5 肛周浸润麻醉七点注射法
每点均垂直穿刺给药

2. 病变周围浸润：多用于肛瘘、肛裂手术。
3. 穿刺路径浸润：适于直肠脱垂直肠周围注射法。一般在左、右中位距肛缘约2厘米左右浸润麻醉。

3.2.3 操作要求
注意无菌操作；注药深浅适度，阻断完全；注药后如局部隆起变形，应按揉注射区，使其复原。

3.2.4 优缺点
操作简便、安全，但对高位或复杂肛瘘注药尚感不便。

3.3 腰俞穴麻醉
此麻醉为骶麻方法之一，即骶裂孔（骶裂沟）麻醉。

3.3.1 适应证
混合痔、环状痔、高位复杂肛瘘、骶尾部肿瘤等肛门直肠各种手术。

3.3.2 常用药物
2%利多卡因；2%普鲁卡因。

3.3.3 麻醉方法

所取体位无特殊选择，若惯于伏卧位手术，则以伏卧位麻醉。伏卧时垫高臀部，暴露手术视野。以碘酒、酒精常规消毒，盖无菌洞巾。按取穴标志顺骶中嵴方向扪得骶裂沟。于穿刺点处先注一皮丘并浸润各层继之垂直深刺，阻力顿然消失施即抵骨，进针深度终止。阻力消失所至空旷感为穿刺成功之指证，此仅表明已刺入骶裂沟内。穿刺成功后回抽无血，推药无阻力，局部亦无隆起时，即可缓慢分次注药 10~20 ml 药应在 5 分钟注完。麻醉剂用量如用利多卡因，一般为 10 ml 左右，最少曾用 4 ml，如用普鲁卡因一般为 20 ml 左右。注药时随时针刺骶尾、肛周皮肤，以该区体表痛觉消失的变化做为麻醉成功的指导。注毕拔针，即可手术。

3.3.4 麻醉效果

20余年来作者经几千例应用，积累了一些经验，获得满意效果。通过不断地研究，麻醉成功率逐年上升，失败率逐年下降，1966年失败率为 5.1%；67年为 2.1%；68年为 1.1%；69年后无一例失败。

麻醉潜伏期亦逐年缩短。66年~67年，为 5~15 分钟。5分钟内奏效者占 50%。68年多为 5 分钟左右。5 分钟内奏效者近占 80%。69年 75% 立即生效。

其有效麻醉时间，采用 2% 普鲁卡因多为 50~70 分钟，如加入 1：1000 肾上腺素 0.1~0.25 ml 或用 2% 普鲁卡因与 0.1% 地卡因混合液，有效期即可延长。此外亦可采用追加法。

麻醉中，病人平妥，较少反应，血压、脉搏、呼吸多无变化。可发生轻微头晕、恶心、心悸、胸闷、血压升高；亦有发生抽搐、痉厥者。前者症状轻微，历时短暂，经片刻休息，即渐消失，可不予特殊处理。后者需注射镇静剂，如安定、鲁米那钠等，即渐复正常。

3.3.5 腰俞穴麻醉临床应用的一些具体问题

1. 关于取穴标志

腰俞为督脉之俞穴，位于第 21 椎及其下宛宛中，即长强上 3 寸和下髎之中心。按现代解剖学即位居第 4 骶椎及其下之骶骨裂孔，为骶管的下进路。骶裂孔与骶管的变异较多，国内外很早已引起重视，并进行了细致考证。尽管其外形不一，但基本是一个长形裂沟。其上被覆坚韧的骶尾韧带，因此骶裂沟之名即能基本代表其实际外貌。

国人骶裂沟的外形，书中记载以三角形为最多。其骨性标志，三角形的上角为骶中嵴末端膨隆处，三角形的两下角即左右骶角。三角形中央为标准骶管麻醉的穿刺点。由于骶裂沟的外形不一，除三角形是取穴的标志外，还发现三角形下有一个正方形（或梯形或长方形）也是取穴的标志，这个正方形上面的标记为两骶角，下面的标记是两尾角。因此体表定位时，这个三角形和正方形的 5 个骨突，不管找到其中几个都能比较容易的找出该穴的部位，而使取穴的定位技能大大提高。

2. 穿刺成功与麻醉成功

穿刺成功的标志是阻力顿然消失。因骶裂沟被覆骶尾韧带，故穿刺时有阻力消失的空旷感。骶裂沟尖端（头端）即连骶管，底部（尾端）紧接尾骨，由底部向上可有深度变化。一般其尖端较其他处为深。常用的穿刺点为骶角间及其前后，此处深度为 1.5 cm 左右。如骶裂沟较长，可将其分为 3 部分，即上部、中部、下部。上部为骶中脊末端膨隆处下，此区穿刺注药易失败；中部为骶角间及其前后，此区穿刺注药易成功；下部为尾角间，此区穿刺注药，只获得部分区域麻醉效果，即后部麻醉，不能满足临床要求。如骶裂沟较短，此 3 部区分即不明显，但穿刺部位，仍以骶角间为标准。

穿刺成功与麻醉成功二者虽有密切关系但并非一回事。就腰俞穴麻醉来说，穿刺成功仅表明刺入骶裂沟内，麻醉效果如何，还要在注药时随时观察。骶裂沟的刺点由上至下不止一处，但并非所有刺点都能顺利成功。及时有效地发挥麻醉作用的刺点，应该严格选择。因骶裂沟在骶管下部，故可推知既往把骶管麻醉的失败，多归咎于解剖的变异，是不够正确的。

3. 腰俞穴麻醉的规律性

临床发现，在骶尾、肛周这个较小的范围内，体表痛觉消失区域是由上至下由后至前逐渐扩大的。这个现象对指导麻醉成功起着决定的作用。注药后如体表痛觉消失区迟迟不降，表明刺点低，应拔出针头向上移位，重新穿刺。如上述区域全无麻醉，表时刺点高，药液及时进入骶管，应拔出针头向下移位，重新穿刺。这种以患者相应部位体表痛觉消失的情况为指导，及时变换穿刺部位的方法，不仅使麻醉潜伏期多不存在，而且保证了麻醉的成功。

4. 腰俞穴麻醉的实质

认识尚不一致。我们数年的细致观察，认为腰俞穴麻醉并非骶管麻醉。如是骶管麻醉，为什么部分患者药液及时进入骶管后反而无麻醉效果？何知进入骶管？根据穿刺成功的指征，药液进入骶裂沟是确切无疑。失败的患者多数其穿刺点在小三角形上部，愈靠上进针愈深，此说明刺入部位愈近骶管，甚或进针区就是骶管下口，故药液的流向自然很易及时进入骶管。骶裂沟的神经鞘膜可能比骶管内的神经鞘膜薄，2%普鲁卡因即能很快阻断。但进入骶管后，因药液穿透力差，故在一定时期内反而无麻醉作用。

因此，我们认为腰俞穴麻醉的实质即骶裂沟的区域阻滞，可有药液侵及骶管下部。全面地说，腰俞穴麻醉即骶裂沟及其上端邻近部位（骶管下端小部分）的区域阻滞。

药液穿透力强，（如利多卡因），穿刺点的选择不若前述严格。在骶裂沟上下刺入，阻断亦可完善并能扩散至骶管。因刺点不当而致的麻醉区别。被药液穿透力部分的弥补了。如果我们开始就用利多卡因，腰俞穴麻醉的实质即被掩盖。

关于其麻醉范围，与低位骶管阻滞的范围一致，如加大剂量阻滞平面更高，这是可以理解的。因骶裂沟在骶管下部，二者无明显间隔，如由此注药，多余药液自然进入骶管或更高部位，再加药液穿透力强，虽然以阻滞骶裂沟为主体但也收到了骶管麻醉的效果，这与将麻药直接注入骶管是有区别的。

其潜伏期的长短，我们认为与穿刺点的选择和局麻药液的穿透力有关。在限量同浓度的用药前提下，如不注意选择刺点，就会产生长短不等的潜伏期。我们应用 2% 普鲁卡因 20 ml，5 分钟注完后多已完全麻醉，手术可立即进行，不必再等一定时间，但最初几年，潜伏期为 5~15 分钟，这主要与穿刺部有关。须待药液扩散至主理肛门、会阴部的主要神经以后，才能完全麻醉。当然时间愈长，阻断愈完善。后以患者相应部位体表痛觉消失的情况为指导，及时变换穿刺部位，使潜伏期在 5 分钟注完药的速度条件下已不存在。潜伏期的消失或甚短，是通过穿刺点的严格选择达到的。而药液穿透力强及药量增大对缩短潜伏期亦起一定作用。

致于用药量，与骶管用量相似，以此证明为骶管麻醉理由亦不充分。由此处注药，如药量多除阻滞骶裂沟外，即可进入骶管或更高部位。大量注药其多余药液之去向亦自然如此。但因药液穿透力不同，进入骶管后亦可有不同效果。骶裂沟之容积到底多大，没有单独这方面的研究。既往所称骶管的容积是否包括骶裂沟在内，尚不明确。

总之，在活体广义来说，此麻醉法为寓于骶管内的特定区域阻滞，如从麻醉学和解剖学观点来看，则称为骶裂沟麻醉，此自然有别于骶管麻醉，就骶管麻醉来说，过去人们只以骶裂沟作为骶管麻醉穿刺的进路，而不作阻滞区域。此麻醉法却将骶裂沟作为阻滞区域，即此区穿刺，此区注药，这不仅是简化了骶管麻醉的操作程序，而阻滞区域偏下，故仅适于肛门部手术。如再掌握体表痛觉消失的规律，可无麻醉潜伏期或甚短。因此腰俞麻醉丰富了骶部麻醉法。

5. 应用时的注意事项

骶裂沟在骶管下部,为硬脊膜外腔的一部分,故此麻醉亦为硬脊膜外麻醉。其与骶管相连,多量注药可进入骶管,因此麻醉注意事项与骶管麻醉相似。

(1) 注药前定要抽吸,无回血方可注药,否则麻药进入血液,可致中毒。

(2) 注药应缓慢,此可避免吸收过速和骶裂沟内压力突然变化所致的中毒样反应。

(3) 严格选择刺点,注意相应区域体表痛觉消失的变化,可使麻醉成功率达 100%,潜伏期全无或甚短。

(4) 刺针宜细短,进针宜浅不宜深。

3.4 其他麻醉

3.4.1 腰麻

小剂量为宜,普鲁卡因用量一般为 60~70 毫克,小剂量腰麻,麻醉范围呈鞍状,故又称鞍麻。

3.4.2 腰骶段硬脊膜外麻醉

效果好,操作技术要求较高。

3.4.3 冷冻麻醉

适于脓肿切开。

3.4.4 静脉麻醉、全身麻醉等

较少应用。

4 肛门直肠手术前后处理与术后反应并发症的处理

4.1 肛门直肠手术前后处理

手术前后处理甚为重要,术前充分准备,术后正确处理,可使患者减少痛苦,治疗过程顺利。

4.1.1 术前准备

1. 宜适当休息,并保持乐观精神,对治疗具有信心。
2. 作好全身与局部检查。
3. 饮食:一般饮食照常,不予限制,必要时可酌情控制。
4. 皮肤准备:有条件时洗澡一次或局部坐浴,术前局部剃毛。
5. 肠道准备

(1) 灌肠:一般不灌肠,术前1日下午2时,用番泻叶6~9克泡水代茶饮,以清除结肠内积粪。亦可服用蓖麻油20 ml,以通便。如行无菌手术,术前清洁灌肠。

(2) 应用肠道抗菌药:痔瘘手术绝大多数勿需作此准备,如行无菌手术,术前3天可用抗生素或化学抗菌药。

(3) 镇静剂:术前15~30分钟应用鲁米那钠0.1克足三里穴位注射。

4.1.2 术后处理

1. 一般注意事项

(1) 手术结束后,应护送患者至门诊休息室或病房,使静卧休息。门诊患者术后休息半小时左右,如无出血即可回家,但不得骑自行车。

(2) 随时询问患者有何痛苦,注意观察其病情。

(3) 按时给住院患者测量体温、脉搏、呼吸和血压。

(4) 术后发生疼痛、排尿障碍、出血等反应与并发症时，应及时处理。

(5) 创口未愈期间，宜适当休息，勿剧烈活动并避免房事。

2. 饮食：一般术后饮食如常，或手术当日略加控制。但不应食刺激性食物。对肉类食品，前人经验忌食狗肉和无鳞鱼。但因个体之差异，术后几日内有人食羊肉后则创口疼痛加剧，有人食鸡肉后则分泌物增多，但食一般无鳞鱼如带鱼则无妨。因此术后几日内宜素食，多吃蔬菜或水果。

3. 调理大便：术后当日勿大便，此后大便如常。如无菌手术须控制大便3~5天，每日可服10%阿片酊1~2次，每次5~10ml。控制大便者，每次排便前除服润肠剂外并应灌肠，术后务使大便通畅并避免腹泻。

4. 换药：痔瘘术后换药有重要意义，因此每次换药必须细心认真。

换药方法：换药前患者先解大便，便后坐浴熏洗。换药时，患者取骑伏位，医者以左手母食二指分开创口，另手取换药镊子，夹盐水棉球清洁创面，创口周围可用酒精棉球擦拭。痔核或肛裂以九华膏（24）换药，可用小棉球外涂九华膏放至创口和肛内，亦可用甘油灌肠器将九华膏注至创口和肛内。瘘管换药，应将创口尽量分开，由外而内拭净创口分泌物，后敷生肌玉红膏（25）纱布块。如创缘易闭合或有窦道时可用药布填塞，后外贴敷料固定。

换药注意事项：

(1) 操作仔细轻柔，尽量减轻疼痛。

(2) 创面肉芽不鲜或腐败组织较多，可用红粉油膏（26）或猫眼草膏（27）换药。

(3) 肉芽组织过长，可用硝酸银棒或硝酸银液腐蚀，亦可剪修。

(4) 换药时,应检查是否有支管遗留,或存在其他妨碍愈合的因素。如有支管残存,当挤压切口边缘时,可有脓液溢出。拭净脓液后,可找到出脓口,然后再以探针检查,了解管道的深浅、长度和方向。

(5) 肛瘘创口深大创缘易闭合者,切口内应予填塞,使创面保持开放状态,新生肉芽可自底部逐渐生长,避免创面粘连,桥形假愈。

(6) 肛门或切口周围皮肤红肿糜烂或形成丘疹、水疱痒痛不适时,必须同时治疗。可用清热解毒祛湿剂内服或熏洗,局部可涂祛湿、止痒药粉或药膏等。

(7) 注意患者全身情况的调理。如身体虚弱或术后创口生长较慢,愈合迟缓,或流脓水较多创面不鲜时,应辅服滋补强壮健脾生肌之剂,如补中益气汤(6)、十全大补汤(28)、生肤汤(29)等。

4.2 术后反应与并发症的处理

肛门直肠疾病术后可发生某种反应或并发症,给患者带来不同程度的痛苦,因此必须注意解决。主要反应与并发症的处理如下。

4.2.1 疼痛

疼痛是痔瘘病术后最主要的反应,因肛门皮肤感觉灵敏,故疼痛易于发生,对患者影响较大。其程度有轻有重,轻者仅觉局部不适,对全身无明显影响,重者坐卧不安,呻吟,身出大汗,影响饮食和睡眠。其性质有胀痛、灼痛、刺痛、坠痛或跳痛等,可为持续性,一般术后1～2日内较重,以后渐缓解。但损伤或刺激时(如大便、换药),可使疼痛一时性加剧或即时发作。

术后疼痛的因素除与肛门区感觉灵敏有直接关系外,患者的精神状况,耐受的程度,术中麻醉方式的适当与否,病变范围大小,损伤的轻重等均有一定的影响。因此消除或减轻术后疼痛,必须从全面考虑和着手。

处理

（1）选择适宜的麻醉方式，注意无痛无菌操作，局麻时深浅适当，阻断完全，可用长效止痛剂，如术后用美兰长效止痛剂（30）封闭止痛效果可持续 7～15 天。

（2）术前术后很好安慰患者，解除疑虑。必要时术前应用镇静剂。

（3）手术、换药应操作轻柔，确保大便通畅，及时消除炎症。

（4）应用镇痛等药物：据疼痛轻重缓急酌情给于镇痛剂。一般只服止痛片，重时可注止痛针，可配镇静药。对病变范围广泛，损伤较重或伴有炎肿等现象者，可辨证服用中药。常用方药为止痛如神汤（31）等。

（5）针刺止痛：镇痛迅速，无副作用。针刺时应注意手法的运用，一般用强刺激法，至疼痛消失或减轻时再予留针，也可用电针。取穴：承山、气衡、长强、八髎、骶侧等。亦可应用耳针，在耳轮找出反应点，用毫针刺激后再埋皮内针固定，或用压豆疗法，平日可随时按压埋针处或压豆点，以减轻疼痛。

（6）磁疗：以磁铁置腰俞穴，胶布固定。如无头晕、恶心呕吐等反应，可带几日。置磁铁后一般约 5 分钟疼痛即渐缓解，如所用磁铁磁场强度较大，则镇痛效果颇为显著，实为痔瘘术后镇痛措施之进展。也可用电磁铁止痛。

4.2.2 坠胀

由刺激引起，如机械刺激、炎症刺激等。患者可觉肛门下坠不适，或有胀满感。因下坠往往引起便欲而使大便次数增多，有时欲便不易排出，或有里急后重感。

处理

（1）去除刺激因素：坠胀为直肠刺激症状，如因手术刺激、损伤，一般术后几日即可缓解。如为痔结扎手术，有时痔块脱落后，坠胀方可减轻。对下坠重者可服秦艽丸（32）或止痛如神汤（31）。

(2) 卧床休息：姿势对坠胀有一定影响，一般站立或蹲踞时间较长，可加重坠胀感，而卧床时则坠胀减轻。因此，如坠胀重时可卧床休息，不要过多活动。

(3) 针刺疗法：收效不如镇痛明显，可结合采用。此外应注意，如将痔瘘术后因坠胀所致便频，疑为肠炎等并取大便送检，则实属错误。如大便检出红、白细胞或脓球，亦非肠道另有炎变，为痔瘘创口之影响，故此时粪检已无实际意义。

4.2.3 排尿障碍

亦较常见，多发于术后当日，亦有持续几日者。其因不一，但主要由于反射所致，肛门区因手术刺激、损伤和疼痛等均可发生反射性排尿障碍。此外肛道填塞压迫，精神因素以及无卧床排尿习惯等亦可引起。有时则为几种因素综合所致。其症状轻者仅为小便费力，排出不畅，或呈点滴状，重者数小时内不能解出，发生一时性尿潴留，而致膀胱膨隆，下腹胀痛，十分痛苦。亦有尿痛者，有时牵及下腹部。此外部分患者，术后虽数小时未能排尿，但检查小腹并不充盈，此种情况并非排尿障碍，乃膀胱尿量尚小，稍待时刻自然解出。

处理

(1) 解除顾虑，饮水多少无妨，可饮茶水。无卧床排尿习惯者，站立排尿。

(2) 热敷或冷敷：小便不能排出可于下腹置热水袋，半小时左右，即可试解，如仍不能排出，可继续热敷，或换用冷敷，亦可先冷敷无效时再热敷。通过温热或寒冷刺激，即可引起排尿，惟冷敷冬季不宜应用。

(3) 针刺治疗：方法简单，收效满意。针刺时注意手法的运用。取穴：三阴交、阴陵泉、关元、水道,可配止痛穴位。

(4) 推拿按摩：可于两大腿内侧自下而上反复按摩数次至有

尿意时为止。亦可指压中极穴（脐下四指）2～5分钟。或用镇江膏药或狗皮膏烤软，掺入0.25克冰片揉合，外贴关元、中极穴。也可用葱熨法，即将大葱捣烂加热，以纱布包之熨脐或小腹。

(5) 如无出血可能，取出肛内填塞物。男性患者亦可用大蒜刺激尿道口。必要时术后当日亦可坐浴薰洗肛门。一般导尿较少采用。

(6) 应用 APC 和 CNB 治疗：卢克杰氏用复方阿斯匹林（APC）0.75克，苯甲酸钠咖啡因（CNB）0.3克，一次顿服，一般排尿障碍者服药后30～40分钟即可顺利排尿。亦可用APC0.8克，CNB0.25克肌注，20分钟小便排出，效果更好。如持续几日排尿不畅者，可辨证服用中药。常用方药为五苓散(33)、八正散 (34)、通脬汤 (35) 加减。

4.2.4 出血

痔瘘术后出血原因较多，但以局部因素为主。其中包括术中止血不良，术后活动过度，干燥粪便损伤，炎症影响等。少数者全身有出血因素。

出血情况根据时间、性质、血量多少可作如下分类：

按时间可分即时性和续发性出血。即时性出血发生于术后当日，主要因术中止血不良所致；续发性出血多发于术后半月内，其中续发性大出血是一严重并发症，目前采用的一些手术疗法尚难完全避免，此多发生于痔块枯脱期。

按出血流向的部位可分向内出血和向外出血。向内出血即血液流入直肠和结肠。因肛门括约肌痉挛和填塞压迫的影响，使肛道阻塞，血不能或不易流出，故向内流入直肠和结肠腔内。其初始因出血量少，患者可无任何感觉。但随流入血量的逐渐增多，患者感到下腹胀满不适，欲大便，或觉肛门灼热。但当不能控制便欲而大便时，肠内积血迅速排出，血液多呈暗褐并有黑色血块。此时因大量积血迅速排除，患者可觉心慌、头晕眼黑、四肢无力、甚至晕倒。其面色苍白,出冷汗,脉搏细弱而数,血压下降。向内出血,初期易于忽略,因出血未能及时制止,常使病情由轻转重,给患者造成严重损失。因此必须特别注意,密切观察病情变化,及时发现及时治疗。向外出血即血液由切口流出,浸染敷料、衣物,患者可觉肛门灼热不适,或觉有水外流,呈阵发性或持续性。此类出血易于发现。

按出血量多少可分大量、中量和少量出血。前二者出血量多,病情较重,多为续发性亦有即时性者,必须及时处理;后者出血量少,可为即时性或续发性,对全身无明显影响。

其症状体征各类出血均有特点,已如上述。总之,大量急性出血,出血量多而急,症状体征明显,严重时可出现休克;少量缓慢出血,出血量少而缓,除向外出血可以及时察见外,一般无明显症状体征。

处理 痔瘘术后出血原因虽多,但以局部因素为主。其防治措施应注意以下几点:

(1) 认真选择适应症,遵循每种疗法的操作原则。术中止血完善。

(2) 术后勿过度活动,确保大便通畅,避免干燥粪便损伤。

(3) 注意消除炎症。

(4) 痔块枯脱期局部避免过热刺激。如熏洗时可用温药水,时间宜短。

(5) 术后少量便血可服止血药物或注意观察不予特殊处理。多量出血应详细观察病情,密切护理,注意血压、脉搏等变化,并迅速作好止血准备。

痔瘘术后出血,其处理要点有3:即及时制止出血,安静卧床休息,控制饮食及大便。

(1) 及时制止出血:制止出血主要采用两种方式,即应用止血药物和局部施以合理的止血措施。

应用止血药物:一般常用维生素K、安络血、凝血质、止血敏、三七粉、中药煎剂等。其用量多少，给药时间及方式，可视病情而定。

局部施以合理的止血措施，根据出血量多少可用不同方法。少量出血，如为渗血，更换敷料后重新压迫包扎，或局部再用止血散（36）、明矾粉等止血药物；渗血快时可重新钳夹结扎，亦可用硝酸银等腐蚀药物涂于出血处；如有出血点须钳夹结扎，亦可烧灼或腐蚀。

大、中量出血，即时性出血者，须缝合出血区创面，或将出血区游离粘膜与粘膜下组织缝着固定。必要时结扎出血创面上部的痔血管。续发性出血者处理较为困难，因多发于痔块枯脱阶段，此期组织脆弱不易缝合。故既往多用填塞压迫止血法。压迫方法有以下几种：

纱卷压迫：取一中空硬橡皮管，长约 8～10 cm，外裹凡士林纱布块，粗细可灵活掌握，如较粗可去掉几层，细时可再加添，一般应略粗些，直径约 5 cm。将纱卷备好后，如凡士林较少可再涂润滑油，取纱卷缓慢放入肛道。为防纱卷滑入直肠上部，在纱卷外端连同橡皮管穿一粗丝线，扎于覆盖的敷料上。

纱布块压迫：取一大纱布块将其缕成条状，亦可外裹一层油纱布，于此粗纱条中央系一粗丝线，以钳夹持纱布一端缓慢送入直肠，注意线留肛外，随即伸入手指触摸纱布送入情况并将纱布推至直肠壶腹。牵拉丝线向外，将纱布由壶腹大部拉入肛管，因丝线牵拉，纱布被折成两股，压迫较紧，为防压迫纱布上滑，将牵拉丝线于肛外再系于小纱卷上。上述 2 法为持续压迫，一般压迫 3～5 天。

气囊压迫：取气囊放入直肠内，然后充气使其膨隆，即起压迫作用，气囊外端以钳钳夹。或用避孕套代替气囊，将此套于一硬棒上，并放入套内一细胶管，于套口端连同细胶管松松扎一丝线，将套放入直肠，由细胶管充气使避孕套膨隆，后将丝线扎紧。用气囊压迫法，可视病情间歇压迫，即压迫一定时间将气放掉，稍待时刻再充气压迫，此可减轻压迫时痛苦。

采用压迫止血法同时须控制饮食，控制大便，应用止血药物，又因局部压迫，给患者造成不同程度的痛苦。有人在出血区上方粘膜下注射硬化剂，虽可获得满意效果，但采用时因麻醉、注射等刺激，对患者亦可带来一定程度的痛苦。

我们根据过去给直肠癌患者灌肠的经验，对内痔便血和痔术后出血，用明矾液（37）灌肛试治，自1965年起，经过反复实践，后又用明矾膏涂布出血区，均获得满意效果。

此种止血法有很多优点，操作简便，效果确实，无痛苦，用费低廉，药源广，不需控制饮食和大便，局部不必再行手术性止血措施，是一简便、验、廉的止血法。

明矾液灌肛方法：取明矾粉若干克，放入盛器内，以温水溶化，制成所需浓度。或以热水溶化，温后再用。以甘油灌肠器吸入明矾液直接缓慢注入肛内。亦可用导尿管插入肛内，以空针缓慢注药。注完药后嘱患者静卧休息，使药液在肠内至少保留半小时以上，至便意窘迫，无法忍耐时，方可排出。灌后无便意，不必主动排便，应尽量延长药液保留时间。

明矾膏涂布方法：取较多明矾粉放入九华膏（24）内，搅匀即可（此简称明矾膏）。以明矾膏涂布出血区，可用纱布块或凡士林纱布块或生肌玉红膏（25）等纱布块布满此药，以钳夹持缓慢放入肛道。但应先行指诊，判定出血部位，以便将药布放至出血区，药布一般应大些，便于覆盖。续发大出血，其出血区多不平坦，创面周边高突，粘膜游离。有时可触得粘膜游离之缝隙。如粘膜游离范围较大，药布放入后可再行指诊，触摸药布放入情况，将堆积折叠处铺平并完全覆盖出血区。如将明矾膏注入肛内，明矾过多时不易由灌肠器推出，应于调整。

临床应用明矾液或明矾膏的几个具体问题：

药物浓度、用量及给药次数：以明矾液灌肠，应据出血不同情况，灵活掌握药液浓度及用量。如仅见出血先兆，可用1～

2%明矾液 100～200 ml。如已大出血，浓度，用量即可增加，一般用 2～3%明矾液 300 ml 左右。我们应用最高浓度为 8%，一次最大量为 500 ml。给药次数亦应视病情而定，一般每日 1 次，可连灌 2 天，必要时可每日 3 次。以明矾膏涂布出血区，因将明矾粉与九华膏混合，明矾用量相对增多。九华膏与明矾粉之比，为 1∶1 或 2∶1 或 3∶1。给药次数每日 1 次，至出血停止。出血当日用药后如已排便，可再给药。

出血制止的观察和预测：灌肠后排出之大便往往血、粪、药液混杂，可观察血粪情况，以便测知出血是否制止。如有较多鲜血，说明出血速度较快，出血一直未停。对此种出血，一次灌肠能否完全收效，尚难判定，仍须密切观察。如血、粪混合物呈暗褐色或紫黑色，说明出血速度较慢，此种出血，一次灌肛可能制止。即使仍有渗血，亦能自行停止。为安全起见，次日可再给药。如粪便已无血色或其中仅有少许褐色积血时，即不再灌肛。以时间推测，灌药大便后如超过 5～8 小时未再排便，出血可能已止。用明矾膏涂布，对出血制止的观察和预测与灌肠法大体相同，但涂布法因给药体积小，可减少刺激，避免或延迟排便，故可避免或延迟续发性大出血休克的发生。

明矾液或明矾膏止血依据：明矾性寒味酸涩，能燥湿祛痿、杀虫、解毒、收敛、止血。此总取其酸涩寒咸之功。

应用注意事项：

a. 灌肛时药液温度不宜过凉，亦不宜过热，应为温药水。因明矾性寒，如药液过凉，对胃肠虚寒的患者，灌后可致腹痛，可做热敷等对症处理。

b. 灌肠器插入肛道时动作轻柔，注药宜缓慢。

c. 灌肠器及导尿管不可插入过深，以注药时，无药液自然外溢为度。一般仅插入 2 cm 左右。

d. 灌后应尽量延长药液保留时间。

e. 涂药前应先判定出血部位，以便将药膏更好地放至出血区。

其他措施的配合：可酌用止血药，但不必控制饮食和大便。如发生休克，应作相应急救。

对术后即时性大出血可做辅助措施。术后即时性大出血即术中由于操作失当致使术后当日所发生的大出血。此种出血在结扎或缝合出血部位后，亦可应用明矾灌肠或涂布作为辅助止血措施。我们曾有一例内痔结扎患者，因结扎线滑脱，当日发生大出血。此例未再结扎、缝合，用8%明矾液200ml，日灌肛3次，出血亦完全制止。此外结扎息肉时，如息肉当即脱落，为防出血亦可应用明矾灌肠。

(2) 静卧休息：大、中量出血须卧床休息，如用压迫止血法卧床有助于减少出血。大出血待出血停止体力大体恢复后即可下床活动。少量出血可适当休息，经即时处理后勿须卧床，便后带血，活动不必限制。

(3) 控制饮食及大便：少量出血且及时制止后，一般饮食，大便如常。大、中量出血如用压迫止血法，应控制饮食和大便。控制时间一般至填塞压迫物取出时为止，约需3~5日。如取出填塞物后因压迫不善仍有出血时，可换用明矾涂布法，饮食、大便亦不再控制。此期间所进饮食视患者体质不同而定，一般食流质，或流质半流质间用。控制大便可服阿片剂，如服阿片片，每次1片，日服2次。

压迫止血结束后，即恢复正常饮食。为防便秘，取出填塞物后可服润肠药。首次大便前应该灌肠。

(4) 大量出血时应据不同情况及时补液或输血，发生休克时应作相应急救。

4.2.5 发热

术后1~3天内发热，白细胞正常或稍高，多为局部刺激反应性发热，亦有因术中出汗多，不慎感冒而发热者，如为低热又无全身明显症状，一般不需处理。如高热可根据全身不同病情，辨证服用中药。如手术几日后高烧，白细胞明显增高，则为感染，可服中药或用抗生素等。

4.2.6　局部肿胀

因感染、静脉及淋巴回流障碍所致。如不注意无菌操作，局麻影响，手术损伤，创口处理不当等均可引起。其创缘红肿或水肿，可影响邻近肛缘皮肤或使整个肛门肿胀高突。亦可激惹未处理内痔急性发作脱垂嵌顿，或肛门皮下片状淤血及形成血栓外痔等。

处理：除术中注意操作外，如肿胀已发生，以薰洗治疗为主。用复方荆芥洗药（38）每日薰洗2～3次，每次半小时至1小时。

4.2.7　湿疹及皮炎

主要因过敏所致，局部炎症及分泌物刺激亦有一定影响。其皮肤红肿糜烂或形成丘疹、水疱，痒痛不适。重者病变不仅限于局部亦可遍及全身。

处理：可用清热、解毒、祛风、除湿剂内服、薰洗和外涂（如青蛤散）（39），或并用其他脱敏药。

4.2.8　创口愈合迟缓

创口久不愈合可能有两种因素，全身虚弱或局部存有不利于愈合之因素。

处理

（1）可服补气血之剂，如十全大补汤（28）、补中益气汤（6）、生肤汤（29）等。

（2）去除局部不利愈合之因素。可选用不同药膏外涂，如红粉油膏（26）、猫眼草膏（27）等。

（3）维生素 B_1 穴位注射。取维生素 B_1 50～100 ml，左右足三里穴交替注射，每日或隔日1次，至创口愈合为止。连用1月时可休药10天。

（4）可用保健针刺激创口周围，每日1～2次。

4.2.9 肛门狭窄及大便失禁

肛门狭窄较为少见。如术中切除肛门皮肤过多，肛管损伤较重，或结扎痔块枯脱期粘膜粘连等则可引起。轻者可予扩肛，必要时切开狭窄区。

大便失禁甚为少见，其形成原因较为复杂。如括约肌严重受损，神经机能失调，直肠压力变化等均可引起。根据失禁轻重一般分为两类：

完全性失禁：肛门全无或几无控制功能，成形粪便自出，自行恢复较难。故又称永久性失禁或不可复性失禁。但临床观察，此类失禁，时日已久亦有部分控制功能恢复。

不完全性失禁：肛门控制功能较差，可慢慢自行恢复。又称部分失禁或暂时性或可复性失禁。

其处理依失禁轻重而不同，轻者可不处理，待其自然恢复。重者可辨证服用中药或针刺治疗，必要时行括约肌成形术。

5 痔

笼统的说，凡肛门内外生有小肉突起，均称为痔，也叫痔核或痔块。两千年前我国古代医学家即认为痔是血管病变。痔为常见病多发病，俗有"十人九痔"之说。

5.1 病因病机

祖国医学对痔的病因论述颇为详尽，认识亦较全面。如《内经》认为痔是血管病变，《素问·生气通天论》说："因而饱食，筋脉横解，肠澼为痔"，此为痔的血管曲张学说世界最早提出者，前人对痔的病因学认识，既重视整体内因，又注意局部外因。下面简要总括历代所述。

5.1.1 整体与内因

阴阳失调，脏腑本虚，气血亏损，情志内伤，以及遗传等因素。

5.1.2 局部与外因

1. 湿、热、风、燥四邪相合而致病。
2. 热邪伤阴、血热妄行及热毒蕴积。
3. 饮食影响：过食炙煿、肥腻、生冷、辛辣，或饮酒过量，或饥饱不均等。
4. 职业及起居影响：久坐久立，负重远行，或房事过度等。
5. 其他：长期便秘，泻痢日久，妊娠分娩等。

综上可知，我国古代医学家认为痔的发病为阴阳失调，脏腑气血虚损，再加湿热风燥等邪之作用和情志内伤，饮食起居职业等影响，致使气血失调，经络阻滞，瘀血浊气下注而成。痔是人类特有的病变,因人是直立行走动物,现代医学对痔的病因认识一向认为,痔的发生主要由于痔静脉丛的静脉内压升高和静脉壁的抵抗力减弱所致。但通过深入研究,对痔的本质问题提出了不同见解。除静脉曲张学说外,又提出血管增生学说,粘膜滑动学说等。

5.2 临床表现

5.2.1 分类

据现代医学结合临床实用,将痔区分如下:

1. 外痔:居齿线以下,被覆皮肤,由痔外静脉丛所形成,多数可直接观察到。外痔又分静脉曲张性外痔、结缔组织性外痔、血栓性外痔及炎性外痔等。

(1) 静脉曲张外痔:此种多见,一般无痛苦,大便或蹲踞努挣时,痔体显露充分,隆起更为明显。触摸时肿物柔软,常与内痔并发。轻者,不大便时局部并无肿物出现。

(2) 结缔组织外痔:此种亦多见,为肛缘增殖的皮垂,大小不等,故形容状如"鸡冠"、"鼠奶"、"莲籽"等。如无急性发炎,一般无明显痛苦。局部可潮湿,有时作痒,因便后不易擦净易污染衣裤。

(3) 血栓外痔:此种较多见,为肛缘皮下小血管破裂形成的瘀血团。由于慢性炎症,皮下血管壁弹性减弱,再受某种因素的影响,如排便用力努挣,饮酒过量等,使血管破裂,血液流溢皮下,当流溢的血液增多时,即可压迫出血处,而使出血自行停止。因出血多少不等,故瘀血团大小不一。一般可发生1个瘀血团,也有时发生2个或几个,甚至10余个,多个瘀血团同时发生时,也可大小不等,且多孤立存在,互不相连。但个别病人可发生特大瘀血团,占居肛门$\frac{1}{3}$或$\frac{1}{2}$或$\frac{2}{3}$,甚至整个肛周。瘀血痔块呈青紫色,稍硬,稍活动,有触疼。合并炎肿时,青紫色即不明显。触摸时有瘀血硬核。其发病突然,病情较急,痛苦较重,也有疼痛不重的。此病有自愈趋向,即数日后,瘀血可自行吸收或成一硬结。因此发病后应及早熏洗,促其吸收。

(4) 炎性外痔:为肛缘皱襞急性炎肿,疼痛较重、触摸时无瘀血之硬核。

2. 内痔:居齿线以上,被覆粘膜,由痔内静脉丛所形成,初期内痔体积较小居肛内,病久时痔体长大可脱出肛外。病情发展一般分3个阶段,即1期也叫初期,2期也叫中期,3期也叫后期或晚期。

1期:便血为主症,痔体小,不脱出,下血多无疼痛,色鲜红,便血量或多或少,出血方式如射如滴,即出血象箭射出或象水从管子里喷出那么快,也可一滴一滴地出血。

2期:便血脱垂并见,下血如前或更重,痔体渐渐长大,便时脱出,能自行复位,即脱出的痔核可自然复回肛内。

3期:脱垂为主症,便血可减少,痔体更大,脱出频,除排便脱出外,行路、站立过久或咳嗽时都可脱出,不能自行复位,需手托复位或卧床休息痔核慢慢纳回。内痔的主症为便血、脱垂,此3期区分,以痔脱垂为主要依据。即1期内痔不脱出;2期内痔能脱出,可自行复位;3期内痔脱垂重,不能自行复位。亦有分4期者,4期内痔脱垂更重。

按痔的病理改变内痔可分3型:

血管肿型:形如杨梅,朱红或紫红色,粘膜菲薄,易出血,触之柔软。

静脉瘤型:痔核表面里丛状或屈曲状隆起,色青紫或暗红,痔粘膜增厚可有光泽,出血较少,触软。

纤维肿型:痔核一般较大,因结缔组织增殖而质韧,色淡红或略呈白色,痔粘膜糜烂、粗糙,或包以纤维膜,不易出血,触之略硬。

此外有人依据痔核外貌之不同,结合发病年龄而将内痔分为两型。即血管型和粘膜型，又称血管痔和粘膜痔。血管痔多见于青年患者，粘膜痔多见于老年患者。

3. 混合痔：居齿线上下，被覆粘膜和皮肤，由痔外和痔内静脉丛所形成，内、外痔间无凹沟存在，而成一痔体。如内痔合并以结缔组织为主的外痔，内、外痔间无凹沟，此亦称混合痔。

5.2.2 症状与体征

痔病的主要病状与体征为便血、脱垂、肿痛、下坠、作痒等。

5.2.3 归经及其关联

痔病与大肠经、肺经、督脉、任脉、膀胱经、肝经、脾经、肾经等经脉有关。

5.3 诊断和鉴别诊断

通过视诊、触诊、窥镜等检查，根据痔的不同外貌即可作出诊断。如内痔则见齿线上有隆起物，朱红或紫红，质软，多个发生时一般彼此分界。临床观察内痔的好发部位为右前、右后、左中3处，此区所生内痔称原发痔或母痔。其他部位所生内痔称续发痔或子痔。根据痔的证候主要应对便血加以区别，可从血出时间、便血特点和血色鲜暗等方面与消化道其他出血性疾病相鉴别。

(1) 血出先后：先血后便此为近血，多为大肠下段出血；先便后血，此为远血，系大肠上段或胃、小肠出血。

(2) 痔便血特点：如粘膜有血性渗出物或擦伤时，则为带血。如痔粘膜糜烂时，每因增大腹压如蹲踞努挣，因压力递增可使痔血管团内压力骤增，而出现逼血外出之征，即便血呈点滴或喷射状。此种出血可称压力出血，为内痔便血的突出特点。

(3) 血色区别：内痔出血，血色鲜红；结肠出血，血色较暗；上消化道出血，便血呈黑焦油状。

5.4 临床治疗

5.4.1 内治法

主要适用于 1、2 期内痔，内痔脱垂嵌顿，血栓外痔，炎性外痔，或年老体弱或合并有其他严重疾病，不宜手术者。其具体治疗，根据历代所述结合临床体会，主要治则和方药为：

1. 辛温和血润燥疏风止痛。秦艽苍术汤（7）或止痛如神汤（31）。此为湿热风燥合而为病的代表治则和方药。如痔瘘肿疼、下坠、便血、局部潮湿作痒等均可服用。

2. 补阴凉血，清热利湿。凉血地黄汤（40）或槐角丸（10）。用治痔疮便血、肿痛等，主要适于实证，如痔病合并高血压、动脉硬化者更宜，唯肠胃虚寒者应少服。

3. 苦寒泻火或清热解毒。黄连解毒汤（41）或犀角地黄汤（42）等。用于热毒炽盛者。

4. 补气升提或气血双补或益气补血等。补中益气汤（6）、十全大补汤（28）、归脾汤（43）等。适于虚证者，此补益之法亦经常应用。

内治法在痔的治疗中起着重要作用，服药消痔是值得研究的内容。目前临床中，一般据痔的常见症状与体证作如下处理。

（1）便血：可辨证服药，根据虚实等病情选用上方。一般出血，可服荷叶丸（44）、槐角丸（10）、化痔丸（45）、脏连丸（46）、消痔片（47）、痔宁（48）、鸡肠散（49）、脏蒜方（50）等止血消痔之剂，或服安络血、维生素 K、维生素 C 等一般止血药。

（2）脱垂：可服补气升提之剂，如补中益气汤（6）等。

（3）肿痛下坠：可服止痛如神汤（31）或秦艽片（32）、秦艽白术丸（14）等。

（4）便秘或腹泻：可辨证服药，或服一般通便、止泻剂。

5.4.2 外治法

方法较多，包括枯痔、结扎、手术、熏洗、烟熏、熨炙、敷药、导便等。此治法亦可分非手术的一般疗法和手术操作的特殊治疗措施。根据临床实用有：

1. 熏洗法：为传统治痔的重要方法，有活血消肿、消炎止痛、收敛止痒等作用。如血栓性外痔、炎性外痔，内痔脱垂嵌顿、术后局部肿痛作痒时，除服药外应以熏洗为主。治疗时，取药煎汤或以开水浸泡，或用散剂冲水，乘热熏洗。可先熏后洗，或将浸药水之纱布挤出过多药液后，敷于患处。每日熏洗2～3次，每次半小时左右。所用方药甚多，上述病症可用复方荆芥洗药（38）或却毒汤（51）等。一般坐浴熏洗可用花椒、艾叶、朴硝、食盐、硼酸、过锰酸钾等直接浸水即可。

2. 敷药法：亦为传统治痔之法，用时将药物涂敷于患处或肛内，因局部和肛内均可直接给药，故效果较好，可与熏洗并用。其作用与熏洗法大体相同，并可用于祛腐、生肌、止血。多适于痔急性发作或术后换药等病情。所用方药甚多，其剂型有膏剂、散剂、栓剂等。可用药膏涂布患处或以棉球、纱条蘸药膏后纳入肛内，如九华膏（24）、明矾膏等，亦可用药膏制成大小不等的纱布块或纱条，敷贴创面。如用散剂可将药粉撒布患处或以水、植物油等调涂。栓剂原为塞药，只能纳入肛肠，不能涂布敷贴。因纳入肛内药栓溶化后，药物即作用于局部，故实为涂药之一种。

3. 灌肠法：将药液灌入肛内，有消炎止痛、活血消肿、收敛止血、除坠等功效。适于内痔血栓形成、内痔出血、肛管炎、痔术后续发性出血等。常用散剂以水调和，使成混悬液或溶液，用甘油灌肠器注入肛内，使主要作用于直肠下段病区，如明矾液灌肛止血即是其例。

4. 还纳法：以手法将脱垂痔体复位称还纳法，适于痔核脱出和脱垂嵌顿。还纳时取一纱块，上涂润滑剂或九华膏，食指或中指戴好指套后，隔此纱块推挤痔核。推送时先抵压痔核一侧，持续施加均等压力。如所压处痔体有所缩小时，可增大压力推送。抵压痔核之手指，可持续加压，勿压压抬抬或频繁移位，抵压一处即需片刻，此可使瘀血逐渐回流，痔体缩小，便于纳入。

如将一处痔体纳入肛内后又复脱出，可重新抵压推挤，至痔核推入肛内时，推挤之手指暂不取出，再抵压片刻，继之用另手挤按第二个欲还纳的痔核，当该痔核被推挤至肛口时，迅速抽出肛内手指，肛外手指继续向内推挤第二痔核，先纳入的痔核因受肛外痔核的挤压，即不再脱出。一般可先推送较大的痔体，小痔体则更易还纳。全部痔核复位后，以楔形纱垫加压包扎固定。其操作要点即以手指静静抵压痔核，两手可交替推挤复位。作者应用此法颇感得心应手，再加还纳时不必嘱患者时时哈气，可听其自然，故患者并不紧张，而医者也似静若无事，操作文雅而不手忙脚乱，实为一较理想的还纳法。

如麻醉后还纳虽较易于纳入痔体，但并不如此法简易，且麻醉时应注意无菌操作，避免感染。如脱垂嵌顿几日后，痔体虽已变黑，但未枯脱时，亦可试行复位。如已枯脱则不必强行推送，可熏洗或敷药治疗。

5. 枯痔法：为传统治痔的主要疗法，因剂型和用药方式不同，又分枯痔散疗法、枯痔丁疗法、枯痔液疗法。所用枯痔药有含砒（砷）和不含砒之别，如含砒枯痔散、枯痔丁和无砒枯痔散、枯痔丁等。枯痔液疗法实为注射疗法之一种，将在注射法中介绍。

(1) 枯痔散疗法

以枯痔散用水或油调涂于内痔表面，使痔核逐渐坏死脱落而痊愈。此法虽以药物涂布敷贴，但其作用与敷药法有别，如内痔能脱垂时则易敷药。如不能脱垂，可用棉球蘸唤痔散（23）塞肛内，激惹内痔变大脱出。涂枯痔散前，先用护痔膏（52）涂于内痔周围或用凡士林等纱条围于内痔周围，以防腐蚀正常组织。根据枯痔散效用大小，涂药次数不尽相同。可每日涂1次或2次或几次,或连涂几日间隔1天,亦可隔日1次。至痔核干枯变黑即可停药,待其自脱。后以另药生肌收口。

此法因疗程长,痛苦较大,目前已较少采用,但内痔脱垂嵌顿已有坏死时或内痔脱垂患者合并有全身某些疾病不能手术时,仍可应用。

(2) 枯痔丁疗法

以枯痔药丁插入痔内使痔萎缩或枯死,又称插药疗法。适于各期内痔和混合痔内痔部分。所用药丁以福建中医药研究所生产的含砒枯痔丁(21)为主。此药丁呈桔红色,为两端尖锐的针状物,长约3 cm,两端均可刺入痔内。药丁插法较多,如以插入药丁排列情况和刺入部位之不同,可分稀插法、较密插法和基底插法。前2法药丁与肠壁呈一定倾斜刺入痔体,后法药丁顺肠壁直接插入痔基部,刺入药丁排列成行,此可使整个痔核由基部坏死脱落。插药方式一般为手持插药,即以拇、食2指捏取药丁,刺入痔内,亦可用器械插药,即以插药枪或枯痔丁投药器。将药丁打入痔内,此适于稀插法和药丁不太尖锐者,下面仅介绍较密插法。

操作方法:取骑伏位或侧卧位,常规消毒麻醉,以手或组织钳将内痔牵出后固定,药丁与肠壁呈15°~45°倾斜,手持药丁向一方旋转插入或直接插入痔内,至适当深度时,一般插入半根或少半根,剪去药丁余端,药丁外露部分应离痔面约1~2 mm。小指端大痔核一般插4~5半根,痔多同时治疗时,用药总量以20~30半根为宜。术毕将痔体纳入,上九华膏(24)或消炎止痛膏(53),后每日换药一次,直至痊愈。

注意点:充分暴露,正确插丁。正确插丁即药丁插入深浅、用量多少、排列疏密必须适当。

6. 注射法

将药液注入痔内使痔萎缩或枯死,适于内痔。因注射药物不同,大体可分硬化剂和枯脱剂(枯痔液)。根据药物的作用,注射疗法可分2种。

(1) 硬化萎缩法：又称注射萎缩法或注射硬化法，即注药后痔块发生硬化萎缩。此法所用药液浓度较同类枯脱药液为低，可称弱性溶液。其注药量少，注射部位较浅，注后痔体略增大，粘膜基本不变色或呈淡白。应连续注药，或隔几日重复注射1次，直至痔块硬化萎缩为止。常用药液有5%鱼肝油酸钠，5%左右的石碳酸甘油或石碳酸植物油，1～5%明矾注射液（54）等。注药方法多在肛镜下进行，即在肛镜窥视下将药液注入痔内，亦可脱出后注药。

山西稷山痔瘘医院在此注射法的研究中提出母痔基底硬化疗法，使硬化萎缩法有了进展。此法主要介绍如下。

操作方法：常规消毒麻醉后，将戴有手套的左手指伸入肛内，仔细触摸右前、右后、左中3母痔区有无动脉搏动，一般选择痔核上动脉搏动处作为注射点。另手持注射针，于此3处肛缘稍外方进针，沿肛管向内穿刺至痔核基部上端，一般约进针3～4 cm。如此处无动脉搏动亦将药液注于此处，用扇形注射法，每处注药约1～2 ml，三母痔区注药量为4～7 ml。此为第一步操作，即母痔基底注药，然后再行痔体注药，此痔体注药与一般硬化法大体相同，唯注药量稍多。可先注较小的内痔，后注较大内痔，注药后内痔核稍有膨隆，一般总量4～6 ml。母痔基底注药和痔体注药总用量每次为8～15 ml。

注意事项

行母痔基底注射时一定将药液注射到内痔核上的痔动脉区，不能注射至括约肌内，以免发生疼痛、水肿和坏死。行痔体注药时，应将药液注至血管丛中，不可注入肌层和齿线下皮肤区。

近年北京中国中医研究院广安门医院、南京中医学院附属医院，根据祖国医学"酸可收敛"、"涩可固脱"的理论，分别应用中药五倍子和乌梅的有效成分柔酸和枸橼酸配制成注射液（55）（56），治疗内痔和混合痔获得良好效果，为注射硬化法的新进展。现以北京"消痔灵"（55）液为例介绍如下。

适应症：各期内痔和混合痔内痔部分

注射方法：取骑伏位或伏卧位或侧卧位，常规消毒、麻醉，肛内放入新洁尔灭棉球后并予扩张，此消毒棉球将被肛镜上推，有阻止污物下流之作用，故不必取出。以广口筒式斜面肛镜蘸滑润剂，缓慢插入肛道，抽出镜心观察直肠下段粘膜、痔核部位数目和大小，以便注射时心中有数。第2次插入肛镜后即可行痔体上粘膜下注射。此区又称高位或高平面注射，即注于痔的上界或痔的蒂部。史兆歧氏称此区为痔上方痔动脉区，即4步操作法的第1步注射区。先消毒注射区粘膜，如有粘液等物，可用纱布拭净。取吸有"消痔灵" 1∶1 稀释液的 10 ml 空针，用5号针头（齿科针头），刺入痔上粘膜下约 3～5 mm 深，注药使之胀满，一般用量 1～3 ml，转换肛镜视野，右后、左中、右前3区注完后，取出肛镜，高平面注射结束。继之以 2∶1 或 1∶1 稀稀液行痔体注射。此区又称低位或低平面注射，亦有叫痔间质注射者。史氏将痔体细分为粘膜下层、粘膜肌板上、齿线稍上方3个注射部位，即4步操作法的第2、3、4步注射处。此区注药时先后于痔中央和痔中部齿线上刺入粘膜下约 5 mm 深，注药后使痔充分胀满，一般用量 3～10 ml。注药后在菲薄的痔表面粘膜上可见微细血管纵横其上，此称红色条纹征，如痔纤维组织增殖较重或注药欠胀满时，此征象可不明显，如痔表面出现红色条纹征，痔体漫肿呈水泡状，为注药充分胀满之标志。若粘膜出现白色圆点，有如皮试丘疹，为刺入粘膜内之征，有表浅坏死可能，应停止注药，更换穿刺部位。如痔体某处仍为原状色泽或略有改变者，为注药不足，即变换刺点于该处刺入注药，使其胀满变色。应注意齿线上，勿遗漏注射区。3母痔依次注药，所余小痔同时注完。痔体注药应分区进行，注完1痔核后，再注另1痔核，因此需几次插入肛镜，而痔上粘膜下注射，仅1次插入肛镜，3区注药时变换肛镜视野即可。注药总量一般为 15～25 ml，大痔体可用至 30～40 ml。注毕肛内放一九华膏棉球或注入九华膏(24)，外贴敷料。此后每日或隔日换药 1 次。如痔未全消，7～10 日后可再次注射。痔体小时，勿需麻醉，可在肛镜下直接注药。

操作注意点：注意无菌操作；穿刺不宜太深，亦不可刺入粘膜内；回抽无血，方可注药；应使注区充分胀满，勿遗漏齿线上注射区；注药后当日勿解大便。

本疗法因用药量大，所用药液应于稀释，即用"消痔灵"原液一份加 1% 普鲁卡因一份配成 1∶1 稀释液，或原液稍多的近于 1∶1 低于 2∶1 的稀释液。注药后痔体迅速增大，每区约比原痔体增大几倍，因痔体被药液充填灌注，成倍增长，可产生直肠刺激症状，下坠不适。由于用药量增大，疗效明显提高，不仅 1、2 期小痔，3 期大痔体亦可消失，为有别于一般硬化疗法，此可称消痔注射法。既往硬化疗法，多用于 1、2 期内痔，3 期内痔痔体较大，血管丛增生扩张较重，并有不同程度的纤维增殖，因此如达到满意效果，即痔消而不致坏死，必用低浓度大剂量之法，取浓度较低之弱性溶液，加大用量，使药液均匀充满痔组织中，方能提高疗效。消痔注射法的要点即在于此。

(2) 枯死脱落法：又称注射枯脱法。即注药后痔核发生坏死脱落，此即枯痔液疗法。此法所用药液浓度较同类硬化液为高，可称强性溶液。其注药量多，注射部位略深，注药后痔体明显增大，粘膜变色，呈灰黑、暗黑、每个痔核一般注药一次。常用药液有内痔枯脱油 (57)，10% 氯化钙注射液 (58)，卤砂注射液 (59) 等。注射方法多需麻醉后将痔牵出注药，亦可在肛镜下注射。此法依据祖国医学枯痔疗法的机理，采用高浓度强性溶液注射，用于各期内痔，扩大了治疗范围，收到了较好效果。其与硬化法注射形式虽同，但实质已异，这给注射疗法开辟了新途径。

操作方法：常规消毒麻醉后，充分暴露内痔，将痔体牵出予以固定。据痔核大小以细针头注入枯痔液适量，至痔核饱满肿胀,痔粘膜变色为度,注毕将痔体纳入上九华膏(24),后每日换药1次。

注意点:注药勿过深。

7. 结扎法

结扎疗法是传统治痔的主要疗法,迄今已近千年历史。如《太平圣惠方》即有"用蜘蛛丝缠系痔鼠乳头,不觉自落"的记载。至明代已普遍采用。最早的结扎法较简单,前人称此法为"系",仅适于基底较细的痔体。如谓:"治外痔有头者,以药线系之"。所用物品有蜘蛛丝、马尾、蚕丝、药线等,现一般应用医用丝线,亦可用胶圈结扎。结扎方法较多,大体可分为以下几种:

(1) 单纯结扎:仅以线系,称单纯结扎。因操作方法不同可分非贯穿结扎和贯穿结扎。

非贯穿结扎。适于2、3期内痔,因操作简单,故有人将此法亦称单纯结扎法。

操作方法:常规消毒麻醉后,将痔牵出,用全牙血管钳于痔基部夹牢,取粗线丝系于钳下,将钳渐渐放松随之勒紧丝线,结扎结束。行此结扎法必需用全牙血管钳钳夹痔基部,以使痔基部变形,便于扎牢。

贯穿结扎法。适于2、3期内痔及混合痔,可用单线或双线系勒,如以扎线所呈状态之不同,可分"8"字结扎、花瓣结扎、套环结扎等。

操作方法:取骑伏位或臀高伏卧位或侧卧位。常规消毒。局麻或腰俞麻醉。以组织钳将痔核钳起,在痔基部穿针引线结扎之。如行"8"字结扎,则引线双股,如行套环结扎即环环相扣,则引线单根。具体结扎法,同外剥内扎法内痔之处理。术后每日换药,直至痊愈。

注意点:切记扎牢,勿使结扎线滑脱;多痔核同时结扎时,其间应保留正常粘膜。

(2) 结扎配合其他措施：即以结扎为主配合注射、切割等。如结扎配合注射称结扎注射法或注扎法，即结扎后又将痔体注药，此可促进坏死。结扎配合压缩称结扎压缩法或压扎法，即扎后将痔体注药，再用全牙血管钳把痔体压成纸薄状。结扎配合切割称结扎切割法，简称切扎、割扎、剪扎，又称外剥内扎、外切内扎等。此法适于环状混合痔的治疗。

操作方法

取骑伏位或臀高伏卧位，常规消毒，局麻或腰俞麻醉。以新洁尔灭棉球放入肛道后，用肛门拉钩暴露痔核，观察痔核部位和数目。用拉钩牵开欲处理痔核的对侧组织，此时内痔部分清楚可见。取组织钳将内痔牵起或牵至肛外，向外牵拉时，通常用两把组织钳先后牵提。于内痔基部稍上处穿针引线。如行"8"字结扎，则引线双股。如行套环结扎，则引线单根。先将穿线处上侧的内痔体轻轻结扎。然后将外痔剪切剥离至齿线稍上处，外痔创面呈梭形或V形。如遇出血点则钳夹止血，一般不必结扎，如需扎线时则留长线头，此可避免术后创面包埋，便于脱线或取线。外痔剥离后，再将穿线处下侧的内痔体结扎，如行"8"字结扎，最后将穿线处上下痔体扎于一起。结扎时牵提痔核的两把组织钳可交替松动，以利痔体扎牢。可剪除部分结扎痔体，修整外痔创缘，后将结扎痔体或痔体残端送入肛内。依法处理其他痔核。如大型环状混合痔，所留皮区因有曲张血管团而高出手术创面时，此可做潜行剥离，去除曲张血管团。如内痔体过大而无分界时，可做分段处理。术毕包扎固定，术后每日换药，至创面愈合。

注意点：同内痔贯穿结扎法，其外痔创面间亦应保留正常皮肤。

(3) 套扎疗法：内痔胶圈套扎疗法始于20世纪60年代，1963年美国Barron氏著文发表此法。我国研究始于1964年，是从祖国医学传统结扎疗法发展而来。20余年来其应用已遍及世界，从临床研究到器械改进都有进展。这种结扎法，操作简便，疗效确实，痛苦小，花钱少，是一值得提倡和推广的治疗方法。

历史发展

国外概况：Holley 氏报告，痔的外科治疗已有许多世纪，Hippocrates 氏即应用结扎、切割和烧灼疗法。但如何结扎却无记载。结扎疗法的实际应用始于19世纪初期，1829年 Salmon 氏曾著文报告，在内痔的基底部予以结扎使痔核枯死脱落。1873年 Allingham 氏实践并描述了内痔结扎结合切割法。1926年 Hirschman 氏推荐混合痔外切内扎之法。

20世纪50年代，结扎疗法有了新发展，1954年 Blaisdell 氏制成一小巧器械，亦即世界最早之结扎器，用丝线或肠线结扎内痔，然而此种结扎法扎线有时会过早松动，偶有严重出血之例，此后 Blaisdell 氏亦改为胶圈套扎。20世纪60年代 Barron 氏首用胶圈套扎法，其应用 Gravlee 氏脐带结扎器的原理，用扩圈圆锥将胶圈套至结扎器套管上，用来结扎内痔，其套扎器由 Blaisdell 氏结扎器改进而成。Mcgivney 氏在前者结扎器的基础上，又有新的改进，故近年 Mcgivney 氏结扎器是最受欢迎的。

20年来此疗法遍及世界各地，如美国、日本、英国、加拿大、德国、澳大利亚以及东南亚国家均有应用。其操作除单用胶圈套扎外，并与注射、切割、冷冻等法结合。以此法治疗千余例者不乏报导。并有远期疗效观察之专文。总之套扎疗法目前在国外颇为盛行。

国内概况：结扎疗法是我国传统治痔的主要方法，迄今已近千年历史。如《太平圣惠方》即有"用蜘蛛丝缠系痔鼠乳头，不觉自落"的记载。至明、清时期已普遍采用。根据祖国医学结扎治痔的原理，山东中医学院附属医院1964年用胶圈套扎内痔。为普及应用所设计的第7型内痔结扎器，1972年曾参加全国科技会议展出。1974年浙江陆琦氏研制成吸引式套扎器。日后福建邓正明氏加以改进，利用拔火罐形成负压的原理将吸引部分由电动吸引器改为类火罐装置，使吸引式套扎器便于普及。1977年上海俞德洪等氏制成吸引式和牵拉式套扎器，天津杜克礼氏、河北芮恒祥氏也制成不同结构的吸引套扎器械。辽宁李润庭氏创用更简易的血管钳胶圈套扎法，此法勿需特制套扎器械，只用血管钳胶圈即可。哈尔滨第三医院的吸引套扎法亦甚简单，用注射器吸引，取材方便。近年韩后基氏研究新型套扎器治疗直肠、乙状结肠息肉，收到较好效果。目前山东牵拉式套扎器又有新的改进。自1964年以来，胶圈套扎法即在我国逐渐推广普及，现应用已遍及全国大部地区。以此法治疗的患者仅以1976年沈阳痔瘘医院、哈尔滨第三医院、浙江医科大学附属第一医院、山东中医学院附属医院4单位统计材料为例，已达4300余例。我国生产内痔套扎器械的工厂也有几家，目前该法正在普遍推广中。

作用原理

本疗法用特制结扎器械将胶圈或胶环套于痔基部，通过胶圈或胶环的紧缩绞勒阻断痔的血运，使产生缺血性坏死，痔逐渐脱落，创面组织修复而愈。

应用方法

器械种类及用品：目前套扎器械已有两种，大体可分牵拉套扎器和吸引套扎器。其前端套管有直视型、斜面型和侧面型。

牵拉套扎器械：以夹持钳将痔体拉入套扎器套管内，然后再把胶圈或胶环由套扎器推至痔基底部的器械称牵拉套扎器。国内外以此型为主。

Blaisdell氏套扎器：有两种，称医院型和诊所型，均为直型，套管为直视。其结构外套管接柄管，内套管比外套管长，内套管前端部分置胶圈，后端与轴心连接，轴心由柄管内通过外形为一整体并长于柄管，轴心末端装一远端帽。以组织钳夹持牵拉痔核，用一般筒式肛镜。

Barron氏套扎器：由Blaisdell氏套扎器改进而成。此结扎器呈膝状，内外套管与轴心柄管连接与按装和 Blaisdell 氏套扎器此部装置完全一样，不能拆卸清洗，但可以握柄外更换长度不同的带有套管的柄管，其内套管直径 11 mm，握柄较美观。其夹持钳亦呈膝状，Maurice 称此钳为把持钩钳 (tenaculum forceps)。所用胶圈为黑色，两端面平整，中央孔为 $\frac{1}{12}$ 英寸。用圆锥体扩圈。使用一般筒式肛镜。

Rudd 氏套扎器：为 Blaisdell 氏套扎器略加改进，其柄管和轴心末端去掉远端帽，柄管末端接有并列的两环，便于握持时伸入食、中 2 指，轴心末端接 1 单环，便于伸入拇指。痔核夹持钳似血管钳样，其柄处略呈膝状。用圆锥扩张胶圈。

Mcgivney 氏套扎器：参照 Blaisdell 氏、Barron 氏套扎器改进而成。结扎器呈膝状，内外套管与轴心柄管连接与按装和 Blaisdell 氏套扎器一样，但柄管与握柄连接处与 Barron 氏套扎器不同，柄管与握柄处可旋转 360°（度），便于套扎痔核，器械容易拆卸，便于清洁清毒。近年又有新的改进，握柄更为美观，握柄与柄管的结合处造形也有更新，如握把柄时内套管退入外套管中，而使胶圈推出。其使用组织钳牵拉痔核，但组织钳握柄近鳃部处略呈膝状。用圆锥体扩张胶圈。

作者之套扎器：为普及推广所设计的普及用第 7 型呈膝状，由套管、柄管、轴心、握柄等结构组成。套管为直视，与柄管连接后称柄头，较短，故器械小巧。内套管与柄管通过螺丝结构旋紧连接，轴心自柄管内通过后经由内套管侧壁长形孔与外套管侧壁圆孔相接而起控制外套管作用。柄管与轴心和握柄相接处结构新颖，可快速更换带有套管的柄管。此套扎器附有 3 支和大小不同口径的套管相接的柄管，即 1 握把 3 柄头，内套管直径各为 12、14、16 mm，适于大小不等的痔体的套扎。套管、套柄均可拆卸，便于清洗。亦用组织钳夹持牵拉痔体。所用乳胶环无明显中央孔可见，即有较大预应力，故套扎后无滑脱可能。使用广口筒式斜面肛镜,暴露痔核充分。如痔核自然脱出,可以肛门拉钩协助套扎。用圆锥体将乳胶环扩张,但此圆锥体之前端有一似锥形的突起,与圆锥体之间成一细颈,作者称此为第2锥体,即有两个锥形的扩环锥体。此结构便于乳胶环向圆锥体按放。为使乳胶环顺利扩张至内套管上,设计了造形美观的胶环扩张器,而取代了手指扩环。

新型套扎器即第8型,为一人操作,可完成钳夹痔核,推动结扎器套管前进和后退,推出乳胶环等动作,仍为1握把3柄头。应用较方便,但结构尚须改进。

此外,李润庭氏不用套扎器只用血管钳和胶圈亦可套扎。

吸引套扎器械:用吸引装置将内痔吸入套扎器套管内,然后再把胶圈或胶环由套扎器推至痔基部的器械称吸引套扎器。

陆琦氏套扎器:呈膝状,套管为直视,内外套管与轴心柄管连接后,套管末端用透明玻璃片封闭,便于套管内形成负压,和观察内痔吸引情况。柄管后接之手柄,为密闭中空,手柄末端再置一中空管,便于连接吸引装置,轴心与板手相接,可推出胶圈,因后接联动弹簧,故外套管推胶管后可自动后缩。用电动吸引器吸引。以圆锥体即装圈锥头扩张胶圈。用一般斜面肛镜。邓正明氏不用电动吸引器吸引,改用类火罐装置形成负压。

杜克礼氏套扎器:按唧筒原理制成直形筒状,前端呈斜面,于吸筒前部放置胶圈。

stille公司套扎器:呈膝状,均为金属结构。握把为丁形,其下端圆状为握部,实心,上端为细管状,中空,尾部接吸引器管。柄管轴心与握把相接,握把处有板手,内外套管与柄管轴心垂直相接,故内外套管为侧面型,其轴心与外套管相接,推环设计新颖。胶圈同Barron氏胶圈,仍有中央孔,扩圈圆锥体有两个锥形,此吸引套扎较为先进。

铺助器械及用品:组织钳等夹持钳,胶圈或胶环,广口筒式肛镜,肛门拉钩,扩环圆锥体和胶环扩张器,吸引套扎应有吸引装置，另外应备消毒棉球、润滑剂、九华膏 (24)、敷料等。

适应症

牵拉套扎法适应症较广，如各期各型内痔、混合痔内痔部分、直肠粘膜脱垂、痔环切后遗粘膜外翻、直肠低位息肉及乳头纤维瘤等。吸引套扎适于1、2期内痔体积较小者。年老、体弱及合并有全身慢性疾病如贫血、肺结核、心脏病、高血压等，可酌情采用。如痔发炎、水肿、栓塞可缓医，一般无禁忌。

套扎方法

该疗法借助器械将胶圈或胶环套至内痔基部，典型操作在肛镜下进行，如内痔核自然脱出也可在拉钩协助下套扎。勿需麻醉。其操作如以痔核如何进入结扎器内，可分牵拉套扎法和吸引套扎法。前者用夹持钳如组织钳、把持钩等直接夹持内痔，能灵活牵拉痔体。有的套扎器能更换套管柄头、适于大小不等痔体的套扎。如混合痔采用外剥内扎时，外痔部分剪切剥离后以此种器械处理其内痔部分，则操作亦较简便。后者即吸引套扎法，用吸引器、吸筒、空针等装置，吸引后套管内形成负压，痔体慢慢自行进入，如吸引力不足则痔体不能进入套管或进入不全。因吸引，内痔周围有时也发生膨隆，影响痔体进入，如混合痔行外剥内扎时，因内痔部分已不规整且术区有血，吸引套扎器即不能应用。

现将牵拉套扎操作方法介绍如下：取骑伏位，不必麻醉。用消毒棉球擦拭肛门，以广口筒式肛镜沾润滑剂，缓慢插入肛道，抽出镜心暴露痔区，观察痔核部位及数目（图6）。消毒痔核及肛道。左手持套有乳胶环的结扎器，结扎器套管口径应与痔核体积大小相适应，右手持组织钳经结扎器套管伸出，一并经肛镜伸入肛道。张开组织钳（图7）于内痔上部将痔夹牢并拉入结扎器套管内（图8），此时亦可将结扎器上推（左手推，右手拉），如结扎器内套管前缘已抵达痔基部时，即可收紧握柄，通过轴心起动外套管而将乳胶环推出（图9、图10），套于痔基部，张开组织钳与结扎器一并取下，结扎结束（图11）。所余痔核依法结扎。如内痔自然脱出显露充分时，以肛门拉钩协助结扎。扎后肛内涂九华膏（24）、盖贴敷料。本疗法操作十分简单，一般结扎仅需3～5分钟。另外如混合痔（图12）采用切扎时，外痔部分剪切剥离后，以此法处理其内痔部分，则操作亦比较简便（图13、图14）。

套扎注意事项

充分暴露痔区；夹持内痔时应钳夹痔核上部，便于整个痔块外牵；牵拉勿过猛，以免痔核撕裂；结扎一处时，注意避开他处内痔；乳胶环外缘应扎于齿线以上，此可减轻扎后痛苦；扎后观察乳胶环是否居痔核基部，如初学者一旦未扎于痔核基底可重新结扎之，以免痔体残留影响疗效，不论痔核数目多少（如环状痔）、体积大小，均可一次扎完，无必要时结扎部位不宜超过3处，如痔多于3个，相邻痔核如有可能亦可扎于一起。

套扎前后的处理。讲明结扎有关事宜，增进治疗信心，解除疑虑；结扎前应先解大小便，使直肠、膀胱空虚；扎后当日勿解大便；保持大便通畅，必要时服润肠剂；定期指诊，及时了解脱环情况，并可避免结扎粘膜粘连，脱环日期应注意观察病情，防止出血；换药日期根据病情灵活掌握，不必每日换药；治疗结束时行指诊及肛镜检查，并作出疗效判断。

治疗的有关问题

牵拉套扎的重要环节：牵拉套扎的操作有两个重要环节。其一，如何将胶圈顺利套于痔基部，这是操作程序的重点。主要靠套扎器和辅助器械的正确使用来完成。其二，扎后痔核枯死彻底与否，这是治愈关键，主要靠胶圈紧缩绞勒的能力，即环的张力。胶圈张力的大小主要取决于环的弹性。我们应用的乳胶环是上海乳胶厂制作，性能较好，扎后痔核能逐渐枯死脱落，即使痔体较小，亦未见自然滑脱者。

一次结扎与分次结扎；国外多用分次结扎法，每次套扎1个痔核，间隔 1 周进行 1 次，通常套扎 3 次。Barron 氏只言每次结扎 1 个痔核，但未谈及间隔时间。Eugene 氏等报告，490 例患者总结扎 1625 次，平均每病人结扎 3.3 次，多为结扎 1 次，最多结扎 9 次，每次结扎 1 个痔核以上者仅占 1.5%，其中 8% 有严重疼痛。此种分次治法可无疼痛，结扎后即可工作或仅作短时休息，但结扎次数多，疗程长。作者自 1970 年以来采用一次结扎法，不论痔核多少，体积大小，均可 1 次扎完，但多数为扎 3 处。有一例患者有 8 个痔核，分 6 处 1 次结扎，疗效甚为满意。临床观察，一次结扎避免了再结扎时窥镜放入之痛苦。第一次结扎后，因结扎间隔期限于 7~10 天，首次结扎痔核如已枯脱但创面未愈，窥镜扩张、损伤等刺激除可引起痛苦外，并增加续发出血的可能。如结扎间隔期较长，则延长整个疗程。但年老、体弱及合并有全身慢性疾病者，可酌情采用延长结扎间隔期的分次结扎法。

胶圈应套于痔核基部，如未套于基底应重新结扎之。

胶圈应扎于齿线上 2~3 mm，如有必要须临近齿线时，可作止痛处理。

乳胶环脱落日期：山东中医学院附属医院在 1970~1973 年系统观察的 694 例，最短 5 天脱环，最长 19 天。7 天脱环者 36 例，有 3 例 7 天脱环者续发大出血，8~10 天脱环者 270 例；11~13 天脱环者 327 例，在此脱环期内有 1 例续发大出血，脱环期为 11 天，14~15 天脱环者 56 例。另有 3 例结扎的个别部位 16 天脱环，19 天脱环者有两个结扎部位 17 天脱环。此处尚有 2 例（均结扎 1 处）各于 13 天 15 天结扎部位垂出肛外，环将脱，枯死组织仅余 4 及 3mm 粗，以剪剪下。此 2 例亦分别列入 13、15 天脱环期内。

疗程。694 例最短 14 天治愈，有 2 例；最长 37 天。有 1 例。15~20 天痊愈者 338 例；21~25 天痊愈者 254 例；26~30 天痊愈者 90 例；30 天以上痊愈者 9 例。疗程的长短与结扎数目、痔体大小、全身状况等有关，一般创面较小，全身健壮，则愈合快。此组大部分患者均结扎几处，故疗程较长。

疗效观察：此法与丝线结扎法相同，是将整个痔核结扎，使其完整枯脱，故治愈比较彻底。痊愈检查时，结扎区颇为平坦。1976年前哈尔滨第三医院以此法治疗的470例，466例治愈，占99%，浙江医大附属第一医院治疗的328例，308例治愈，占93.9%，好转13例，占4%；沈阳痔瘘医院治疗的2517例、山东中医学院附属医院1970年～1973年系统观察的694例，近期全部治愈。David氏等随访125例，随访期为3.5～6年，平均4.8年，89%远期效果满意，44%完全无症状。

反应与并发症：本疗法痛苦较轻或无痛苦，如发生疼痛、坠胀、便血及排尿障碍时，可按一般方法处理。如续发大出血，可用明矾液灌肠或明矾膏涂布出血区。

主要优缺点

优点。操作简便，容易掌握，便于在基层单位推广普及；疗效好，治愈比较彻底；痛苦少，并发症少，由于操作简单、痛苦小，扩大了适应范围；多数在门诊治疗，勿需住院，费用低廉。

缺点及存在的问题。少数患者仍有疼痛、坠胀、排尿障碍等反应及续发大出血的可能，通过研究，必要时应用长效止疼剂或以明矾膏换药，并注意观察，上述反应与并发症已基本解决。

如上所述，由于本疗法有许多优点，在痔的预防没有取得重要突破以前，今后的应用中套扎疗法仍不失为内痔的重要治法之一。

8. 手术疗法

手术疗法是现代医学治痔的重点内容，而我国直肠学家也积累了自己的经验。手术种类繁多，按创口缝合与否可分创面开放和创面闭合两类。现将应用方法介绍如下。

(1) 血栓外痔切除术：血栓外痔经熏洗治疗仍无吸收时，可手术切除。

操作方法：消毒麻醉后，在痔表面作一放射状切口，切开皮肤后，如见瘀血块包以纤维膜，剥离后将其完整取出。如瘀血块有大小几个，可将其一一取尽。如瘀血块剥破，将瘀血拭净即可。创缘可作修整，压迫止血，术毕创口挤压对合或缝一针，术后不必换药。此外可试行挤压法，即麻醉后将血栓痔块慢慢挤压，压迫包膜，瘀血流溢组织间，后用中药熏洗，促进瘀血吸收。

(2) 静脉曲张外痔及结缔组织外痔切除术。

操作方法：静脉曲张外痔可作梭形切口，剥离静脉丛并予切除，剪修创缘，创面间应留有正常皮肤。结缔组织外痔作 V 形切口，将隆突痔块剪除即可。所成创面均不逢合。后每日换药，直至痊愈。

(3) 痔血管丛摘除术：适于较大的孤立内痔和混合痔。此法可将曲张之血管团完全摘除。使术区肛、管修复平整。

操作方法：常规清毒，局麻或腰俞麻醉，以肛门拉钩牵开肛门，暴露术区痔核。于痔基部两侧各作一切口，在齿线处两切口相连，由此向内剪切，剥离曲张之血管丛至痔上端仅有较小蒂时，用钳将蒂部夹住，以丝线于钳下贯穿缝扎，后将痔块剪除。如为混合痔，痔基部两侧切口须延至皮区，并超过外痔下端约 1～2cm。所成创面粘膜创口部分开放，皮区创口全部开放。术后每日换药，直至痊愈。

Howard 及 Turner 氏所倡导的痔切除术，与上法相似，其操作法如下：

消毒麻醉后，扩张肛管至容 4 指。此可充分暴露痔核并能最大限度减少术后括约肌痛性痉挛。探查并验证 3 组痔块，将每组内外痔以钳钳起，于内痔上面痔血管周围用缝合肠线贯穿粘膜结扎之。再于外痔基部作一"V"形切口，并向上剪切至成一细茎时为止。然后在此基部钳夹，于钳上面将内、外痔切除。保留的粘膜及皮肤，以肠线对缝。近肛缘处只留几处引流。术后每日换药，直至痊愈。

(4) 痔孤立剪除分段钳夹结扎术。

适应症：适用于2、3期内痔及混合痔。

操作方法：取骑伏位，常规消毒，局麻或腰俞麻醉。麻醉充分后，先将两食指蘸滑润剂伸入肛内，进行扩张。再以两手拇指按压在肛门两缘，并向两侧牵拉，同时嘱患者屏气努挣向下进气，如排便样增大腹压，以使痔核脱出，或术前蹲踞努责，使痔自然脱出。

手术时重新消毒术区。以组织钳将痔核夹住提起，除混合痔须先将痔区皮肤切→"V"形切口至齿线区然后再予钳夹外，单纯内痔可直接取一弯形或直形全牙血管钳，根据每1次钳夹位置的高低钳夹于第1道全牙钳的下面或上面，两钳紧密相靠或留有较小间隙，其上下完全平行并排，或仅全牙钳的钳夹部分上下并排，两钳尾各居两方。钳夹的深度应至痔核基底，但不能损伤过多粘膜。然后剪去上道全牙钳上面的痔组织，并将上道钳子去掉，继以血管钳将上道全牙钳夹扁的组织，分段钳夹，去掉下道全牙钳，用盐水纱布拭净血迹，查看有无出血。如有明显出血时，应更换钳夹部位，至不出血为止。最后以丝线由外而内分别结扎。内端2~3个钳夹点为重点处理区，应予重复结扎或贯穿结扎。术毕复查确无明显出血时，再以止血散（36）、凡士林纱布填塞切口，包扎固定。后每日换药，直至痊愈。

操作注意事项

全牙钳必须顺痔的原来位置钳夹。由于痔的位置不同，全牙血管钳与后位肛沟所成的角度即有所不同。如痔居左右中位，钳应与肛沟垂直；居于前后中位，应与肛沟平行；居于右前右后或左前右后。则与肛沟近平行或成一定角度。无论痔的位置居于何处，钳夹的方向必须顺痔原来位置的方向，即垂直该痔区的肛管壁，否则会损伤较多的粘膜。

分段钳夹结扎，创面内端必须作为重点处理区。痔剪除后，这种结扎法仅能扎住对应区的粘膜和粘膜下较浅部位的出血区，较深部位的出血是不易扎牢的，而初学者又常钳夹过上，因此当术毕检查时往往发现结扎区高达直肠环上。必须强调指出，直肠粘膜是血运旺盛的多血区，如损伤范围广泛，再加结扎不牢，最易发生因粘膜大片游离，多量持续渗血而造成的大出血现象。为此，钳夹结扎的内端即创面的上部，必须重点处理。处理方法，即在创面内端留有2~3个钳夹点，予以重复扎牢或贯穿结扎。

混合痔同时剪除几处痔核时，创面间必须留有健康皮肤。此能使创面愈合增速，同时亦可减少因大片疤痕而引起的肛门狭窄。

(5) 内痔原位缝闭术：适用于2、3期内痔，此法较简单，基本无出血。

操作方法：常规消毒，麻醉后，以拉钩牵开肛门，暴露术区，钳起痔核，将全牙血管钳夹于痔基部，以无损伤针，用细肠线将钳夹痔组织连同血管钳一并贯穿连续缝合，抽出血管钳拉紧缝线，痔核即被缝于原处，术后不必换药。

(6) 痔切除连续缝合术：适用于3期内痔和混合痔。

操作方法：常规消毒，麻醉后，以组织钳将痔核提起。用血管钳于痔基部钳夹，切除血管钳上痔组织，以0~1号肠线或细丝线连续缝合，将钳抽出时缝线随即拉紧。如混合痔，外痔切口开放。

5.4.3 针灸与磁疗

1. 针刺疗法：适用于痔肿痛等急性发作，处理方法与术后疼痛的针刺治疗相同。如有便血、脱垂可加足三里等穴。

2. 挑治：适用于痔肿痛、便血、脱垂等。

操作方法：在背部或腰部找出痔点，常规消毒，用三棱针挑出白色纤维，挑尽后涂碘酒，盖贴胶布。

3. 灸法：多用于便血的治疗，可灸足三里、中脘、气海、长强等穴。

4. 磁疗：适用于痔肿痛等急性发作，处理同术后疼痛的磁疗法。

6 肛门直肠周围脓肿

凡生于肛门直肠周围的化脓性疾病，祖国医学可总括为肛门直肠周围痈疽。据现代医学，结合临床实践，肛周脓肿应与疖肿等区别。以此观点来看，祖国医学所称的肛周痈疽，实际包括肛周脓肿、疖肿等病，或现代医学所称之瘘管性脓肿和非瘘管性脓肿。

6.1 病因病机

总由湿热下注，热毒蕴积所致。实证多因醇酒厚味，湿浊不化；虚证多因肺、脾、肾亏损，湿热乘虚下注。现代医学认为，多为肛隐窝感染，炎症扩散至肛周组织而成。其发病自内而外，肛隐窝为感染源进入门户。其发病过程可分3期，即肛隐窝感染期；肛管直肠周围组织反应期；局部病变即脓肿形成期。此3期演变，先有肛隐窝炎，导至肛腺炎，然后炎症通过血流或淋巴或肛腺崩解后，侵犯至肛直肠周围组织使其发炎，最后炎变区形成脓肿。肠道病菌较多，但多为大肠杆菌致病。

6.2 临床表现

脓肿可侵犯不同部位，浅层者有皮下脓肿、肛门后脓肿，较深部位有坐骨直肠窝脓肿，如穿通盆隔蔓延至骨盆腹膜外间隙，可引起骨盆直肠间隙脓肿和直肠后间隙脓肿。盆隔上脓肿病变范围广泛且深，不易早期诊断。骨盆直肠间隙脓肿和坐骨直肠窝脓肿，可由一侧蔓延至对侧。直肠粘膜下脓肿虽距肠腔表浅，但不居体外，可属深部范围。其症状与体征按虚实述之。

实证：患处疼重。浅者局限高突，皮肤红热，有触痛，脓成时软而应指。溃速、脓稠、臭秽。深者患处漫肿、肤热，或为常色。全身可有寒热交作等中毒症状。

虚证：患处疼轻。平塌，肤色暗红或如常，不热、溃迟、脓稀、臭味小。

不论实证、虚证，肛内指诊时，可触及发炎肿胀之隐窝，即肛周脓肿之内口，此可与肛周疖肿等区别。

6.3 临床治疗

6.3.1 内治法

可辨证服药，实证，应清热解毒利湿，内服三黄汤（60）合三妙散（61）加减或黄连除湿汤（62）。虚证，应滋阴除湿，内服滋阴除湿汤（63）加减。可并用抗生素或消炎药。

6.3.2 外治法

1. 局部坐浴熏洗或热敷，熏洗用复方荆芥洗药（38）或解毒洗药（64），每日洗2～3次，每次半小时左右。热敷用热水袋等，可持续热敷。

2. 局部敷药：以蒜硝糊剂（65）、黄醋糊剂（66）交替敷用，或涂消炎止痛药膏。

3. 手术疗法：脓成未消时，切开排脓，术后继续熏洗敷药，待炎肿消退成瘘时，再按肛瘘处理。或行肛周脓肿一次切开法，此术切口较一般脓肿切开为大，可由脓肿波动区切至肛缘，并将内口切开，如深部脓肿，切至肛缘后，肛内部分可予挂线。术后常规换药，创面逐渐缩小而愈合。此术不后遗瘘管。但应注意控制感染。

7 肛瘘

凡孔窍内生管，出水不止者为漏。生于肛门或直肠下部称肛瘘，又称痔瘘，亦为常见病多发病。

7.1 病因病机

祖国医学认为，肛瘘的病因与痔病大体相同，是在脏腑虚损的情况下，湿热下注，热毒蕴积而致病。根据临床实践，肛瘘为肛周脓肿所后遗，也就是说为肛周脓肿的自然结局。肛周脓肿实为肛瘘的急性初发期，而肛瘘则为肛周脓肿的慢性阶段，即炎肿消退瘘管形成。因此肛周脓肿与肛瘘为一种疾病的两个不同阶段。肛周脓肿的病因即本病的病因。肛瘘形成后为何不易自愈，有以下几种因素：

1. 脓肿自溃或切开后，脓水由外口引流，因内口继续感染，故瘘管不愈。
2. 肠道粪便等物继续污染。
3. 瘘管外口较小或时封时溃，脓水排出不畅。
4. 瘘管弯曲或者深在腔道，脓水贮存，难以排出。

7.2 临床表现

7.2.1 分类

现代医学对肛瘘的分类较为复杂，今据临床体会结合有关文献，将其分类归纳如下。

1. 以管道和溃孔多少而分类

(1) 单纯性肛瘘：1管1外口称之。

(2) 复杂性肛瘘：2管2外口以上者称之，但内口仍只有1

处。

2. 以管道深浅而分类

(1) 低位肛瘘：亦称浅在肛瘘，管道表浅可触及。

(2) 高位肛瘘：亦称深在肛瘘，其判定标准以瘘管通过括约肌何部而区别之。此法在临床检查时尚感不足。作者临床实践，将高位肛瘘的特点总结以下几点：a.管道沿肛道方向走行，即瘘管平行或近平行肛管。b.管道深不居表浅组织，故检查时仅触得溃孔区局限硬结或部分硬索。c.探针检查除证实上述瘘管方向外，一般深约 4 cm 以上。d.探针指诊复合检查，肛内手指可于直肠环上管道内端对应区之肠壁感触探针冲撞。e.直肠环纤维化。

3. 以瘘管内外口是否相通而分类

(1) 全通瘘：又称全瘘或内外瘘，有内口，管道和外口 3 部分。

(2) 不全通瘘：有单口内瘘和单口外瘘，单口内瘘为肛瘘未溃破皮肤，单口外瘘，为穿刺外伤感染而得。

4. 以管道的曲直而分类

(1) 直形瘘：管道行径直，多居肛门前位。

(2) 弯形瘘：管道行径弯曲，多居肛门后位。如弯形瘘管道较长时，则称长管弯形瘘，长弯瘘外口可居肛门前位，而管道弯曲部分居肛门后方，内口多居后中。因管道弯曲，可呈镰形或钩形。两侧弯形瘘于后位相通则构成后位蹄铁形瘘。

5. 以内口多少而分类

(1) 单发性肛瘘：内口 1 处；管道 1 支。此即单纯性肛瘘。

(2) 多发性肛瘘：内口 2 处以上，管道 2 支以上。典型多发瘘，管道无分支。

6. 以管道与括约肌的关系而分类

(1) 括约肌间瘘：即低位肛瘘。瘘管只穿过内括约肌，外口 1 个，距肛缘较近。

(2) 经括约肌瘘：瘘管穿过内括约肌和外括约肌浅部与深部之间，外口常有数个，并有支管。

(3) 括约肌上瘘：瘘管向上穿过肛提肌，然后向下至坐骨直肠窝开口于皮肤。

(4) 括约肌外瘘：瘘管穿过肛提肌直接与直肠相通，临床甚为少见。

7. 以瘘管的病理性质而分类

(1) 非特异性肛瘘：即一般炎症性肛瘘，此类肛瘘最多。

(2) 特异性肛瘘：目前常指结核性肛瘘而言，其他特异感染如梅毒性等则甚为少见。

肛瘘的分类虽有多种，但有时一种分类法尚不能说明其实际病情，须几种分类法结合应用。为便于临床，尽量简明实用，经我国有关单位研究，根据瘘管多少和深浅制定统一标准而分4类：

(1) 低位单纯性肛瘘：管道1条，通过外括约肌浅层。内口1个，居齿线肛隐窝处。

(2) 低位复杂性肛瘘：管道和外口2个以上，瘘管通过外括约肌浅层，内口1个或几个，居肛隐窝处（包括多发瘘）。

(3) 高位单纯性肛瘘：管道1条，行于外括约肌深层以上，内口1个居肛隐窝处。

(4) 高位复杂性肛瘘：管道2条以上或有支管空腔，主管通过外括约肌深层以上，外口两个或数个，内口1个或几个居肛隐窝处（包括多发瘘）。

7.2.2 症状与体征

以流脓流水为主症。新形成的瘘管，脓多而稠；时间较长时，脓少而稀，或时有时无。有时瘘管外口可在一段时间内自然封闭，貌似愈合，但不久又发炎肿痛，重新溃破，流出脓液。如不从原口出脓，即形成1新管。如此反复发作，延成痼疾。患者平时多无疼痛，但瘘口封闭脓液排出不畅时，则肿痛不适。此外，由于分泌物经常刺激，也可发生肛门瘙痒。局部体征因管道多少、深浅而不同。单纯者，外口1个，管道孤居，或直或弯，复杂者外口多个，管道数生，行径弯曲。低位者，多能触得硬索通肛；高位者，亦有其临床特点，已如上述。如以虚实辨之，实证外口呈凸形，脓水稠厚，皮色如常，有硬索可触及；虚证外口凹陷，有潜行性创缘，脓水稀薄，皮色暗褐，或无硬索。

7.3 诊断和鉴别诊断

肛瘘的初步诊断并不困难，通过病史的询问和局部观察，即可得出。但欲进一步分清肛瘘的类型，查明内口的位置，管道的行径、深浅、分支状况及与括约肌的关系和直肠环是否纤维化，以及肛瘘属于何种性质等，则须通过各项细致的检查，方可得出明确的诊断。此为肛瘘的诊查重点。检查时必须细心认真。其具体诊查方法，分述如下。

7.3.1 问诊

多有肛门直肠周围脓肿的历史。在询问中，应问清发病的时间，典型症状，如肿痛，自溃或切开，脓水从肛门流出或从外口流出，量多或少，色黄或白，浓稠或稀薄，臭味大小，持续性或间歇性。如脓水忽然增多，病情多有加重。另外，有无气体及粪便等由瘘孔排出。肛旁有无硬结和硬管，如有多管应问清发生的先后。

7.3.2 视诊

检查时注意肛门外形，病变范围，外口的数目、部位、形态及其周围组织的变化等。

1. 肛门外形及病变范围：注意肛门有无移位、凹陷或缺损。病变范围大小，占居肛周几个象限。

2. 外口的数目、部位及形态：如只有1个外口，一般多为单纯性肛瘘。如2外口左右分居肛门后位而两口之间亦有条形隆起时，常为蹄铁形瘘。但有不少患者两口之间条形隆起并不明显,亦有管道贯通2口之间;有时即使隆起显著,却无管道存在。前位外口左右并存常不为蹄铁形肛瘘。但前位肛瘘其外口距肛门较远者,常有向阴囊皮下侵及的可能,结核性肛瘘多有此特征。因此在诊视前位外口的同时,应注意阴囊与股根部皮肤的变化,观察有无与外口相关的条形隆起或结节肿块。

如较多外口居于肛门一侧或两侧,则管道复杂。复杂性肛瘘病变广泛者,皮肤表面可凹凸不平,外口数目不一,形貌各异。

外口距肛门的远近,对考察管道的深浅亦可提供参考。一般外口近肛门者,管道较浅;远肛门者,管道较深。但有不少患者,外口距肛门较近,管道却深;外口距肛门虽远,管道却浅,仅于皮下蔓延不向深部穿凿。

外口形态的观察,对了解肛瘘的性质及病程可提供参考。新生之瘘管,外口处常无增殖结节;患病已久,外口处常形成肉芽组织的突起,或纤维化的结节或疤痕性凹陷,结节或凹陷的中央有瘘口存在。有时外口开于结节根部的一侧或闭锁,有时瘘管与结缔组织性外痔并存,无外口,如不细查常被忽略。

一般炎症性肛瘘的外口多有结节形成,结节的大小、外貌以及突起皮肤的高度不尽相同。结核性肛瘘外口不规则,常无突起小结,外口边缘向内凹陷卷曲,其肉芽组织可呈灰白色。

3. 肛瘘病变区的皮色变化:复杂性肛瘘尤为结核性者,外口周围常有褐色圆晕。如管道区皮肤呈现弥漫的暗褐色,或变化的皮色间有正常皮色,显有明显或暗淡的褐色圆晕时,其皮下常有空腔,腔隙可为单个或几个,或呈蜂窝样。

7.3.3 触诊

十分重要。一般通过此法即可直接辨别肛瘘的不同体征。如瘘管的行径是笔直或弯曲,蹄形或钩形;单管孤存或分支蔓延;内口的位置、数目;直肠环的情况,以及管道与括约肌的关系和括约肌的功能等,均可通过触诊获得。触诊的方法大体可分以下几种:

1. 肛外触诊：慢性炎症性肛瘘常可触及硬韧的条索状物，由瘘的外口通向肛门。初发、短小的结核性肛瘘，常无硬索触及。

如几个外口距肛缘较近时，并应触摸外口间的组织，以区别管道与纤维性变的括约肌束，后者不如管道硬韧。如数个外口居于肛门同侧或异侧，管道可有分支，应细细触摸分支状况。但复杂性肛瘘，因病变区常较硬韧并凹凸不平，故不易确切触知管道的分支及行径。

低位肛瘘，硬索与周围组织界线较为明显，容易触摸。但高位肛瘘其主道多与肛道平行或近平行，因而行肛外触诊时，常不能触及明显硬索，而仅能触及外口区的孤立硬结。

在肛瘘的触诊中，作者应用加压移动触诊法和复合触诊法。加压移动触诊法，即于管道区施加一定压力，并顺管道做垂直往返移动或垂直管道做垂直往返移动。此法对触诊浅深管道确有一定的帮助。因管道较硬，其周围组织较软，往返触摸管道及其两侧的组织，给区别管道提供了更有利的条件。此法不适于复杂性肛瘘的触诊。

2. 肛内触诊：手指伸入肛道后，应由外而内先后触摸。粘膜下脓肿及瘘管可触及包块和硬索。内口应于齿线区寻找。可触及突起或凹陷小结，但内口闭锁且无明显结节时，不易触清。直肠环区的变化亦应重视，注意环区纤维化的程度和范围，纤维化与管道和内口的关系等。如触摸直肠环区上部应使指曲为钩形。高位肛瘘常有一明显体征，即行探针指诊复合检查时，肛内的手指可于主道顶端对应区之肠壁感触探针之冲撞。另外并应检查括约肌的收缩力如何。

3. 复合触诊：即肛肠内外的手指于病变区同施压力，加压移动互应触摸。这样更有助于诊查管道的情况。

7.3.4 探针检查

此法虽甚重要，但因穿插管道易引起疼痛，患者有时不愿接受。因此在检查前应充分说明其重要性，取得患者合作。

检查时，将戴有指套的食指沾润滑剂伸入肛道，触于内口处，然后另手取适宜的探针由外口缓慢而轻柔地插入管道，肛内手指与探针由外口缓慢而轻柔地插入管道，肛内手指与探针呼应，检查行径至穿通瘘管为止。如内口闭锁或管道平行、近平行肛管时，探针与手指的呼应检查，亦可测知瘘管与肛管间的距离厚度，并与内口处及管道顶端感触探针之冲撞。在检查中不可用力过猛，只凭主观想象勉强硬插，否则可造成假道，加重了患者的痛苦。对于复杂性肛瘘，可同时插入几根探针，探查各管道是否相通和内口部位是否同处。如探针于管道某处碰触，则瘘管于此处分枝。探针由几处探入肛道时，内诊的手指即可发现通入的不同部位。

7.3.5 肛镜及隐窝钩检查

这种方法可清楚地观察内口的位置和形状，并能探查内口是否闭锁及鉴别内口与隐窝。

1. 肛镜检查：检查前将肛镜前端涂足润滑剂，然后于后位肛沟内上下往返滑动，当发现患者的注意力已不太集中于肛镜的检查时，即在某次的往返中用力下压肛门后位，继之慢慢将镜插入肛道。因下压肛门后位，可使该部后移，故易于插入。此法可减轻或消除因突然插入而引起的精神紧张和括约肌的痉挛。

肛镜插入后，抽出镜心对好灯光即行窥查。然后徐徐外退，随镜视野的外移注意观察肠粘膜的变化。一般肛瘘患者，齿线区可充血肿胀，或见有红肿发炎之隐窝及突起之结节。由于扩张肛管，挤压瘘管壁，有时可见脓水自内口向肠腔流溢。如瘘管注入染色剂，可看到内口着色区。

2. 隐窝钩内口定位：是检查内口是否存在的重要措施。检查方法是以二翼镜扩开肛门，取钩长不同的隐窝钩，予以先后钩探。常用的隐窝钩有两种，钩长各为 0.5 cm 和 1 cm。先取钩小者，首先钩探所窥见的明显病变区，再沿齿线慢慢检查。如遇内口则一钩即入，但内口闭锁时不易钩入。如肛隐窝因发炎变深，必要时可取钩长者予以鉴别。如为隐窝仅可钩入一定长度；如为内口常可顺利吞没全钩，且钩得的方向与肛外触得的瘘管方向一致，这是因为隐窝钩经内口钩入管道之故。低位瘘管再以探针自外口插入，二者相遇时即有碰触之感。

7.3.6 管道液体注入法

1. 美蓝染色法

(1) 纱卷填塞：取窥镜涂润滑剂插入肛道，抽出镜心，再把卷好的纱卷放入肛镜内，或用二翼镜扩开肛门将纱卷放入，然后缓慢取出肛镜，使纱卷留于肛道。亦可直接挟取纱卷放入肛内，如用此法，纱卷必须保持一定硬度并须涂足润滑剂，否则不易放入。

(2) 美蓝注入：取空针吸 1%～5%美蓝溶液适量，由瘘管外口慢慢注入。所取针头以钝针头为宜，如外口较大可去掉针头直接注入。当患者感觉胀痛时，迅速将空针抽出，用手紧堵管口，按揉 1～3 分钟再将纱卷取出。

(3) 着色区的观察：内口着色区的观察可分直接观察和间接观察。于注射药液的同时，扩开肛门直接窥视着色的部位称直接观察，而纱卷着色区的辨识则为间接观察。当由肛道取出纱卷后，首先观察有无着色。如发现蓝色圆形或不规则的着色区时，则证明有内口存在。同时可借助着色区的部位及与纱卷外端的距离，测知内口的位置，但着色范围广泛时，辨清内口位置即有困难。如内口闭锁，管道迂曲或括约肌痉挛时，染色液常不易或不能通过内口染及纱卷。故纱卷没有着色并不能否定没有内口。

此外亦可应用 2%龙胆紫进行检查，此药着色力强，无副作用。

2. 普鲁卡因溶液加压注入法：此法简单易行，但应直接窥视。取空针吸入 0.25%普鲁卡因溶液适量，由外口加压注入。未注前取窥镜插入肛内，注射、窥查同时进行。如药液由肛内某处射出或溢出，此处即为内口。

7.3.7 X线摄片

欲进一步明确肛瘘管道的深浅、方向、分支状况、空腔的大小及其与肛肠周围脏器组织的关系等，可采用此法使瘘管显影。常用的造影剂为碘油，因浓度高注射后可发生疼痛，故拍片后应予冲洗。如用次硝酸铋或次碳酸铋糊剂（次硝酸铋或次碳酸铋1分，凡士林2分，加热溶化搅匀，待温后应用），或硫酸钡糊剂（用硫酸钡粉以水调成稠糊），均可获得密度较深的影象。

方法是先将1链状金属条（每节长1 cm）放入肛道，再取适量造影剂由瘘管外口注入至管道内压力较大或由其他外口溢出时，即停止注药，此时造影剂已将管道或空腔充满。亦可在X线下观察其充盈程度，至充盈满意时即可拍摄。此法不必做为常规检查。

7.3.8 了解内外口关系和管道曲直的有关规则

1. Salmon氏定律：于肛门中央画一横线，如瘘管外口位于此线前方，且距肛门不超过5cm时，则管道较直，内口居同位齿线上，与外口相对；如外口位于此线后方，则管道多弯曲不直，内口多居肛门后中位齿线上，不与外口对应。

2. Goodsall氏规则：于肛门中央画一横线，如瘘管外口位于此线前方，或肛门横线上，且距肛缘在2.54～3.81 cm（1～1.5寸）以内时，则管道较直，内口居同位齿线区；如外口位于此线后方，则主道弯曲，内口居后中位齿线区。如外口距肛缘超过2.54～3.81 cm。无论外口居此线前后，则主管均弯向后中位。

上2法相似，有时称索-哥氏规则，但对长管弯形瘘尚感不足，作者根据临床体会。参照上述2法提出修订的索-哥氏规则：

以肛门中央横线为基础，以外口离肛缘的距离为范围，在横线之前者，如其管道短于5 cm或外口距肛缘5 cm内，则管道多直，内外口多相互对应；在横线之后者，则管道多弯曲，内外口多不对应。如后位管道超过肛门中央横线之前，其外口虽距同位肛缘不超过 5 cm，但管道亦较弯曲，内外口亦不对应（图15）。

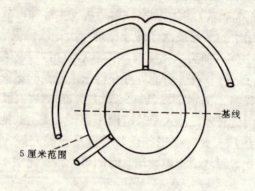

图 15 修订的索-哥氏规则

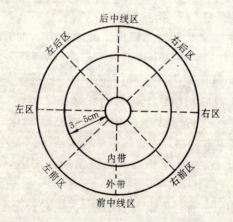

图 16 Parks 分区图

3. Parks 分类

Parks 按自然解剖标记，以肛门为中心将肛门会阴部分为 8 区。即：前中线区、左前区、左区、左后区、后中线区、右后区、右区和右前区。肛门皱襞外 3~5 cm 的范围内称内带，3~5cm 以外与肛门有关的区域称外带（图 16）。病变根据所在部位而定名，如右外带瘘、左后内带瘘等。如瘘管外口位于内带者，其管道方向呈放射状垂直肛口，大多数内口位于相应的肛隐窝处，内带之肛瘘多局限于肛门前区。如瘘管外口位于外带者，其管道弯曲，内口大多数位于后中线区。

7.3.9　病理切片检查

此项检查是确定肛瘘性质的最可靠方法。但须注意如何取得正确的标本。所取标本应包括瘘管壁及与管壁相连之组织或特异变化之组织。

肛瘘的鉴别诊断亦较复杂，现仅就其主要者鉴别如下：

1. 肛周疖肿所成之窦道：较少见，无管道通肛，无内口。

2. 坐骨结节滑囊炎感染溃后：溃孔居左右两侧坐骨结节附近，距肛缘较远，管道较深，无内口，直肠环无纤维化。

3. 骶尾部窦道：窦孔在骶尾部多距肛缘较远，窦道较浅，无内口。

4. 骶尾部畸胎瘤溃后：病变在后位，溃孔在骶尾部或肛周，管道特深，无内口，直肠环无纤维化。造影摄片，局部有占位病变。其内有时有毛发、骨质，有时有腺体，病理切片可证实。

5. 骶尾部骨质破坏而成之窦道：如骨结核、骨髓炎等，摄片骶尾骨有骨质破坏或有死骨。有时可从溃孔排出骨性硬物，或有骨片卡在窦道内。

6. 由腹盆腔炎变而来：腹盆腔脓肿并发肠瘘，由肛周或臀部溃破，如克隆氏病并发肛瘘，此等患者全身情况较差。

7. 由腰部寒性脓肿而来：如腰椎结核并发寒性脓肿后侵犯至臀部，必要时可行腰椎 X 线摄片以明确诊断。

7.4 临床治疗

7.4.1 内治法

历代对肛瘘的内治较重视，通过服药使炎肿消退，溃孔闭塞。其治则及用药与痔病近同，唯更强调补益。前人对肛瘘的内治法积累了丰富经验，治愈者亦不乏例，但亦有愈而复发者，故对此法仍需深入研究。如对闭管主方胡连追毒丸（67）、黄连或胡连闭管丸（4），象牙化管丸（5）等应进一步观察其闭管作用。但目前对内治法的应用，常限于一般体虚患者，用以改善全身状况，增强体质，创造手术条件，或急性发作期控制炎症，消肿止痛，或用作润肠通便等一般对症处理，具体可辨证论治。

7.4.2 外治法

1. 一般疗法：保持局部清洁，如急性发作除服药、熏洗外可结合涂药等法。

2. 脱管疗法：又称脱管锭疗法，通过药物的腐蚀使瘘管壁坏死脱落，新生肉芽逐渐生长，瘘管愈合。此法操作简便，不需手术，适于低位直形瘘。弯管和管道较深或有较大空腔时，治疗则感不便。

操作方法：先应脱管，后将内口封闭。脱管，先以探针探查瘘管是否畅通，同时大体测量管道长短，如脓水较多，可冲洗管道。然后取红升条（68）等腐蚀药条，缓慢插入瘘管内，药条插入适当长度，不能插过内口，以免腐蚀内口使其扩大。药条外端略露出外口，后贴敷料以胶布固定。应用红升条（68）可隔日将溶化的药条连同坏死组织取出，取出腐物后冲洗管道，更换新药条插入。一般连插 3~5 次再换祛腐生肌药条，至腐去新生瘘管闭合。内口封闭，瘘管腔道新肉生长时封闭内口，即以硬化剂注于内口周围，以使内口闭锁。操作时先用肛镜暴露内口，以消毒棉球擦试内口区，将少量低浓度明矾或鱼肝油酸钠液注于内口周围粘膜下，一般仅注 1 次。此法或许能使内口变小，但不能使其确切闭塞。传统脱管法无此操作步骤，复杂性肛瘘其支管处理可配合脱管疗法。

3. 手术疗法：手术治疗肛瘘，祖国医学亦早有记载，如《五十病方》、《外科图说》等均载有肛瘘之切割法，后者并载有一些比较切合实用的痔瘘手术器械图谱。近年经各地研究，均称此法疗效高，痛苦较小，疗程较短，与挂线疗法各取所长，在该病的治疗中起着重要作用。对高位肛瘘，一向认为不宜直接切开，如须手术应分次进行。但作者临床体会，如遵循一定原则操作，既可顺利治愈，亦很少发生不良后患。其操作方法根据瘘管深浅和多少分述于下。

(1) 低位肛瘘切开术

操作方法：取骑伏位，术区常规消毒，局麻或腰俞麻醉。将探针由外口探入，沿管道自内口穿出，肛内手指可作引导，并将探针拉出肛外。沿探针切开瘘管。如系弯管，可边探查边切开，逐步找到内口后全部切开之。如管道通畅，可用探针刀切割，取探针刀先插入前端探针部分，通过内口插入肛道。肛内手指掀起探针刀前端并牵出肛外，另手推刀向内，两手呼应，随将管道切开，或往返推拉剖开管道。如无外口或外口闭锁，但可触及硬索通肛时，可与管道外端的触硬区或闭锁外口处作一切口，并将探针通过切口深入管道，然后再行瘘管切开术。亦可将探针的一端弯成钩状，用肛门拉钩牵开肛管暴露术区，在隐窝钩引导下，将钩形探针探入内口及管道，沿探针将瘘管剪开。或在隐窝钩引导下由内而外直接剪开。如有支管，须一一切开，然后剪修创缘，刮除腐败组织，肛瘘管壁勿须剪除，或仅部分修整。切口开放呈"V"形以利愈合。术毕细心检查，如无出血点或多量渗血时，即以止血散（36）纱条填压切口，包扎固定。术后每日换药1次，直至痊愈。

操作注意点：探针探查时，勿盲目乱探，避免人工假道形成；必须沿管道切开；遵循括约肌切开的原则，如垂直切断括约肌束，不宜斜切，切开范围宜小，损伤宜轻等；注意出血。

(2) 高位肛瘘切开术

操作方法：取臀高伏卧位或骑伏位，常规消毒，行腰俞麻醉或鞍麻。充分麻醉后用探针探查管道深度，另手指伸入肛内触摸直肠环硬变情况，以便作出合理的切割计划。如高位单纯性肛瘘，管道单个孤存，在切至管道内端时，可与此区垂直切开肛管壁，切开的创面必须能使引流通畅，创面的外形呈"△"形（三角形）或"Γ"形（半 T 形）。由于外口距肛门的远近，管道的深浅和管道与肛道并行的角度不同，创面的大小、深浅和下缘的长度即有所不同，因而创面所呈现的三角形或半"T"字形可明显或不明显。如高位复杂性肛瘘，在切开所有支管时，亦须切开与主道内端对应的肛管壁。切断肛管壁创面的大小，必须根据直肠环区纤维化的程度酌情而定。一般肛门切口应切至齿线或稍上，而直肠环区一般不全剪断。其剪切方法即以钝直剪刀在主道内端向里慢慢剪切，逐渐剪断直肠环肌束。而另手食指最好放入肛道内，抵于手术区内侧，剪开的程度，以探针能由创面基底沿切口近肛门端顺利划出为度，此时肛内之手指极易感触探针之冲撞。如此区直肠环已全部纤维化，可将该区全部切开，使直肠环于此区呈一凹陷缺损，亦无失禁之后患。但内口对应环区无纤维化或硬变甚轻时，不能轻易剪切。在切断肛管壁前，如管道有腐败组织应予刮除，肛瘘管壁仅部分清除，修整创缘使创面对合整齐，勿使一侧皮缘与对侧创面抵触。术中注意止血，术毕以止血散（36）纱布块填塞切口，包扎固定。术后注意护理，无必要时饮食大便照常。每日换药 1 次至创口愈合。

手术治疗的有关问题

a. 直肠环区硬变是手术治疗高位肛瘘的局部基础。高位肛瘘如何一次切开，曾是研究的重点，因此种手术有时须广泛切断肛管壁包括全部直肠环，故既往很少取得成功。作者通过临床观察，发现直肠环纤维化现象，高位肛瘘由于脓肿范围广泛，直肠环区发生硬变，1963年作者发表的1250例浅深肛瘘的治疗中，高位肛瘘360例，330例直肠环发生了轻重不同的硬变，占91.6%。其硬变程度有轻度、中度、重度之别，后位多较前位明显。而硬变的范围可在内口同位对应环区，或波及少半环、半环、多半环和全环。纤维化的程度和范围与管道的单纯与复杂，管道距肛道的远近和病程的长短有关，一般如管道复杂，主道距肛道稍近而病程又长者，硬变重范围广。

高位肛瘘给直肠环带来的硬变损害，改变了其富有弹性的特点，减弱了它的括约功能，但硬变的本身却给手术准备了有利条件。此时若将其切断也不会引起肌纤维的回缩而使大便失禁。因此使高位肛瘘的内口区及管道内端的处理不会遇到更多的困难，给手术的成功提供了更大的可能性。关于直肠环区硬变后对手术和严重并发症的影响，有两点必须弄清。

(a) 纤维化的程度与环区剪切范围的关系：切开直肠环区的多少，决定于该区纤维化的程度。环区硬变较重时，可将此区大部或全部切开。如仅轻度硬变。只可部分切开。对于纤维性变甚重触摸甚硬而其范围又较广泛者，可彻底切开，使直肠环于此区成较大缺损，也无失禁的后患。如无硬变，不可轻易剪切，可并用挂线或分次手术。

(b) 肛管壁广泛切开与严重并发症的关系：高位肛瘘常需切开与主道内端对应区的肛管壁，这也是治疗成败的条件之一。一般应切至齿线或稍上。如直肠环区硬变较重，可由肛缘一直剪至管道内端对应之环区。这种在环区硬变基础上的肛管壁的广泛切开，少有大便失禁之后患。如环区无纤维化而管道又距肛门甚远时，管道区仅切至探针经由创面基底向近肛门端划出为度，肛管壁可暂时或永久保留完整。必要时部分切开。否则易致大便失禁和引起因粘膜大片游离，多量持续渗血所造成的大出血现象。此时内口对应区直肠环可予挂线或分次切开。总之，直肠环纤维硬变为手术治疗高位肛瘘的局部基础，应该正确掌握这种变化。

b. 切割的重要区域和非重要区域：肛瘘手术可分重要和非重要区域。非重要区域即远离肛门的病变区，如瘘管外口、管道外端大部、支管等。重要区域即近肛门的病变区，如管道内端和内口区等。非重要区域对手术成败关系较小，处理时较为灵活。重要区域为手术成败的关键，因切割内口和管道内端，故应格外慎重。高位肛瘘有时须切开肛管壁，其重要区域的处理，即如何使外端创腔与肛管交通。而此操作须具备直肠环纤维硬变的局部基础。

c. 内口和管道内端在浅深肛瘘治疗中的意义：切除内口和消除管道内端均是肛瘘治疗成败的关键。低位单纯性肛瘘其内口与管道内端居于同一位置。但大部分高位肛瘘其内口与主道内端，不居同处。在低位肛瘘和少部分高位肛瘘的治疗中，内口的清除与否和治疗成败的关系是极为密切的。即内口如不切除，肛瘘不易治愈，愈后易致复发。但高位肛瘘内口与主道内端分居两处时，切除内口固然重要而消除主道内端亦不容忽视。作者认为，切除内口与消除主道内端均具有重要意义。低位单纯性肛瘘切除内口对治疗成败的作用虽然显得更为突出，但实际上因内口与管道内端同居一处，在肛瘘的整个切割过程中，管道内端的切除无疑也包含内口的切除了。两种不利愈合因素的同时去除，当然显出了它对治疗成败的突出意义。

在高位肛瘘的治疗中，由于瘘管内口与主道内端不居同处，治疗就比较复杂。经验证明，如内口并未闭锁，去除内口与去除管道内端均属重要。不能只切除内口而遗留管道内端的盲腔，或仅消除管道内端而遗留内口。因而在后位蹄形或单侧弯形肛瘘的手术中，应先由外口沿管道切至内端，再由管道内端切至内口处。不应仅于内外口间作一直形切口，只切除内外口和外口端的部分管道，将管道内端遗留。如内口闭锁，其管道内端相距较远，其间又无直接联系时，消除管道内端则是重要的。它的实质即如何获得合理的外科创面，消除死腔，去除腐败组织，使引流更为通畅，以利愈合。而切除内口则是去除肠内污秽物质进入瘘管的必经孔道，杜绝肠内感染源继续污染的机会。显然这些因素在治疗中都具有重要意义。因而作者认为，内口不除瘘不愈的论断，是不够全面的。

d. 高位肛瘘手术治疗的原则：

（a）术前必须查清直肠环区纤维化的程度和范围及与管道的关系。

（b）一次或分次剪切环区的选择：环区纤维化者一次剪切，唯切开的范围因硬变程度的轻重和范围的大小而不同。有必要切开而无纤维化者，应分次切开或一次手术切开与挂线并施。

（c）管壁剪除的多少和皮肉损伤的程度：肛瘘管壁不必完全去除。应据创面不同情况适当剪除不利于愈合之部分。但结核性肛瘘管壁的腐败组织必须清除彻底，否则不易愈合。创口健康皮肉在保证创面对合良好的条件下尽量少剪，近肛门端的创缘更应珍惜，否则易引起肛门变形或狭窄，也可影响控制功能。

（d）必须正确处理内口区和管道内端，严格掌握肛管壁切开的程度。

（e）管道切开应尽量彻底，必须使引流通畅。

（f）换药应注意：引流通畅，尽量保持创面外紧里松，使肉芽由基底部逐渐增生，避免桥形假愈。

(3) 肛瘘内口切开术：为了进一步缩短疗程，减轻痛苦，在一般切开疗法的基础上，应用内口与管道内端切开术，简称内口切开术或称截根疗法，治疗低位肛瘘获得满意效果，现将此术介绍如下。

适应症：低位单纯性肛瘘，特别适于低位蹄铁形和长管弯形瘘。

操作方法：患者取骑伏位或臀高伏卧位或侧卧位，常规消毒、麻醉。用肛门拉钩牵开肛门，暴露内口区，以隐窝钩轻轻钩探内口，确定内口位置。在隐窝钩引导下，以剪刀剪开内口和管道内端，切开范围约 1 cm 许，如内口腔隙较大，切口应长些。切开内口和管道后，搔刮腐败组织，创缘略加剪修。如后位蹄铁形肛瘘两侧管道较长时，于后中内口区切开后，可在两侧管道弯曲处各作 1 cm 长切口，分离皮下组织并刺破瘘管，取刮匙由此切口插入瘘管向肛门切口处和瘘管远端搔刮，以去除管道更多腐败组织，全部切口均不缝合，但左、右后位管道切口一般不放引流条，使其尽快闭锁。长管弯形瘘除切开内口外，管道切口按上法进行。

如高位肛瘘需挂线时，内口可不切开，外端大部管道亦不切开。先由外口伸入刮匙，刮除部分腐败组织，然后以弯血管钳由外口插入瘘管至管道弯曲处，抵压血管钳握柄，因钳尖部撬起而使皮肤高突，在此高突处作 1~2 cm 长之切口，用血管钳向深层分离，直至刺破瘘管，此钳与由肛瘘外口插入之血管钳发生碰触。取探针由此切口探入肛瘘管道，并探至管道内端，于管道内端人造内口插穿直肠壁，由直肠引出橡皮筋条，完成挂线操作。此种手术虽没有切开内口，但较一般切开配合挂线法创口缩小，组织损伤减轻，有利愈合。术后内口区创面每日换药，直至痊愈。

治疗机理：低位肛瘘的治疗，关键在于去除内口。此术由于切开内口和与内口相连的管道内端，使此区成一新鲜创面，改变了原内口和管道内端周壁皆硬不易粘连自愈的条件，而新鲜创面愈合过程中，引流通畅，创面与瘘管外端通连之空腔可粘连闭合。待创面平复愈合后，感染源已无进入门户，故远端旷置瘘管闭合后无溃开之虑。

优缺点：此法较一般切开术和切除缝合术操作更为简便，疗效较好，疗程缩短。复杂性肛瘘和高位肛瘘，可据此术原则结合不同病情灵活运用。如切开内口不能解决所有管道闭合时，可配合部分管道切开。管道深需挂线时，虽其内端处理大致相同，但肛瘘外端大部管道却免于切开而旷置。如肛瘘炎症期或管道内端有空腔时，不宜采用，高位肛瘘亦有愈而复溃者。

(4) 挂线疗法：此是祖国医学治疗肛瘘的传统方法之一，早在明代已被采用，此后至今均较重视并有所发展。所用挂线器材亦较完备，如药线、探针、挂子等。近年所挂之线有橡皮筋、药线、丝线，但以橡皮筋应用方便。其治愈机理，为缓慢勒开管道，使逐渐愈合。故可称其为慢性切开法。根据所挂不同线材，可分重力挂线和弹力挂线，前者多用药线或丝线，因无自缩张力，如欲加速其勒开过程，须于线外悬吊铅锤达此目的，此即称重力挂线；后者即用橡皮筋类胶圈或称胶线，拉紧敷于挂线处，借其自身之张力，勒开管道，勿需再借助外力，此即称弹力挂线。主要适于单纯性肛瘘。

操作方法：取骑伏位，常规消毒，局部麻醉，用一端系有橡皮筋的探针由外口探入，沿管道经内口拉出，橡皮筋亦随之引出肛外，肛内手指可作引导，切开挂线区皮肤，将橡皮筋收紧，然后以丝线将橡皮筋结扎，使橡皮筋嵌于皮肤切口内。高位肛瘘之挂线，参见切开配合挂线法。关于胶线或药线引入管道之方式有两种，即由外而内或由内而外将线引出。前者将线从外口经管道由直肠引出体外，后者将线从直肠经管道由外口引出体外。作者习用前法。关于紧线，如挂胶线，一般术中系紧后，术后勿须再次紧线，此即一次紧线法，术后约10～15天挂开。如挂药线或局部病情需缓慢勒开者，术后须再次紧线，此即分次紧线法。术后每日换药，直至痊愈。

(5) 切开配合挂线法：即外切内挂法，适于高位肛瘘，如高位单纯性肛瘘和高位复杂性肛瘘等。

操作方法：取臀高伏卧位、骑伏位或侧卧位，常规消毒，腰俞麻醉或鞍麻。外口、主管大部、支管、空腔一一切割，剪修搔刮，使创面开放，然后用系有橡皮筋的探针，由剩余管道轻轻插至管道顶端并人造内口穿通直肠壁，如此处有续发内口，可由此内口通入直肠，最后将探针连同皮筋引出肛外，切开肛门左右或左右处皮肤，将橡皮筋沿皮肤切口收紧后结扎。根据所挂组织的多少，必要时可双重挂线，如橡皮筋与丝线结合或与药线结合等。高位肛瘘因管道较深，由外而内的引线方式探针不易由直肠翻出，故操作常感困难。如橡皮筋引出程序改为由内而外，则需借助另外器械。以此法处理高位肛瘘主道内端，因缓慢勒开肛管壁，可避免大便失禁。高位复杂性肛瘘，应尽量一次手术成功。如后位蹄铁形瘘两侧瘘管的主道皆深时，可用抓主要矛盾之法处理。最深侧切开主道大部，为防肛门变形和创口张开过大，在切口近肛门端留一宽 1 cm 左右的皮桥或皮肌桥，然后于近后中位将主道内端挂线，缓慢勒开，创口开放。较深侧处理，偏于保守。即将主管大部切开后，于其内端挖掘隧道，经后中肛尾韧带下与对侧挂线创口相通。术后隧道内填塞纱布块，2~3 天取出，以使创腔成形。术中注意出血，术后每日换药，直至痊愈。

(6) 切除疗法：适用于浅短小瘘。

操作方法：常规消毒，麻醉后，以探针缓慢探入管道并由肛内牵出，后将整个瘘管包括周围变硬组织全部切除，修整创缘，使成一平坦创面，术后每日换药直至痊愈。亦可采用切除缝合法，即将整个瘘管切除后予以缝合，亦有只切除部分管壁而缝合者。缝线不宜贯通创腔，应由创面基底通过，术后 7 天拆线。采用此法应注意：术前清洁灌肠，应用肠道消毒剂。术中注意无菌操作。术后控制饮食和大便。

8 肛裂

肛裂为肛管皮肤的纵行裂疮，居肛缘与齿线之间，以疼痛为主症。多发于肛门后位和前位，作者观察结合普查资料，发现肛裂多为单发，男女均多发于后位，而前、后中位单发和前后中位并存为肛裂发病部位的3种主要类型。患者多为青年和成年，小儿老人少见。此病因发病率高，痛苦重，故可列为肛门3大主病之一。

8.1 病因病机

多由血热肠燥，大便秘结，排便时猛力努挣所致。如《医宗金鉴》说："肛门围绕折纹破裂便结者，火燥也"。据现代医学结合临床实践，肛裂的发生除与肛门直肠解剖学因素有一定关系外，主要病因为局部炎症损害和机械性损伤，且二者又互为因果。其病因总括如下。

8.1.1 解剖学因素

1.肛门前后弹力小血运差：因外括约肌等的起止分布关系，使肛门前后浅部组织形成弹力小血运差的三角区。有人认为，肛门后位内括约肌缺乏外括约肌的有力支持，而在肛门侧方，外括约肌与内括约肌紧密包绕。

2.肛门后部重力负担大：因肛管由前下至后上与直肠形成的自然角度，使肛门后部增加了排便时的重力负担。此二因素说明该病易发于前后位，尤为后位。

8.1.2 炎性因素

因炎症的变化，组织弹性减弱，脆性增加，若再蒙受机械损伤，最易破裂。

8.1.3 机械性损伤

损伤为本病致病的直接因素，而裂伤可视为该病的初期病变，如继续遭受炎症损害，即形成慢性肛裂。其中主因为便秘，此外肛肠异物损伤，肛门直肠检查及手术操作的撕裂等，亦可引起。由此可见，损伤和炎症为肛裂的主因。炎症造成的组织脆弱，给皮肤的破损提供了可能性，而机械的损伤更易使脆弱或正常的组织遭受炎症的损害，二者互为因果，致使患处不易愈合或愈后又易复发。

8.1.4 其他因素

有人认为肛裂与栉膜带有关，所谓栉膜带，即生长在齿线与白线之间变形皮肤下的纤维膜状组织，缺乏弹性。由于这种组织的形成，使肛管经常处于紧张状态，妨碍括约肌的松弛。

通过研究，亦有人认为肛裂与内括约肌关系密切。并指出肛裂是位于内括约肌上。慢性肛裂病人在裂缘下之基部可见到内括约肌的纤维化，而急性肛裂患者，局部无此征象。通过肛门压力和动力的测定，发现肛裂患者肛门压力明显增高并出现极慢波形。认为这是由于内括约肌功能异常所致，似乎内括约肌处于一种慢性过度活动状态，此与肛裂何为原发或继发尚不明确。

此外，因结核等所致的特异皲裂或溃疡，临床甚为少见。

8.2 临床表现

8.2.1 临床分期

为了更好的治疗，临床分期是有必要的。在这方面有人主张分急性期和慢性期两个阶段。急性期即初期所呈现的炎症现象。继裂损而起的炎症损害，使裂隙的边缘充血肿胀，疼痛剧烈，而炎肿的结果又是裂缘结缔组织增殖的主要因素。慢性期即后期阶段，或称陈旧性病变。裂疮愈发交作，病变区结缔组织增殖，边缘隆起，形成一具有特征性的皮肤赘生物——裂端皮垂。既往曾称前哨痔、哨兵痔、前哨片等。

作者观察，肛裂的急性期并不完全发于初期阶段，而初期的裂损发展至慢性阶段亦有从无炎肿的过程。因而将该病分为初发期和慢性期及一个特有的急性发作病证。初发期即初期损伤，肛门因受机械损伤而破裂。有人将此病征称为肛门擦伤而与肛裂区别。作者认为，尽管名称不同，然此期肛门的病理损害确属是裂疮发病的开端，不管裂隙的多寡均给炎症的发生或加重提供了条件。此期容易治愈。慢性期同前所述。至于急性发作，在肛裂发展过程中则可加重局部病变，可发生于由初发期至慢性阶段的任何时间内。如遇急性发作，可称肛裂炎症期，但其意义仅表明裂疮处于急性的炎症损害状态，并不意味着发病时间。另外亦有分1、2、3期者。

8.2.2 症状与体征

1. 主症

(1) 特殊性疼痛：该病虽仅限于肛门局部，而裂损范围亦较局限，但其疼痛却较严重。故疼痛为其主要痛苦，且具特殊性。疼痛之发生与大便有直接关系，可放射至其它部位，便干时尤甚。典型疼痛者，便时疼轻，便后疼重，先轻后重中有间歇，呈一特殊的疼痛周期。其疼痛之特殊突出表现为排便后片刻发生之疼远较排便时剧烈。而剧痛来临之前常有一小息，称疼痛间歇期。继轻疼后的间歇为何又起剧疼，乃括约肌痉挛之故。排便时的初疼是直接损伤或刺激的结果，而继此初疼所引起的括约肌痉挛，却强力挤压着裂损，使肛门处于较长时期的紧张状态。

(2) 便血：部分患者于排便肛痛的同时有少量或较多便血，与内痔的无痛性便血不同，如痔裂并存，检查时可以查清。

(3) 便秘：由于大便干燥，可引起裂损，而患者惧怕排便时疼痛，不敢大便，因此使便秘加重，形成恶性循环。习惯性便秘者易患此病。

2. 局部体征

一般初发时裂浅新鲜，边缘整齐，无皮肤赘生物。如病期已久，裂深色暗，裂缘及基部纤维组织增殖，裂疮外端皮垂，尤其居前后中位者，常为慢性肛裂的典型标志。

8.3 诊断和鉴别诊断

肛裂的诊断并不困难，结合病史及局部体征即可确诊。其症状多有便秘史，主症为特殊性疼痛，如有便血，与内痔无疼性出血容易区别。检查时一般牵开肛缘即能发现裂损，多发于前后位，应注意观察局部状态。个别患者如不能自然查及裂损处，可麻醉后检查。

8.4 临床治疗

治疗总则为通畅大便，消除裂疮。肛裂的特点大体可总括为病变轻，疼痛重，可治愈，易复发。了解此特点，对其辨证论治颇有俾益。肛裂初发，以润肠通便、止痛止血、促进裂损愈合为主，一般不必手术。如病期已久，长期不愈，裂缘高突赘生皮垂或有其他并发症时，可手术治疗。

8.4.1 内治法

以润肠通便为主，在大便通畅的前提下，再结合其他治疗。因此本疗法在肛裂的治疗和预防中甚为重要。临床时应强调调理大便，务使通畅，避免只着眼于裂损局部。调整大便可采用综合措施，具体方法如下：

1. 饮食调理：是最主要的方法。食物和水分要适量，如进食过少，水分缺乏，或食物纤维素少，均可引起便秘。故平日应多吃蔬菜和水果，多饮开水或喝有通便作用的一些饮料，即可使大便通畅。现将常吃的蔬菜、水果等食物及一些饮料介绍如下：胡萝卜、白萝卜、芹菜、韭菜、菠菜、大白菜等均有通便作用，胡萝卜又富含维生素应多吃。香蕉：通便作用较大，进食时间和量不必一致，多吃、少吃、何时吃均可，也可每晨空腹吃，以大便通畅为度。脾胃虚寒者便秘时，可将香蕉带皮以热水浸泡，使其烫热后再吃，以减少腹疼。梨：通便作用较大，并有润肺、止咳、化痰之功。可生吃或煮熟吃，量多少不限。蜂蜜：通便作用较大，并有润肺、止咳作用。以开水冲调后即可饮服，清晨空腹喝效果更佳。香油：有清热通便作用，取适量以开水冲调后空腹饮。红薯、山药：均能润肠通便，可煮熟当点心吃或做菜吃，量多少不限。荸荠（马蹄）：能清热、润肠通便，可生吃或煮熟吃，量多少不限。也可用荸荠粉以沸开水浸冲或煮粥，空腹喝或每日喝几次。花生米：宜生吃或煮熟吃，但炒熟或油炸后无通便作用。胡桃肉：有补肾、润肺、通便等作用，可生吃。芝麻、黑芝麻：有补肝肾、润肠等功效，可生吃或炒熟研末，加蜂蜜调服。松子仁：含有丰富的维生素 E，并有润肠作用，每次吃适量。银耳、黑木耳：有滋阴润肺通便作用，可单食或做菜吃。有通便作用之饮料有：梨汁、红枣蜜汁、山楂蜜汁等，饮时取汁适量以开水冲兑，每日饮几次。桔汁有理气、开胃助消化作用，能帮助排便。

在便秘的治疗过程中，可据患者不同的体质，灵活掌握调治方法。每天可吃一种蔬菜和水果或吃几种蔬菜和水果，也可与其他办法结合应用。如晨起空腹先喝蜂蜜或香油适量，上午约9～10点钟吃香蕉或梨，下午约3～4点钟吃荸荠或荸荠粥，午、晚餐时再结合吃些有通便作用的蔬菜，这样调理，一般大便都能通畅。如仍干燥再吃点药物，大便通畅后，即停用药物，仍以饮食调理为主。

2. 药物调理：可服一般润肠通便药，如果导、双醋酚汀、三酸酚汀、通便灵、液状石蜡、润肠丸（69）、麻仁丸（70）、麻仁滋脾丸（71）、润肠片（72）等，也可用炒草决明、番泻叶泡水代茶饮。蓖麻油通便作用大，适于大便干结时，一般不要用。以栓剂等药物纳入肛内，也可通便，如甘油栓、导便栓、开塞露等均可用。另外也可针灸或按摩。

关于大便的时间，以早晨起床后为最好，晨起后胃肠可发生大的蠕动,有助于排便,当然每人有不同习惯,但必须定时,对习惯性便秘可辨证服药,如大便干结不能排出者,亦应及时治疗。

肛裂疼痛重可服止痛剂。便血少不必处理,多时可服一般止血药。

8.4.2 外治法

1. 熏洗与敷药:熏洗药物不必强求一致,可用复方荆芥洗药(38)或花椒、艾叶、过锰酸钾、食盐等熏洗局部,每日1~2次,并涂九华膏(24)等消炎止痛生肌药膏,亦可应用具有同类作用的肛门坐药,以促进裂损愈合。

2. 腐蚀疗法:病期虽久但无皮垂者可以采用此法。可用红升丹(68)、红粉、硝酸银等腐蚀药物,腐脱裂疮表面陈旧组织,使成新鲜创面,再用生肌药物,如生肌玉红膏(25)、牛黄散(73)、珠麝散(74)、收口散(75)等。

3. 照射疗法:以紫外线照射肛裂,效果良好。紫外线除有杀菌作用外,能刺激细胞的代谢过程,促进上皮生长,使裂损愈合。此法操作简便,无副作用,主要适于新鲜肛裂。

操作方法:患者取一定体位,暴露局部病变。将紫外线弯导子。用酒精或新洁尔灭消毒后,直接接触裂损处。一般首次照射6秒钟,每次递增3秒,每日1次,4次为1疗程。合并感染者,首次照射11秒钟,每次递增4秒,每日1次。

4. 烧灼疗法:即以高热烧焦裂疮,然后焦痂脱落渐成新鲜创面而治愈。前人曾用烙铁或金属丝加热后烙烫,现用电灼器电灼。烧前先麻醉。

5. 封闭疗法:以普鲁卡因溶液于病灶周围注射,可切断恶性循环的刺激,即解除疼痛和括约肌痉挛,有利于裂损的修复。常用方法即以 0.5~1% 普鲁卡因溶液于裂疮两缘各注入 5~10 ml,治疗期间应保持大便通畅。

有人推荐应用普鲁卡因酒精封闭治疗肛裂,此法是于裂损处先后注射普鲁卡因和酒精。由于酒精对神经组织的影响，解除了疼痛和括约肌痉挛，增进了组织营养，兴奋了再生过程，因此收到应有的效果。

10~96%酒精可引起神经纤维形态上明显的退行性变化，因此该法为一完美的化学"神经切断术"。

操作方法：局部以5%碘酒消毒后，取空针用细针头于距肛裂外端0.5~0.7cm处刺入，注入1~2%普鲁卡因10 ml，浸润于肛门皮下组织和部分括约肌内。针头不必取出，继而将70~96%酒精1 ml注于裂损下0.8~1 cm深处。

封闭后应保持大便通畅。此法对肛裂初发期效果显著，近年应用类蓝长效止痛剂封闭，获得满意效果。亦可用其它局部长效止痛剂或麻醉剂封闭。另外，也可用酸敛或活血化瘀药注射，效果亦好。

6. 扩肛疗法：又称肛门扩张术，即以手术扩张括约肌，此法简而有效。

操作方法：常规消毒麻醉后，将戴有手套之食指沾润滑剂伸入肛道，两食指各向对侧扩张肛管，即右指外推左侧肛管壁，左指外推右侧肛管壁。待肛管开大后随之伸入两中指，两手以食中2指再按上法继续扩张，此时肛内已容4指，注意用力应均匀。亦可用两食指或食中2指各向同侧扩张，即手指掌侧面向外，扩拉两侧肛管壁，肛管前后方向亦可扩张。一般扩张至容指4指，Lord氏操作程序扩至6~8指。有人主张须扩断粘膜下部分组织，可能为内括约肌，使粘膜下环状组织于某处断裂。扩张时间不限，一般仅几分钟。经此治疗即可减轻或解除括约肌痉挛。扩肛时如将裂损撕大，愈合亦快。此时局部可换药。

7. 手术疗法：

肛裂的手术疗法，很早已被推荐，但因种类不一，操作各异，疗效亦不一致。又加医者对肛裂的病因病理缺乏充分和全面的了解，使不能收到满意的效果。作者认为，应针对肛裂不同病期给予合理治疗。如慢性肛裂，已有明显裂端皮垂或虽无皮垂但久不愈合者，可手术治疗。常用手术有肛裂扩创，括约肌松解及栉膜带切开等。

(1) 肛裂扩创术：即单纯切除增殖的裂缘、皮垂、发炎之隐窝及肥大的乳头等，对裂疮基部稍加剪修，创面不必缝合。但有人认为不缝合之创面与肛裂并无本质的区别，主张用切除缝合法。而缝合之方式有纵切纵缝，纵切横缝及纵切横缝粘膜，皮区创面仍然开放等几种。其中纵切纵缝法有时能使肛门狭小，易再裂损。

(2) 括约肌松解术：所谓括约肌松解，即剪断括约肌部分肌束以消除或减轻括约肌的痉挛。

操作方法：单纯扩创后再予后中位以血管钳分离出部分括约肌束并垂直剪断，或不作分离直接垂直剪切，所成创面不予缝合。术毕敷止血散（36）包扎固定，术后每日换药，直至痊愈。

注意事项：

a. 剪切括约肌前，应先切除肛裂陈旧组织，即应先行单纯扩创。

b. 此术仅于后位实施，前位不宜采用。女性患者前位施术尤应慎重。

c. 切口大小及括约肌剪切的多少：切口过小，容易复发，切口过大，可延迟愈合。一般切口长约 2 cm，深约 1 cm，仅剪断部分括约肌束。如增殖皮垂较大，裂损较深，可适当延长和加深切口。

d. 切口开放不予缝合。

(3) 栉膜带切开：其作法即行单纯扩创的同时于裂疮基底作一"V"形切口，切断纤维薄膜及少许括约肌。创面可予缝合或不缝合，或仅缝合皮肤及粘膜，其下留有桥形空腔，以使结缔组织充分修补填充。

(4) 肛门后切或侧切法：此法对裂疮本身不加处理，而在肛门后位或侧方作一切口,并剪断切口下组织,而使裂损治愈。

操作方法:常规消毒麻醉后,在肛门后中或左、右侧,约距肛缘 1~2 cm。作一放射状切口,长约 0.5 cm,深达皮下,将血管钳入切口内挑出部分外括约肌予以切断,创口挤压对合或缝一针。

如于肛裂同位处施术,切口距裂损外缘约 1~2cm,在向深层组织剪切时,切口不应与肛裂通连。

如慢性肛裂在行此术时,可对裂损略加剪修。术毕不必每日换药。

(5) 侧方皮下内括约肌切断术:1969 年 Notaras 氏首先采用此法。裂损 3 周痊愈。此术仅切割内括约肌,内括约肌断离后仍被皮肤和外括约肌包绕,此时断离处构成桥形,肛门无疤痕凹沟,能完全闭合,故肛门轻度失控亦明显减少,因此他认为是肛裂治疗方法的新进展。

操作方法:患者取侧卧或截石位,局麻或一般麻醉。局麻时须等待局麻隆起处消失,方可手术。先用二叶镜插入肛管并扩开,受检处肛门轻度扩张。此时觉得内括约肌像一紧带围绕于二叶镜之叶片,其下缘最易触及。取一钳向上轻轻挤压进括约肌间沟,增厚的内括约肌下缘即能显露。内括约肌被识别后,用一窄片刀在肛门左右中位 (3 或 9 点) 通过肛周皮肤插入。刀片在内括约肌与肛门皮肤之间平行刺向头端,直至齿线,然后刀片之锐缘转向内括约肌,向外侧切约 0.5 cm,内括约肌即被切开,当内括约肌完全离断时,解剖刀所遇之阻力减弱,肛镜叶片之张力立刻解除。于此插入点退出解剖刀,继之收紧肛镜握柄,使肛门轻度扩张。此时常以外面小创口流出少许血性物,但取出肛镜和外括约肌麻醉恢复后,血性物即可停止。外边创口通常小于 1 cm,不予缝合,以便血液由创口引流。

肛裂本身不加处理,如有肥大乳头或大的皮垂时,须予切除。此时用一尖头剪刀剪切,留一小的创面,外括约肌皮下部无损伤。术后肛内不放敷料，用纱布盖于会阴部以吸收创口血性物。

为简化操作，作者以肛门拉钩代替二叶镜，切断内括约肌后，用手指扩张括约肌，同时触摸内括约肌断离处，发现刚切断时皮下有较小凹沟，手指扩肛后，则凹沟明显变深延长，向上可至粘膜下。此沟即内括约肌创口，痊愈时凹沟平复，触摸时可有硬感。术中用手扩肛，较二叶镜扩肛更为灵活。如陈旧肛裂，除采用此术外，可于后位加作外括约肌切断术，则效果更好。

(6) 挂线疗法：常规消毒麻醉后，先行单纯扩创，于创口上缘稍外再剪一小口，以探针由此探入，从肛门拉出，即于裂损下人工造瘘，予以挂线。通过敷线之绞勒，阻断血运，使此区组织逐渐枯死而成开放创面。以后每日换药。因所挂组织较少，可挂丝线和橡皮筋单条。

8.4.3 针刺与磁疗

磁疗同痔病之处理。此外局部亦可针刺，即麻醉后用三棱针直刺裂损处，一般可刺几行，刺后可换药。

9 直肠脱垂

直肠脱垂为直肠肛管甚至部分乙状结肠移位下降外脱的病理现象。多发于小儿、老人、经产妇及体弱的青壮年。

9.1 病因病机

祖国医学对本病病因之记述颇多，但主要为气血不足，脏腑虚损，致使气虚下陷，固摄失职，而发生本病。其局部功能之异常主要为固涩不牢，升提无力，收缩弛张。现代医学认为，全身机能状况尤其是神经系统机能减退，对脱垂发生有重大作用。但局部因素如解剖结构缺陷和机能不全、肠原性疾病、腹压增高等，亦是造成脱垂的重要条件。成人完全性直肠脱垂的发生，有两种主要学说。

9.1.1 滑动疝学说

有人认为直肠脱垂是直肠膀胱陷凹或直肠子宫陷凹腹膜的滑动性疝，此陷凹又称腹膜陷凹或腹隐窝，在腹腔内脏的压力下，腹隐窝的壁逐渐下垂，后将复盖于其下的直肠前壁压入直肠壶腹，最后肠管脱出肛外。作者认为小肠或网膜于腹压增大时，坠入腹隐窝所成的腹膜囊内，并挤压直肠壁由肛门脱出的现象，与滑动性疝极为相似。如果把肛门称做脱出肠管的疝孔或疝环的话，则腹隐窝与其内容物连同直肠壁的脱出，可称为大疝中孕有小疝，大疝即脱垂之直肠，小疝即脱垂的腹隐窝内容物，腹隐窝所成之腹膜囊就是小疝的疝囊，此脱垂平面为直肠前壁腹膜返折之高度，因腹隐窝可下移，脱垂平面亦下移，但均在直肠环上。

9.1.2 肠套叠学说

有人认为直肠脱垂是乙状结肠与直肠套叠，并发现套叠始于乙状结肠、直肠交界处，脱垂平面较高。套叠后此部下移，直肠逐渐被推向远端，由于反复套叠，肠管向下移位，再加直肠侧韧带功能减弱，直肠即由肛门脱出。作者认为，如以套叠而言，常为上部较活动的肠管套入下部固定的肠管，即乙状结肠套入直肠，如患病已久，直肠脱出，则为乙状结肠脱垂牵及直肠外脱，直肠脱垂已成次要矛盾。临诊时如肛管不脱出反折沟不会触及上界，但临床发现直肠脱垂如肛管不脱出时反折沟上界均能触清。因此认为对脱垂较长的患者如乙状结肠已有脱出时，则为直肠脱垂牵及高位肠管下降。虽然近年国外对此学说较多提倡，但仍值得研究。此外亦有人认为此2种学说并无实质差别，只是脱垂程度不同而已。

9.2 临床表现

9.2.1 分类

本病分类方法颇多，迄今尚未统一。常用的分类方法有以下几种。

1. 完全脱垂和不完全脱垂：这是根据脱垂组织的不同而分类的。脱出为肠壁全层，称完全脱垂或全层脱垂；脱出仅为粘膜称不完全脱垂或部分脱垂或粘膜脱垂。有人把累及直肠壁层的全降又称真性脱垂。亦有人认为无论粘膜脱垂或肠壁全层脱垂，如下降外脱之组织波及肛肠周壁时则称完全脱垂，仅限于肛肠某侧而并非全周者称不完全脱垂或部分脱垂。此种分类观点狭义。因肠壁全层的内翻下降可首先始于某侧，他侧随之下移，同时或先后脱出肛外。单纯一侧脱出他侧并不下移者，临床甚为少见，30余年来作者仅见1例。粘膜脱垂虽有全周和部分脱出之别，如将其分为粘膜完全脱垂和粘膜不完全脱垂，也仅能说明粘膜脱垂的范围。此外有人把粘膜脱垂称为翻肛，肠壁全层脱垂称为脱肛。亦有人将全层脱垂称为直肠脱垂性脱肛，粘膜脱垂称直肠粘膜脱垂性脱肛。

2. 内脱垂和外脱垂：这是根据脱垂肠管于肛外是否自然察及而分类的。

(1) 内脱垂：肠管虽然移位下脱，但肛外不能自然察见者称之。发生这种现象有两种可能。其一，即虽有脱垂但脱垂较轻，肠管下移较短，未能脱出肛外。其二，即脱垂发生平面较高，肠管于高位下降套入直肠壶腹，但并未脱出肛外。上述现象实际上是直肠脱垂发展过程中的初期表现。但亦有患者，患病虽久，内脱垂并无加重而致脱出。故有人将其称为直肠套迭。

(2) 外脱垂：肠管下移能够脱出肛外而自然察见者称之。临床所见几乎全属此类。

此外有人以可视性和非可视性即隐匿性之名来分类，以说明脱垂组织的可见与否。

3. 3级或3度分类：这是根据脱垂的轻重及脱垂反折沟的存在与否而分类的。所谓脱垂反折沟即指脱出肠管与肛管直肠间的环状凹沟而言。

1级（1度）直肠脱垂：直肠粘膜与肌层分离脱出肛外者均属此级范畴。此级病变较轻，仅为粘膜脱垂，并未累及肠壁全层。有人根据肠壁全层脱垂和粘膜脱垂的主要病因不同，认为二者并非程度上的区别。因此不主张将粘膜脱垂列为第1级脱垂而将全层脱垂列为第2或第3级脱垂。

2级（2度）直肠脱垂：脱垂部分为肠壁全层，脱垂反折沟存在或大部分存在。

3级（3度）直肠脱垂：脱垂为肠壁全层，反折沟消失或大部分消失。这说明不仅直肠而且肛管亦脱出或大部脱出，另外或有部分乙状结肠外脱。此类患者肛门常松弛较重。

有人以脱垂的长度作为分级的主要依据。脱垂较短者称直肠轻型脱垂或轻症脱垂，包括1级和2级。脱垂较长者称直肠重型脱垂，或重症脱垂，即3级脱垂。作者认为脱垂较长固然说明病变较重，但反折沟是否存在也是病变轻重的标志。

4. 3型分类法:

脱肛型: 脱垂仅限于肛管部分。如仅粘膜外脱称肛管粘膜脱垂。脱出之粘膜可波及肛周或仅位于某侧。如完全脱出,称肛管完全脱垂。反折沟消失或大部分消失。

直肠脱垂型: 脱垂始于直肠环上,脱出为肠壁全层,反折沟存在。

混合型: 肛管和直肠完全脱出,反折沟消失。

Altemeir氏3型分类为:

(1) 粘膜脱垂型: 为一种假性脱垂,成人常合并有内痔或混合痔。

(2) 肠套叠型: 不合并肛管脱垂及滑动性疝。

(3) 滑动疝型: 直肠及肛管全部脱垂,是一种真正的直肠脱垂,此型多见。

5. 单纯性脱垂和非单纯性脱垂: 脱垂不伴有会阴正中疝者称单纯性脱垂,如有会阴正中疝伴发称非单纯性脱垂。直肠脱垂伴有痔脱垂时,亦可属此范围。

9.2.2 症状与体征

1. 主要症状: 本病发病缓慢,初始全身局部常无明显不适。病久可觉肛门坠胀,或有里急后重,欲便不能解除之感。

2. 刺激症状: 初期常不明显。病久由于长期脱出和纳入,刺激肠粘膜发生病变,使粘膜充血肿胀、糜烂或形成溃疡,可致便血。其下血色红或暗褐。如无内痔、息肉伴发,多数便血较少或不便血。粘液流出亦较常见,有的便时排出可与粪便混杂或布于粪便表面,粘稠或稀薄,量多或少。有的粘液可自行外溢,浸渍肛门,污染衣裤。由于肛周经常受分泌物的刺激,皮肤变湿,皱壁增殖肥厚或成湿疹,此时可觉作痒,有时因搔抓皮肤破损。

患者肠道功能可能失调,发生腹泻或便秘。有时虽无腹泻,但因坠胀大便次数可略增多。亦有排便不易控制,大便轻度失禁者,少数者偶有下腹疼痛、尿频等症候。如无嵌顿,一般无疼痛。

3. 肠管脱垂

(1) 脱垂发生程序：肠管下移外翻究竟何部为先，临床观察尚不一致。滑动性脱垂由于腹压的直接作用或腹腔内小肠、网膜坠入牵引之影响，直肠前壁可先下脱，他壁随之下移。而套叠性脱垂则周壁同时下降。

(2) 脱垂大小：脱出肠管长短不一，粗细亦非同样。初发脱出较小，病久脱出较大。如伴有会阴正中疝，则脱出较粗。

(3) 脱垂发生的时间及次数：多发于大便时。有些患者刚一蹲厕，粪便未解肠管先出；有的粪出肠亦出；少数者于粪便即将排尽时肠才脱下。患病已久脱垂即较病初频繁。除便时脱出外，劳动、行路、久站、久蹲甚或小便咳嗽时亦可脱垂。

(4) 复位难易：脱垂轻者便后肠管自行缩回，重时须手托纳入。有时脱出后静卧少息，也可自然复位。有时脱出不能及时送回，须卧床休息较长时间方能慢慢回缩。肠管纳回后，有的患者感觉肛门瘘胀不适，休息片刻才能继续活动。脱出后纳入之难易取决于脱出肠管的大小，如脱出较长较粗，还纳较难；脱出较短较细，还纳较易。

(5) 脱垂嵌顿：脱出后如不及时送回，可嵌顿肛外。因瘀血肠管肿大，肛门可疼痛不适。亦可发生绞窄坏死，应及时处理。

4. 肛门弛张：多见于病久患者。轻者仅指诊时方可发现，其肛门仍可自然闭合。重者肛门自然开张而成一洞腔，这也是稀便自溢的因素之一。

5. 脱垂对全身的影响：由于该病可常年不愈，除局部病痛外，对精神影响颇大。可引起其他疾病或植物神经功能紊乱。近年国外注意到直肠脱垂常伴有精神疾患，有人统计伴有精神病者高达 50% 以上。此外亦可导致全身虚弱或邻近器官子宫的脱垂。

9.3 诊断和鉴别诊断

9.3.1 诊断

该病的诊断并不困难,但欲分清何种类型则应细致检查。

1. 病史:多有腹泻病史,且泄泻时日较久,未能及时治愈。亦有便秘者或便秘腹泻交潜发作。询问时应问清脱垂发生的时间和发病的可能因素及典型症状等。

2. 视诊:通过脱出物外貌的观察,即可区别脱垂的不同病变及其轻重和肛门松弛情况。检查前令患者用力努挣,或蹲踞排便或用吸肛器吸引,使肠管脱出肛外。检查时应注意以下几点。

(1) 一般外貌:如脱垂仅为粘膜,则脱出较短,或仅外翻肛口,可居某侧或全周。全层脱垂则脱出较长,如小肠、网膜坠入,脱出甚粗,前壁特别膨隆,脱出肠管向后弯曲,状如弯牛角。如病期较短,肿物表面粘膜平滑,色泽鲜艳,淡红光亮。如患病已久,因反复脱垂和纳入,粘膜肥厚粗糙,色暗无光,或见结节溃疡等。但检查前如脱出时间较长,因血运障碍而致瘀血,粘膜可呈紫褐色,此非为肿物之真实色泽,故脱出后应及时检查。

(2) 皱壁形态:如脱出物有明显或不明显的放射状皱壁时,则脱垂组织为粘膜。典型者放射状之凹陷沟纹,由肛门周壁汇向脱出部分的中央腔隙,而呈一菊花状。如直肠全层脱垂,可见明显或不明显环状皱壁,层层折迭。如有增殖结节,皱壁表面可见大小不等的结状隆起,此区有时可能充血。

(3) 肛门松弛状况:轻度松弛者,肛门自然闭合,视诊不易分辨。重度松弛者,于膝胸位或骑伏位检查时,肛门可自然开张而形成一洞腔。松弛愈重,洞腔愈大。

3. 触诊及量度:通过此项检查,可以查清脱垂反折沟的有无,脱垂部分的长短粗细,括约肌力如何,以及肛门直肠或附近器官的其他病变等。

(1) 肛外指诊：首先触摸脱垂组织的软硬，一般柔软无坚硬肿块，全层脱垂则有弹性。然后细心量度并作记录。检查时着重以下几点：

a. 触摸反折沟的有无：反折沟消失标志着肛管完全脱出，反折点高度亦可作为治疗的指志，其对诊断和治疗都有一定意义。检查时应细心触摸，以了解此沟是否完全消失或部分消失。如未消失应测量反折高度，此即由肛缘至反折点的距离。

b. 测量脱垂的长度和厚度：脱垂长度应从反折沟量起，至脱出物顶端为止。如反折沟消失，应从肛缘量起，前后左右4壁均应测量。多数患者前壁长于后壁，左右两侧壁大致相同。一般长度在15cm以内。测量直肠脱垂之长度，历来以外露肠管为标准。然直肠脱垂为肠壁双层下降，外壁为下段肠管，内壁为上段肠管，故其真正长度应以测量之数加倍算之。以脱垂15cm为例，则实际是30cm，乙状结肠已经外脱了。其厚度应于脱出物顶端测量，各壁厚度大致相同，约0.5～1cm。如伴有会阴正中疝而使脱垂肠管典型后曲时，则各壁厚度即有明显差异，前壁格外膨隆，整个脱垂部分亦较粗大。遇此病况应将"子疝"纳入，重新量度，以兹比较。当小肠或网膜纳回后，整个脱垂部分顿时缩小，脱垂轴线变直，各壁长厚可无明显差异。挤压子疝时有时可闻肠鸣声。

c. 测"同心圆"孔大小：所谓"同心圆"孔即脱出肠管顶端内外周壁所形成的中间孔腔。由于内外周壁顶端基本处于同一水平面，因而可称为同心圆孔。测量同心圆孔的内外径，可知脱出部分顶端的粗细和大小。此为测量厚度的方法，一般各壁厚度相差较少，另外并测同心圆孔可容几指。如伴有会阴正中疝时，则同心圆不居中位而偏向后侧，此时前壁甚厚。亦可将手指伸入同心圆内，触摸两侧脱垂之肠壁或其包含的腹内容物。

(2) 肛内指诊：首先检查括约肌力并作脱垂重演等。当手指伸入肛道后，如觉肛门紧缩有力，则括约肌功能无明显减退。如手指极易伸入肛内且无明显紧缩感或以手指挤压肛管壁肛门即开张成一洞腔时，则表明括约肌张力减退。然后可令患者有意缩肛，进一步了解括约功能。如了解脱垂发生情况，可做脱垂重演试验。即令患者加大腹压用力努挣，肛内手指可触及脱垂下降之肠管。滑动性脱垂，前壁先降。如以手指抵压前壁，努挣时，即不再脱垂，但压迫他壁，努挣时脱垂仍可复现。套迭性脱垂，周壁多同时下降，以手压迫任何一侧肠壁，努挣时均不能使脱垂终止。内脱垂者有时可触及折迭之皱壁，如折迭较大，触时有壅肿或阻塞感。此外触摸肛内有无肿瘤，男性患者注意前列腺是否肿大。如伴有痔瘘等病可按该类病的指诊要求检查之。

4. 窥镜检查：检查时操作应轻柔缓慢，不可用力过猛。切实注意窥镜检查原则。当放入窥镜取出镜心后，宜慢慢外抽，随着视野的外移，仔细观察肠壁变化，注意皱壁或隆起的情况，如肠壁全层下移，环状折迭有时可充满全部视野。内脱垂者窥镜检查更为重要。

9.3.2 鉴别诊断

直肠脱垂的鉴别诊断，主要为粘膜脱垂与痔脱垂区别。

1. 多发性或大型内痔脱垂与粘膜脱垂的区别：内痔脱垂各痔块间多有明显分界，痔粘膜常充血，色鲜红或暗紫。因肿物内为曲张之血管团，故其表面有时呈桑椹状。单纯粘膜脱垂，可见放射状皱壁，脱垂粘膜多平滑光亮，色淡红。如脱垂为全周时，肿物无明显分界，如局限于某侧，因其内无曲张之血管团故亦可区别。有时粘膜脱垂伴发内痔脱垂，或内痔脱垂牵拉部分粘膜下移外翻，二者何为先发，须据不同病史，症状和体征区别之，但有时尚难确定。

2. 肛周皮下静脉高度曲张与肛管脱垂之区别：肛周皮下静脉高度曲张，因病变范围广泛当努挣时肛管虽显著下移，然此种下移为肛管外端变长的表现，并无外翻现象。患者可误认为有物脱出。临床所见的肛管脱垂，肛周皮下静脉无明显曲张，努挣后肛管外翻，可察见齿线并有粘膜翻出。

9.4 临床治疗

9.4.1 内治法

服药治疗直肠脱垂是祖国医学的主要治法，可使症消肛复。其主要治则和方药为补气升提固摄，以补中益气汤（6）加减，可重用黄芪、党参、升麻等。作者应用枳壳复肛汤（76）亦收到一定效果。但内治法取效较缓慢，对重症完全脱垂，疗效欠佳，亦可愈而复发。另外并注意调理大便，勿使便秘或腹泻。

9.4.2 外治法

1. 熏洗：多用收敛固涩之剂，如石榴皮、五倍子、枯矾、乌梅、枳壳、苦参等，单方或几味合用，煎汤熏洗，每日1～2次。

2. 敷药：所用方药甚多，仍以收敛固涩为主。常用药物如赤石脂、五倍子、乌梅、诃子肉、煅龙骨、浮萍草、鳖头等，上药为细末多几味合用，干撒或水油调涂，亦可用鳖血涂布。

3. 熨灸：此法简而易行，多用于小儿脱肛。现多以砖块烧热后外包毛巾或布，热敷局部，每次约半小时。

4. 封闭疗法：以普鲁卡因肛周或骶前封闭，可切断恶性循坏而使脱垂终止。一般每次用量，0.25～0.5%普鲁卡因60～100 ml，小儿酌减。每周可注1次，至不脱出为止。

5. 烧灼疗法：以器械烧灼脱垂粘膜，因烧灼区焦痂脱落后疤痕形成，使该区粘着固定，适于粘膜脱垂。可用高频电灼器或二氧化碳激光。

操作方法：常规消毒，局部麻醉，应使括约肌松弛，或予扩肛，便于粘膜外牵。以组织钳将粘膜牵出后，于烧灼区两侧固定。拭干粘膜表面，于脱垂粘膜顶端与齿线之间，由内而外，或由外而内作4～6条放射状线形烧灼，深至粘膜下层，至该区组织焦黑为止。注意烧灼勿过深。术毕移去固定之组织钳，将粘膜纳入。肛内放一凡士林小纱条或注入九华膏（24），术后每日换药，至创面愈合。

6. 结扎疗法：适于粘膜脱垂，可结扎右前、右后、左侧3区粘膜，方法同内痔结扎。

7. 注射疗法：本疗法操作简便，痛苦较小，安全，容易普及。其疗效与所用药物和给药途径有关。所用方药较多，大体可分硬化剂、收敛剂、平滑肌兴奋剂等。如明矾、酒精、石碳酸甘油或植物油、鱼肝油酸钠、盐酸、盐酸尿素、麦角、葡萄糖、中药复方制剂等。给药途径有粘膜下注射和直肠周围注射法。

(1) 粘膜下注射：将药液直接注于粘膜下层，如点状注射或柱状注射等。适于粘膜脱垂或轻症全层脱垂。

操作方法：一般需使肠管脱出肛外，消毒粘膜，以细针头穿刺粘膜后将药液直接注于粘膜下层。多由远端分点孤立注入药液，注药量依所用药物之不同而不同。如用5%鱼肝油酸钠，每点可注0.5 ml，注药点环绕肠管呈轮状，每轮可注4～6点。由远而近间隔穿刺时，各轮刺点相间而不平行，注毕将肠管纳入。亦可不使肠管脱出而用窥镜扩开肛肠，将药液按上法注于粘膜下，此即通常所称的粘膜下点状注射法。近年我国重庆用粘膜下直接给药方式，以长针头沿肠管纵轴平行刺入几处，注入较多药液，注药区呈纵行片状隆起，药液分布较点状注射广泛，收到较好效果。注毕肛内涂九华膏（24），包扎固定。后不必换药。

(2) 直肠周围注射：刺针不直接穿刺粘膜而经肛周刺至直肠周围，再将药液注于粘膜下层和肠壁周围。注药时肠管在复位状态，勿需脱出。现将明矾液（77）直肠周围注射法介绍于下：

适应症：主要为直肠全层脱垂。

药液制备：所用明矾为纯明矾，又称试剂明矾，即硫酸钾铝，勿用一般明矾。因其含杂质较多，注药后易致反应。常用浓度为6～10%，作者习用7%的浓度。制液时加枸橼酸钠稳定剂，或加适量普鲁卡因，按要求封装安瓿，高压灭菌。明矾液能耐高压，但不能耐长时间的高压，作者常用 15 磅压力 15 分钟，如高压灭菌时，发生沉淀，则不能应用。

器械及用品：本注射法所用器械甚少，可按一般外科准备消毒物品、空针等，应备 8 cm 长封闭针头，用于明矾注射。如用纱卷填塞，可备 8～10 cm 长中空硬橡皮管一段和凡士林大纱布块，以制做压迫纱卷。

疗效判定：关于直肠脱垂的疗效判定标准，历来以自觉症状消除与否再加医者视其局部，见无脱垂时，即谓痊愈。如由外脱垂变为内脱垂时，则不能视出。因此确切判定其疗效，尚有一定困难。作者通过多年临床实践，除上法外主要采用直肠脱垂重演试验，使疗效判定更为可靠，现将判定标准介绍如下：

痊愈：自觉或令其努挣时无肿物脱垂，做脱垂重演试验，直肠中下段肠腔无下垂肠壁存留，肠腔较空旷，括约肌力增强。

基本痊愈：自觉无明显肿物脱出，努挣时肠粘膜可部分或全部外翻肛口，做脱垂重演试验，直肠中下段肠腔无下垂肠壁存留，肠腔或较臃肿，括约肌力如前。

好转：自觉脱垂减轻，努挣时仍见有部分环状皱壁之肿物外脱，括约肌力如前。

注射方法：取臀高伏卧位，常规消毒，局部浸润麻醉。以右手持吸有明矾液之空针，于左、右中位距肛缘约 1～2cm 处刺入，刺针应先平行肛道，当穿过直肠环后使针斜向外侧，穿刺时另手食指伸入肛道以作引导。如发现针头距直肠粘膜较远不易触及时应重新穿刺，刺入部位适当时与刺针仅有薄膈之隔，触得明显。进针一定深度，一般 4～7cm，回抽无血，缓慢注入药液的 $\frac{2}{5}$，退针向外继续注完。但勿将药液注入括约肌内，否则可引起疼痛，亦可减低疗效。刺入点离肛缘过远，刺针距粘膜远，固定作用差；刺点离肛缘过近，刺针可穿透肠粘膜。一般只注射左、右中位，必要时加注右前、后中两处。严重者除上述几刺点外，右后、左前、左后亦可穿刺注药,但前中位不宜穿刺。通常采用一点穿刺,一处注药,故刺点较多。轻症患者,只注左右中位亦可治愈。如重症患者,也可采用一点刺入多处注药之法,即行扇形注药。其用量如 7% 浓度,成人一般为 20~60 ml,20~30 ml 为中等偏低量,60 ml 为中等偏高量。个别患者曾用至 80 ml 和 100 ml,亦无不良反应。注毕可按揉注射区,如注射药量较多,该区粘膜膨隆突起,应按揉至平坦,以使药液浸润较大面积。最后将一裹有硬橡皮管的凡士林纱卷放入肛肠中,以压迫固定。所用纱卷的粗细应据肛肠腔道大小和肛门松弛程度而定。一般成人所用,其直径约 3~4 cm,小儿适当减细。为了不使该填塞物进入直肠上段而造成取出困难,可先予橡皮管一端穿 1 系线,将线留置肛外扎于敷盖的敷料上。注射次数一般 1 次成功,必要时可注 2 次。

操作注意事项:严格无菌操作;刺入厚度与刺针仅有薄膜之隔,触得明显;前位不宜穿刺;回抽无血,缓慢注药;注药量应足够。

注射前后处理:术前 1 日进软食,注射当日饮食略加限制,必要时控制大便两天,注射前清洁灌肠两次,一般于手术日前晚用温生理盐水 800 ml 灌肠。注射前 3~5 小时再灌 500 ml 左右。注射后卧床休息 1~2 天,全身或局部如有不适,应及时处理。纱卷压迫,有助于固定,对疗效有一定影响。作者倡导纱卷压迫可作为注射后常规处理之法。压迫时间一般为 24~48 小时,有的压迫 60 小时以上,压迫时间较短能影响疗效。待压迫结束取出填塞物时,可观察肛门收缩情况,以予判断疗效。如肛门收缩较快,收缩停止时又不易牵开,这往往表示注射成功,而其固定亦比较牢固。如肛门收缩迟缓无力,收缩停止时又易牵开,这往往表示固定较差,但不能证明注射是否失败。对肛门极度松弛自然开张而成一洞腔者,填塞物取出后如肛门闭合,则说明括约肌张力增加。此现象可称为固定征兆,必须说明,固定征兆应在填塞物取出时观察。填塞物取出后,用 50% 甘油或蓖麻油 60~100 ml 灌肠排便,并嘱病人不可下蹲和过分用力努挣,排便可取站立躬身式。明矾液注射能固定肠管,但括约肌力常无明显增强,因此还需采用其他措施,进行综合治疗。如根据患者不同体质配合服药,调理大便勿使便秘或腹泻,局部热敷,经常进行缩肛等辅助运动,必要时针刺缩肛或手术紧缩括约肌,如仍有粘膜外翻肛口,可做粘膜结扎等。

明矾注射治疗直肠脱垂是我国肛肠学科取得的一项突出成就,对成人完全性脱垂尤为适宜,与开腹等较大手术相比,有许多优点。但对其疗效之评价有不同认识。有人认为注射疗法,包括明矾注射,对成人完全性脱垂不可能治愈。作者发现一次多量注射法,较分次少量注射法,疗效大为提高,只要用量足够,疗效甚佳。实践证明,此法可完全治愈直肠脱垂。但应用方法不同,疗效可有明显差别。

8. **手术疗法**: 手术疗法对直肠脱垂的治疗曾起到重要作用,一向为国内外学者所重视。其操作方法甚多,有人统计有 50 多种,有人统计有 80 多种,但基本可归纳为:(1) 紧缩肛门加强括约肌;(2) 脱垂组织的切除或修整;(3) 肠管固定;(4) 骨盆底加强;(5) 闭锁直肠膀胱或直肠子宫陷凹以及几种手术的综合应用等。手术之进路有经会阴部、经骶部、经腹会阴部等几种径路,操作简繁不一,疗效亦不一致。其中紧缩肛门加强括约肌手术能矫正肛门松弛状况,对直肠脱垂并有肛门极度松弛者,可予实施。一般说此类手术只能治疗肛门松弛,加强括约肌张力,对脱垂肠管无固定作用。然因肛门松弛而部分肠粘膜外翻者,通过紧缩肛门,外翻粘膜可不再脱出。此术可分两类,即生理性缩肛术和非生理性缩肛术。直接紧缩括约肌或把具有活力的皮瓣、筋膜植于肛周皮下,此类手术符合生理功能的要求,称生理性缩肛术。后者是把无活力的金属或非金属线状或带状物,扎于肛周皮下,多不附合生理要求。此类手术可按操作的异同分为三种：

(1) 外括约肌紧缩术：可单纯紧缩外括约肌或配合肛尾间沟缝闭。

操作方法：常规消毒，局麻或腰俞麻醉。于肛门一侧或两侧常在左右中位距肛缘 1 cm 左右，作一放射状切口，切开皮肤，分离皮下组织，使外括约肌暴露后以血管钳垂直插入肌束内，予以分离。挑起分离之肌束，以细丝线或肠线于其基部贯穿缝扎，约紧缩全周$\frac{1}{3}$。扎线上端组织，可剪除或包埋皮下。切口缝口或不缝合，术毕包扎固定。如为开放创口，术后每日换药至创面愈合。如配合肛尾间沟缝闭，其操作方法：常规消毒麻醉。在肛门后位距肛缘 2 cm 处作一"∧"形切口，切口一般应大些，切开皮肤及皮下组织，分离皮瓣至肛缘，显露肛尾韧带和外括约肌。括约肌分离与缝扎同上，或不作分离于创缘两侧将括约肌贯穿，拉紧后缝合 2 针。肛尾间创口拉紧后缝合，游离皮瓣剪除后其余端略呈"△"形。并与后位创口两侧皮肤对位缝合。术毕肛门闭合有力，指检时有紧缩感。术后楔形纱垫压迫，包扎固定。

(2) 真皮埋藏括约肌成形术：此术将富有活力的有蒂皮瓣埋于肛周皮下，术后能加强括约功能。其操作方法大体有 3。

第 1 法：常规消毒，腰麻。于肛门左后或右后距肛缘约 10 cm 处，向近肛门端作一前窄后宽的剑状切口，切至离肛缘 1 cm 许，将皮瓣游离，剥去表皮及脂肪层，使成长 8 cm 宽 1 cm 厚 0.2 cm 左右的有带皮瓣。再于前中位作一长约 1.5 cm 的纵切口。用弯血管钳由此处插入，经肛门一侧至皮瓣部穿出，夹持皮瓣远端牵至前中位切口处。另取 1 血管钳，由皮瓣蒂部的另一侧穿至前中位切口，挟持皮瓣，并牵拉使其绕肛门另一侧由皮瓣基部穿出，后拉紧之。用肠线或丝线将皮瓣游离端与基部缝合固定，剪去皮瓣余端，以丝线间断缝合皮瓣切口。前中位切口可缝合或不缝合。如欲加倍紧缩肛门，可以同法于肛门另侧切取皮瓣并移植于肛周皮下。

第2法：于肛门两侧左右后位距肛缘5cm处，向近肛门端各作1剑状切口，游离皮瓣各为第1法的1半，其宽度厚度相同。然后仍于前中位作一同长纵切口，依法用弯血管钳将2游离皮瓣沿其同侧牵出前中位切口，并予拉紧。以丝线将2皮瓣紧密缝合，剪除余端，并用肠线或丝线将皮瓣缝接处与其下面组织缝合固定。皮瓣切口间断缝合，前中位切口处理同前。

此法与第1法大致相同。唯皮瓣较短且在肛门两侧切取，游离皮瓣并不环绕肛门一周，只沿其同侧至前中位缝接固定。故后中位肛缘皮下无皮瓣贯通。所以在肛门左右后位切割皮瓣并使其于前中位缝接固定，其目的着重在于加强肛门前部收缩作用。

第3法：于肛门左右中位各距肛缘5 cm处，依法切取2剑状皮瓣，其长亦各为第1法的1半，宽度相同。再用弯血管钳先后挟持皮瓣各绕肛门半周，并于对侧切口处牵出拉紧。将两皮瓣各与对侧皮瓣的蒂部缝接，剪除余端，并将缝接处与其下面组织缝合固定，皮瓣切口断间缝合。

此法与前2法基本相同，唯切取皮瓣于左右中位。两皮瓣各绕肛门半周，肛周皮下都有皮瓣贯通。以上3法应严格无菌操作，避免感染。

(3) 扎肛术；以金属或非金属线状或带状物扎于肛周皮下，其缩肛作用较小。

金属丝扎肛法：用不锈钢丝扎于肛周皮下，轮状紧缩，肛门松紧以通过食指为度，如为小儿仅容小指尖即可。由于肛门皮下异物刺激，结缔组织逐渐增殖，有助于缩肛。所扎金属丝于数月后取出或不取出。亦有用肠线或粗丝线代替金属丝者。

橡皮管扎肛法；用柔软有弹性的橡皮管扎于肛周皮下，其操作方法与金属丝扎肛法相同。所扎橡皮管2～3月后取出。此法除能短时缩肛外，亦可刺激形成疤痕组织，但疼痛重，易感染。

筋膜等扎肛法：切取大腿阔筋膜条，亦可用丝制或尼龙网带扎于肛周，紧缩肛门。操作与前法大致相同，但应注意无菌操作。其缩肛作用较线状物为好。其它手术因损伤较大，国内采用已趋减少。

9.4.3 针灸疗法

针刺取穴：百会、足三里、长强、承山、环门（肛门左右中位赤白肉际分界处）等。中等度刺激，留针 3~5 分钟，隔日 1 次，一般 10~15 次为 1 疗程。挑治方法，同痔病处理。同时灸百会、足三里、中脘、长强等穴。

10 直肠息肉

直肠内生有大小不等的赘生物称直肠息肉。包括在祖国医学痔病范围内，称息肉痔、葡萄痔等。可单发或多发或几个散在，小儿常单发，青壮年可多发。有蒂或无蒂。

10.1 病因病机

多认为是湿热下迫大肠，使肠道气机不利，经络阻滞，瘀血浊气凝聚而成。现代医学认为，直肠息肉是直肠里的新生物，属直肠良性肿瘤范畴，发病原因尚不明确。

10.2 临床表现

10.2.1 分类

根据息肉有无蒂部可分有蒂息肉（又称蒂型息肉）和无蒂息肉（又称广基型息肉），根据息肉多少可分单发和多发，多发性息肉严重者又称息肉病。小儿息肉多生于直肠下部，且常单发，如有蒂时可称低位单纯蒂型息肉。此分类有一定临床意义，可说明息肉一般特点。然而临床中有蒂无蒂有时并存，故辨明蒂之状况和单发、多发或散在时，常须细致检查。按息肉的病理变化可分以下几种：

1. 腺瘤：又称腺瘤性息肉或管状腺瘤，为直肠息肉较多见的一种。故临床有时将直肠息肉笼统称为直肠腺瘤。此病各种年龄均可罹患，是直肠粘膜下腺体过度增生而成。既往认为是癌前期病变，故有人将其增长曾分 4 期。初期，腺体上皮细胞过度增殖；第 2 期，腺体细胞增生成一突出肿物，即息肉形成；第 3 期，瘤向周围组织浸润，即已癌变，第 4 期，瘤侵犯周围严重，与周围组织固着。但经多年观察,此种息肉仅有癌变可能。

腺瘤初发时,肠粘膜生一小隆起,如米粒或粟粒大,渐渐长大成形,凸入肠腔。其大小不一,小如豌豆、樱桃,大如杨梅、胡桃,直径一般为 0.5~1 cm 左右。有蒂或无蒂,蒂长短不等,粗细不均。蒂内不含腺体组织,为粘膜、粘膜下组织和血管。如多发时息肉大小和生长集密程度亦不一致,小者为粒状突起呈片状,大者为丛生如葡萄,多为大小相间。息肉体质嫩,色红,表面光滑。如因粪便磨擦或反复脱出,息肉表面可发生糜烂出血,此时色变暗红。有时息肉可由蒂部自行折下而排出。如蒂部纤维硬化,血运减少,息肉体颜色变淡。

2. 幼年性息肉:亦较多见。其形状与腺瘤不易区别,表面可呈细粒状。多为单发或几个散在,通常有蒂。儿童、青年多患。常生长于直肠下部。尚无癌变者。

3. 乳头状或绒毛状瘤:此种息肉小儿少见,多见于年长者,为肠粘膜上皮组织所生。先由粘膜表面生长,渐累及肠腺。息肉色暗红,表面有甚多乳头或绒毛状突起物,故息肉形状差异很大。有的为圆形,仅表面不平,呈粒状突起;有的分叶,呈海绵或海蛰状。其多为单发,体积较大,临床所见巨大息肉此类者居多,为无蒂广基,如将粘膜牵下,则可有蒂,唯此蒂较粗,蒂之肠壁端粗于蒂之息肉端。如息肉由肠管上部坠入肠腔而脱出时,则其游走活动度大。其血管丰富,易于出血,常有恶变。有人统计,成癌率高达 30%。近年研究,此瘤细胞能分泌一种物质,刺激肠粘膜充血肿胀而使肠道分泌增多引起腹泻,甚或引起脱水酸中毒或低血钾症。

4. 增生性息肉:为粘膜增生所致,多见于中年,无明显症状。息肉可退化自行消失或脱落,无癌变。如多发时,息肉体大小一致,一般如豆大。

5. 炎性息肉:又称假性息肉,为炎症刺激所致。多同时伴有肠道炎变,如慢性溃疡性结肠炎、慢性痢疾、血吸虫病等。

6. 大肠息肉病：息肉生于全大肠内，以直肠、乙状结肠、回盲部为多发区，多见于青壮年，可有家族遗传因素。

10.2.2 症状和体征

可便血脱垂。一般便血量少，为带血，或粪便有血迹，亦有出血多者。血色鲜红或暗褐，有时带粘液。绒毛状瘤常排出较多粘液血性物。血色较淡，有时血液积存肠腔可有黑血便。重时亦可腹泻。

息肉蒂长时可脱出。息肉脱垂有时仅露肛口，有时连同部分蒂部脱出肛外，如息肉较大，脱出后须手托还纳，偶可嵌至肛外。其大小形态，单个孤存或丛状生长等已如上述。高位息肉不能脱出时，如其表面无充血、糜烂，可无症状。多发性息肉病久时，可引起全身虚弱如贫血、消瘦等，青少年可影响身体发育。

10.3 诊断和鉴别诊断

低位单纯蒂型息肉，诊断多不难确立。患儿有便血史，肛门脱出物有细蒂牵连。

如息肉不能脱出，可作指诊检查。儿童息肉大部可以触及。触摸时应细心，由肠壁一处慢慢摸至他处，肠管周壁手指所及范围内均应触至。勿左1指右1下，此因触区不连贯，息肉可被遗漏。触摸时亦可令患者用力努挣，此时高位息肉可下移而被触及，或下垂时碰触手指。如肠腔有粪便积存，排出后再行触摸。有时须变换体位检查。直肠镜检查可予实施，此可直接窥视息肉外貌和观察直肠上段息肉病变。如多发时可行乙状结肠镜或纤维结肠镜检查，以查清息肉生长区域和范围。

直肠息肉钡剂灌肠一般意义不大。如疑结肠生有息肉等病变时，可采用之。钡灌肠前，先以温生理盐水清洁灌肠，清除结肠内粪便和气体，灌后可多排几次，尽量使粪便气体排尽，以免与息肉影象相混。为使诊断较为可靠，洗肠后可嘱患者休息1小时左右，洗肠所致肠管刺激此时已恢复。所灌钡剂应较稀薄，钡剂灌肠可作3步观察,即钡剂灌入时,先行检查;钡剂排出后复查对照;最后肠管充气双重对比。钡剂排出充气后拍片,可获得清晰影象。

直肠息肉的鉴别诊断,主要为多发性息肉初发期与肠道炎性病变如慢性直肠、结肠炎相鉴别。二者均可出现成片的粒状突起区,但前者还可发现成形之息肉突入肠腔,即各区息肉生长之速度多不呈一致性。

10.4 临床治疗

10.4.1 内治法

服药治疗直肠息肉,疗效尚难确定。各地都在不断研究。可用清热利湿、酸敛等剂试治。炎性息肉,通过服药则可消失。多发性息肉粘膜充血肿胀时,服药后能使炎症减轻或消退,亦有息肉消失者。可服椿皮酒醋煎(78)、复方乌梅丸(79)、秦艽苍术汤(7)等。

10.4.2 外治法

1. 灌肠法:直肠多发性息肉可用复方乌梅汤(80)保留灌肠,每日1~2次。

2. 结扎疗法:如能脱出,可在自然脱垂下单纯结扎或贯穿结扎。结扎后息肉不必剪下,纳入肛内使其自行脱落。如欲剪除,应防止结扎线滑脱。不能脱出时,麻醉后结扎。如息肉位置较高不能察见时,可用几把组织钳将息肉区肠壁先后向外牵提,将息肉拉出肛外。如为广基息肉,将息肉基部连同部分直肠粘膜一并钳起,用细丝线于基部正常粘膜处贯穿结扎之,后将息肉剪除,并将标本送检。或单纯缝扎使息肉自脱或萎缩。

如为多发息肉,可将生长密集区之息肉连同部分正常粘膜一并结扎之。结扎时将丛生息肉提起,于其下正常粘膜处穿针引线即可。此法可同时结扎几处,愈后再结扎他处,至结扎完为止。此外亦可应用套扎器将乳胶环套至息肉蒂部,待其自行枯脱。

3. 注射疗法：如用硬化剂应将药液注于息肉部，使息肉硬化；如用枯脱剂应将药液注于息肉蒂部，使息肉自蒂部脱落。

4. 电凝疗法：蒂型息肉可烧灼蒂部使其脱落；广基息肉较小者可直接烧灼。但应注意，勿烧灼过深而致肠壁穿孔。可用高频透热圈套勒除器或纤维结肠镜圈套电凝装置，圈套电凝勒除。

5. 指掐疗法：能脱出之息肉用手指直接掐其蒂部而使息肉脱落，此法简单可行，如蒂部较粗血运较好时，不宜采用，否则有时可致大量出血。

6. 手术疗法：息肉位置较高或多发息肉、广基息肉可手术切除。距肛缘 8～12 cm 的直肠中上段息肉，经肛门切除时，因位置较高，不易操作。如从腹部手术，需切开肠管，因息肉位置低操作亦较困难，同时给病人增加了痛苦。赵硕氏对直肠中上段息肉提出了新的切除法。操作方法：患者取截石位，常规消毒，硬膜外麻醉或再加用局麻。以手指扩张肛管，新洁尔灭棉球擦拭直肠，用 2～3 根 30 ml 的 Foley 氏导尿管捆在一起，插至息肉部位上方，分别注水后，将此导尿管向肛端牵拉，则息肉亦随之下移，用肛门拉钩拉开肛管直肠，从肛门以血管钳夹住息肉基底部粘膜，先以肠线缝扎钳夹之粘膜，依次切除息肉，如有渗血，再行缝扎，观察无出血时，手术结束。

此法将 Foley 氏导尿管插至息肉上方，向下牵拉肠管使息肉距肛缘的距离明显缩短，便于从肛门切除息肉。方法简便，安全可靠。

如息肉基底较大，麻醉充分后以肛门拉钩牵开肛门，充分暴露手术区，再作切除缝合术。如息肉位置很高，直肠下进路不能将息肉牵出时，必要时可考虑切开直肠后壁，结扎或切除。

11 肛肠疾病的预防保健

11.1 痔病的预防保健

痔病的调护与预防甚为重要。《疮疡经验合书》说："少劳，戒怒，远色，忌口，斯能愈矣"此对预防亦有指导意义。痔是人类特有的疾病，其病因是多方面的，因此预防应采取综合措施，使不发病或发病后控制其发展，或患病痊愈后不再复犯。可注意以下几方面：

11.1.1 加强锻炼，增进健康

应积极参加各种体育活动，如做操、打太极拳、跑步、爬山等，久坐久站工作的同志，要定时活动下肢和臀部肌肉，如两腿交替伸屈，臀部肌肉按摩等，能减少局部血流瘀滞，使气血通畅，则不易患痔。

11.1.2 精神调养与起居

保持精神愉快，不可过于忧虑；工作要劳逸结合，过劳可促使发病；要节制房事，病时或治疗期间，应杜绝房事；

11.1.3 注意饮食调节

不暴饮暴食，也不要过饥过饱，少吃或不吃辛辣等刺激性食物，如辣椒、酒等，可多吃蔬菜和水果，并注意多喝开水，饮食不宜过分精细，要食五谷杂粮，平日荤素搭配，犯病或治疗期以素为主。

11.1.4 保持大便通畅，养成定时大便的习惯

最好每天一次。排便时，不要看书、看报或吸烟，每次大便时间应尽量短些，排完即起，不要久蹲。应保持大便正常，及时调治便秘和腹泻。妇女妊娠期和分娩后，应确保大便通畅。

11.1.5 保持肛门局部清洁，减少刺激

可常洗澡，勤换衬裤；便后不要用不清洁或过于粗糙的手纸拭肛内；坐浴熏洗是重要的防治方法，除能使肛门清洁外，可改善局部血液循环，犯病时或手术后坐浴可使炎肿消退，减轻痛苦，促进创口愈合。

11.1.6 按摩与提肛

按摩是定时按摩肛门或骶尾部，提肛是有规律的收缩提升肛门。古云"谷道宜常撮。"实践证明："肛常提痔能愈。"这种方法可改善局部血液循环，增强肛门括约肌功能，促进肠道蠕动，有利排便，是防治痔疮的有效方法。

1. 按摩：常用方法有两种。一种是睡前用手指隔衬裤按揉肛门局部。按摩时先将下肢屈曲，把手掌放在臀部一侧，食、中、无名指3指微曲靠拢，用指尖（主要是中指尖）在肛外抵压后进行按揉，手指向一方旋转或前后移动，旋转或移动手指一下为1次，可连续按揉100次。每晚睡前按摩1回，或隔日隔几日按摩1回均可。另一种方法是睡前用手掌按摩骶尾部和肛门后方，从骶尾向肛门后方长强穴，上下来回按摩50~100次。使局部感到发热。两种按摩法可结合应用。

2. 提肛：又叫缩肛，主要有3种练法。1种是按着广播操式的练习，即按拍节缩肛，这种缩肛又叫肛门保健操。第2种是与呼吸结合的提肛法。第3种是缩肛与臀部、会阴等肌肉收缩同时进行，也叫提肛综合运动。

（1）肛门保健操：浙江王耆德设计的肛门保健操要求便后操练。先备置一盆温水或冷水，便后将臀部和肛门浸在温水里，先清洗肛门，然后用右手食指尖轻轻推肛门向上或使食指尖进入肛内一半，此时可采用广播操的节拍（约每秒钟1拍）有节律的收缩肛门，4次为1小节（口令节拍为1234、5678、2234、5678）。每次要求连操8节结束。操练时注意力要集中在肛内。每日便后练1次，也可只作缩肛运动，不将手指伸入肛内。这种方法更简单，每日晚上或早上各作1次，按着广播操的拍节收缩肛门，每次操练8节。

(2) 与呼吸结合的提肛法：此法实为气功之1种，气功防痔治痔效果很好。值得提倡，但应遵法练习，现据功法之易难介绍如下：

a. 一般功法；坐、站、卧式均可练，吸气时腹部鼓起，肛门放松，呼气时腹部塌陷。上缩肛门，如此1呼1吸，1松1缩，有节律的进行，每次练15～20分钟，每日1～2次。如腹部和肛门有温热感则更好。也可配合"吸、舐、撮、闭"4字诀进行。练时全身放松，配合吸气，舌舐上腭，同时向上收缩肛门，提肛后稍闭气，然后呼气，肛门放松，如此反复练15次，每日早晚各练1回。

b. 南京林先德设计的提肛加按摩法，于每晚睡前和晨起练习。取仰卧位，意守肛门，慢慢吸气提肛，以意引气入丹田，待丹田气满，再慢慢吐气松肛。如此约10分钟后，双膝屈曲，两手指轻轻按摩肛旁约5分钟收功。白天不管行、坐、常常提肛，此法可防治便秘，痔疮。

c. 燕子杰功法：山东杨泽等从学于"佗南侠"韩其昌老人之高足、五式梅花桩第15代传人燕子杰老师，结合自己的练功体会，用于防治痔疾的功法如下：

功法： 患者取仰卧位，头垫高，全身舒松自然，舌抵上腭，双目微启，壹志凝神，意守丹田，自然呼吸。

提肛： 呼气时用全力提肛，意念引气上行，尽量使会阴和丹田相接；吸气时松肛，肛门与丹田一起松弛，一紧一弛，反复做27次。

揉丹田： 意念放在两手掌内劳宫穴，将两手搓热，左手压住右手，按于丹田，作逆时针方向揉腹81次。

通阴阳； 两手中指相叠，点按百会穴1分钟，后点按会阴穴1分钟，意守丹田，呼气时提肛，吸气时松肛。

和带脉； 取盘坐位，两手身前相握，两少商穴相接，上身自左至右转9次，复自右向左转9次，自然呼吸。

要求：心情轻松恬淡，动作平稳缓慢，呼吸细匀慢长。按穴时用力刚柔适中，口中津液宜慢慢咽下，用意念送至丹田，每天做两次。此功之提肛、揉丹田两法，配合深长呼吸，有利于改善肛周气滞血行不畅，及括约肌松弛现象，增强胃肠蠕功。丹田真气充实，能健脾补中、升阳举陷。配合点按督、任二脉之百会、会阴穴，以引阳气下行，导阴气上达，带脉和则诸经得以约束，筋不得以纵，气不得以陷，诸法共奏补气升阳，行气和血，祛淤止痛之功。

(3) 提肛综合运动：

a. 坐式：先坐于椅上或凳上，两脚交叉，两手插腰，两腿保持交叉站起，同时收臀、夹腿、缩肛，持续5秒钟后再坐下，全身放松。

b. 站式：两手插腰，两腿交叉，足尖起立，同时收臀、夹腿、缩肛，持续5秒钟后全身放松。

c. 仰卧式：两腿交叉，足跟和肩部着床，收臀、夹腿、同时缩肛，持续5秒钟后全身放松。以上3式动作可重复10~20次，每日早晚各练1回。

d. 仰卧屈膝式：两腿屈曲，两足跟靠近臀部，两手放在头下，足蹠和肩胛部着床，收缩会阴部肌肉并上举骨盆，使躯干呈拱桥样，同时吸气，持续3秒钟，放下骨盆，全身放松并呼气。根据体力可反复进行10~20次。

e. 下蹲式：先自然站立，然后下蹲，同时收臀、缩肛，持续5秒钟后再起立，全身放松。如此可连续作1分钟，每日练1~2次。

11.1.7　导引法

《诸病源候论》养生方云：导引法有补养宣导之功，可治痔疾，其功法为："一足踏地，一足屈膝，两手抱犊鼻下，急挽向身极势，左右换易四七，去痔五劳，三里气不下"，此法即1足踏地，1腿屈膝，屈膝后两手抱于膝下，尽力将膝部靠近前身。片刻后抱膝停止，腿落地还原，继之另腿抬起，抱膝，如此左右交替抱膝动作 28 次。如常人练此法则可防痔。

11.2 肛瘘的预防保健

肛瘘是肛门直肠局部发炎的结果。由于直肠下部特定的地方，细菌容易侵入，造成直肠周围感染化脓，最后形成此病。如何使局部不发炎化脓，目前尚无较好的预防疗法。预防痔疮的综合措施，能改善局部血液循环，增强局部抗病能力，可能会减少发病。患病后应注意局部卫生，每日坐浴熏洗很重要。得病初期或肛瘘发炎时，应适当卧床休息，减少活动，并注意饮食调摄，保持大便通畅。

11.3 肛裂的预防保健

该病合理治疗容易治愈，但常复发不易根除。为此，如何预防肛门不致破损和愈后的复发，确属重要。根据肛裂的主要病因是局部炎症损害和机械损伤，且 2 者又互为因果，因此消除或减轻肛道炎症和避免机械损伤是其预防原则。常用方法有：饮食调摄，起居注意，局部按摩，提肛气功等预防措施与痔病相同。肛裂的预防最主要的是确保大便通畅，切勿便秘。因此应养成定时排便的习惯，每日 1 次。如 2、3 日或更长时间才解 1 次，由于粪便在结肠和直肠内停留时间长，水分易吸收而发生便秘。如大便干燥，应及时调理，使在最短的时间内大便正常。如已发生裂损，大便应稀软，不要成形，大便头稍干也不可，尽量减少对局部的刺激，减轻痛苦。大便干燥时排便应注意，不要猛然用力，因括约肌松弛不全，最易裂损。可用手指反复轻揉肛门，有助于括约肌的扩张。当大便排出部分时，不必急速完全排出，可再将干便缩回肛内，如此排出缩回反复几次，也能使肛门更快扩张。如仍不能解下，可将排出的部分干便用力挤掉或隔手纸挖掉，如此慢慢清除干燥粪头,可减少裂伤的可能。平日应经常保持大便通畅,妇女怀孕和分娩后更应注意。经常保持肛门局部清洁;及时治疗肠道炎性病变。腹泻亦能增加痛苦,应及时调治。

11.4　直肠脱垂的预防保健

该病虚证为多,除幼儿随着身体的生长发育而有自愈可能外,成人老年不易自愈。其调护和预防应采取综合措施。腹泻是儿童直肠脱垂的主要病因之一,其所以能影响肠管使发生移位脱垂,系由于神经营养机能障碍。因此,如能预防和及时治疗腹泻,则直肠脱垂的发病率,当可大为减低。患病后亦应避免腹泻,以免加重病情。平日保持大便通畅,便秘也可使脱垂加重。排便时间宜短,可采用站立躬身式排便。脱出后及时还纳,经常保持局部清洁。提肛和气功对该病的防治有较好效果,可按法练习,并注意饮食调理和起居等。

11.5　直肠息肉的预防保健

直肠息肉为良性肿瘤,目前尚无较好的预防方法。根据祖国医学整体调治的观点,应加强锻炼,增进健康,增强机体的抗病能力。气功疗法是强身保健祛病的最好方法,能否预防息肉发生,可以试练。

THE ENGLISH–CHINESE ENCYCLOPEDIA OF PRACTICAL TCM
(Booklist)
英汉实用中医药大全
(书目)

VOLUME	TITLE	书名
1	ESSENTIALS OF TRADITIONAL CHINESE MEDICINE	中医学基础
2	THE CHINESE MATERIA MEDICA	中药学
3	PHARMACOLOGY OF TRADITIONAL CHINESE MEDICAL FORMULAE	方剂学
4	SIMPLE AND PROVEN PRESCRIPTION	单验方
5	COMMONLY USED CHINESE PATENTMEDICINES	常用中成药
6	THERAPY OF ACUPUNCTURE AND MOXIBUSTION	针灸疗法
7	*TUINA* THERAPY	推拿疗法
8	MEDICAL *QIGONG*	医学气功
9	MAINTAINING YOUR HEALTH	自我保健
10	INTERNAL MEDICINE	内科学

11	SURGERY	外科学
12	GYNECOLOGY	妇科学
13	PEDIATRICS	儿科学
14	ORTHOPEDICS	骨伤科学
15	PROCTOLOGY	肛门直肠病学
16	DERMATOLOGY	皮肤病学
17	OPHTHALMOLOGY	眼科学
18	OTORHINOLARYNGOLOGY	耳鼻喉科学
19	EMERGENTOLOGY	急症学
20	NURSING	护理
21	CLINICAL DIALOGUE	临床会话

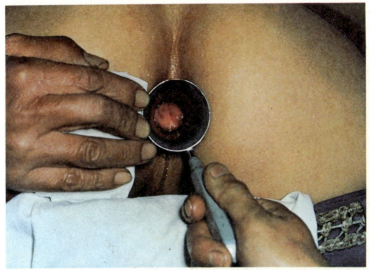

Fig. 6　Expose hemorrhoid
图 6　暴露痔核

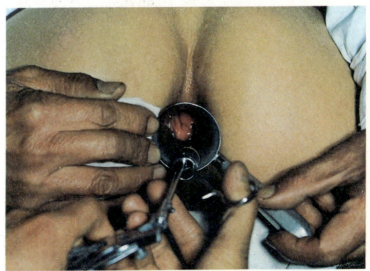

Fig. 7　Open the tissue forceps to grip the internal hemorrhoids
图 7　张开组织钳准备夹持内痔

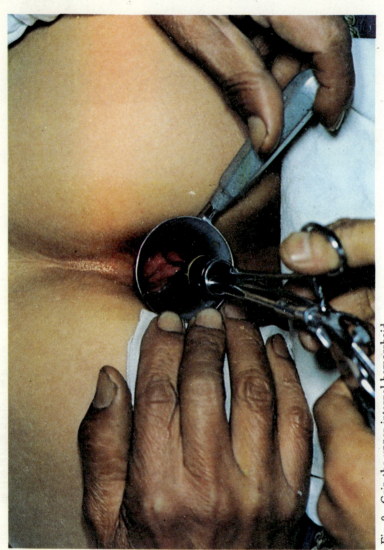

Fig. 8 Grip the upper internal hemorrhoid
图 8 于内痔上部将痔夹牢

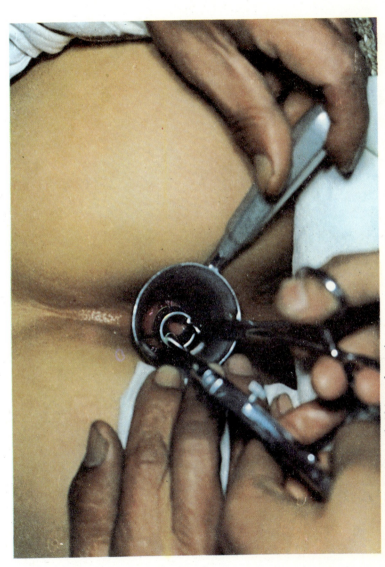

Fig. 9　Pull the hemorrhoid into the casing

图 9　将内痔拉入套管内，内塞管前缘已抵达痔基部

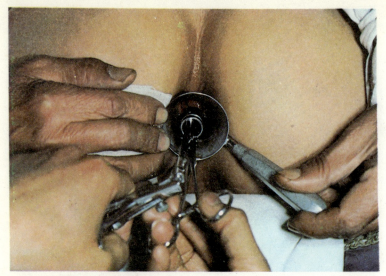

Fig. 10　Push the emulsive ring
图 10　推出乳胶环

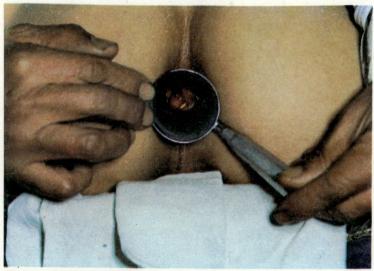

Fig. 11　Complate the ligation, the emulsive ring is at the base of the internal hemorrhoid
图 11　结扎结束，显示乳胶环套于内痔基部

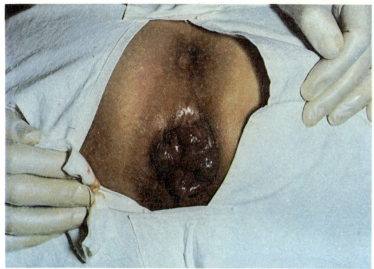

Fig. 12 Mixed hemorrhoids
图 12 混合痔

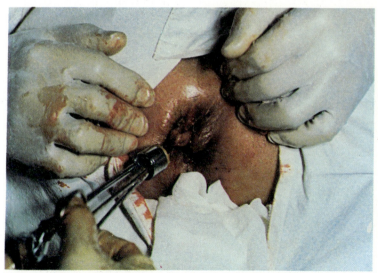

Fig. 13 The emulsive ring is at the base of the internal hemorrhoid after incision of the external hemorrhoid

图 13 外痔部分剪切后将内痔部分拉向套管

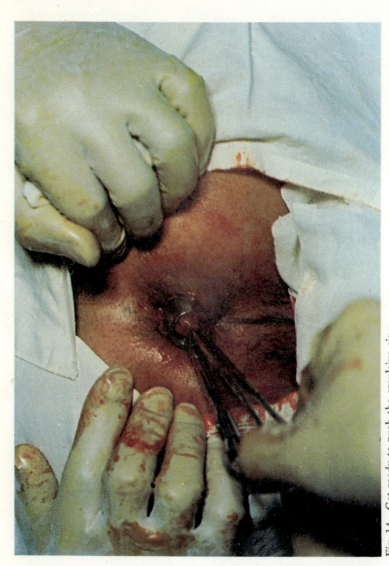

Fig. 14　Get ready to push the emulsive ring

图 14　准备推出乳胶环